Rehabilitation and palliation of cancer patients

Springer

Paris
Berlin
Heidelberg
New York
Hong Kong
Londres
Milan
Tokyo

Hermann Delbrück

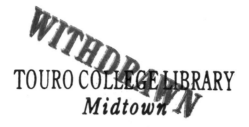

Rehabilitation and palliation of cancer patients

(Patient care)

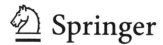 Springer

Hermann Delbrück

Lehrstuhl für Klinische Rehabilitationswissenschaften
der Fakultät für Medizin an der Universität Witten/Herdecke
Germany

Professorship for clinical
rehabilitation sciences at
the faculty of medecine,
University of Witten/Herdecke

ISBN-13 : 978-2-287-72826-6 Springer Paris Berlin Heidelberg New York

© Springer-Verlag France, Paris, 2007
Imprimé en France

Springer-Verlag France est membre du groupe Springer Science + Business Media

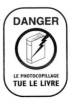

Design of cover : Jean-François Montmarché
Cover illustration: © Matthias Rating - contact: dr.rating@t-online.de

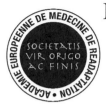

Members of the European Academy of Rehabilitation Medicine

Pr ALARANTTA Hannu
Helsinki (Finlande)

Pr ANDRE Jean-Marie
Nancy (France)

Pr BARAT Michel
Bordeaux (France)

Pr BARDOT André
Marseille (France)

Pr BARNES M. Ph.
Newcastle upon Tyne (Grande-Bretagne)

Pr BERTOLINI Carlo
Rome (Italie)

Pr CHAMBERLAIN M. Anne
Leeds (Grande-Bretagne)

Pr CHANTRAINE Alex
Genève (Suisse)

Pr CONRADI Eberhard
Berlin (Allemagne)

Pr DELARQUE Alain
Marseille (France)

Pr DELBRÜCK Hermann
Wuppertal (Allemagne)

Pr DIDIER Jean-Pierre
Dijon (France)

Pr EKHOLM Jan
Stockholm (Suède)

Dr EL MASRY Wagih
Oswestry Shropshire (Grande-Bretagne)

Pr EYSSETTE Michel
Saint Genis-Laval (France)

Pr FIALKA-MOSER Veronika
Vienne (Autriche)

Pr FRANCHIGNONI Franco
Veruno (Italie)

Pr Garcia-Alsina Joan
Barcelona (Espagne)

Pr GATCHEVA Jordanka
Sofia (Bulgarie)

Pr GOBELET Charles
Sion (Suisse)

Pr HEILPORN André
Bruxelles (Belgique)

Pr LANKHORST Gustaaf J.
Amsterdam (Pays-Bas)

Dr MAIGNE Robert
Paris (France)

Pr MARINCEK Curt
Ljubljana (Slovenia)

Pr McLELLAN Lindsay
Hampshire (Grande-Bretagne)

Dr McNAMARA Angela
Dublin (Irlande)

Pr MEGNA Gianfranco
Bari (Italie)

Pr MICHAIL Xanthi
Athènes (Grèce)

Dr OELZE Fritz
Hamburg (Allemagne)

Pr RODRIGUEZ Luis-Pablo
Madrid (Espagne)

Pr SJÖLUND Bengt H.
Umea (Suède)

Pr STAM Hendrik Jan
Rotterdam (Pays-Bas)

Pr STUCKI Gerold
Munic (Germany)

Pr TONAZZI Amadeo
Saint-Raphaël (France)

Pr VANDERSTRAETEN Guy
Gent (Belgique)

Dr WARD Anthony
Stoke on Trent (Grande-Bretagne)

Dr ZÄCH Guido A.
Nottwil (Suisse)

CONTENTS

PREFACE OF THE AUTHOR

To improve quality of life for cancer patients has been the endeavour of the author for the past 25 years in rehabilitation and palliation. This goal is the guiding theme throughout the book. The book contains experiences of the author and specific instructions how to assess, treat, and evaluate rehabilitation and palliation in cancer patients.

During the last two decades improving the "quality of life" has been the focus of attention in the medical oncology community. It has increased in importance because it has a significant affect on the patients over all well-being. In fact quality of life is now the second parameter after survival used to evaluate the effectiveness of new potentially curative first line oncological therapies. The invasiveness of some of the current therapies and the restricted life expectancy of many patients led to the change in therapeutic paradigms. Rehabilitation and palliation have become an essential part of modern comprehensive cancer care. There are many excellent textbooks in cancer management which provide therapeutic recommendations thereby influencing the disease. However, this book focuses on improving well-being of cancer patient versus curative measures.

The author would like to emphasize that well-being and quality of life must not be confounded with wellness. Well-being in cancer patients simply means: "To extend the patient's ability to perform the daily life activities, as long as possible". Quality of life includes subjective and objective aspects as well. To maintain quality of life is an important challenge not only for health aftercare service, but also in palliative and terminal situations. It is easy to confuse the true meaning of rehabilitation and palliation health care. Rehabilitation does not focus on prolonging survival but rather on improving the patient's quality of life. However, this is also the goal of palliation. But the difference is rehabilitation attempts to re-establish impaired functions, while palliation focuses on the alleviation of symptoms. Another way to understand the difference is: "The worse the prognosis for the patient, the greater the importance on palliative measures."

The establishment of quality assurance measures and guidelines has been a driving factor in improving cancer therapy in last decades. However there are very few quality measures and guidelines pertaining to rehabilitative and palliative oncology. Perhaps the primary reason is due to the subjective interpretation of such measures regarding quality of life. Few publications exist which discuss quality and how to secure it in rehabilitative and palliative treatments. An important aspect of this book actually provides and discusses objective criteria and parameters which can be used to evaluate the effectiveness of such measures.

Outcome assessment in most clinical trials is affected by a purely medical and somatic understanding of the disease. This is reflected in the predominant use of oncological symptoms as the content of outcome measures. However, the assessment of other health aspects like psychological symptoms, interpersonal or social or vocational consequences of the disease, seems to be similarly, if not more, important and should be considered in quality of rehabilitation. It has been the concern of the author to accent the need for a holistic approach in management of cancer after care.

Management of cancer appropriately focuses on prevention, early diagnosis, and cure but following effective treatment, most cancer patients will experience some significant symptoms and complications during the course of their illness or treatment. In addition to their physical symptoms, patients and families are burdened with psychological, social, vocational, and spiritual difficulties. In consideration of the impressing therapeutic progress, we often forget the costs we pay for prolonging our lives. The price is not only subject to money, but has to be understood in terms of chronic functional deficits following "successful" therapies. One of the author's goals was not only to specify possible unwanted side effects and sequelae of "successful" cancer therapies, but also to give instructions and help prevent, reduce and compensate these sequelae and handicaps. As the prognosis for most types of cancers improves, it becomes more important to ensure that all cancer patients regain maximum function and are able to live their life in a manner which is acceptable.

It has been the utmost concern of the author to point out that rehabilitation and palliation is a complex discipline that involves the interaction of many diverse medical health care providers. As a result it is important to understand that for a total optimum health care management solution a multi-discipline approach is required. Therefore, this book has been written not only for oncologists, but for all members of the rehabilitation and palliation teams.

A number of collegues helped by reading parts of the manuscripts on which they had expert knowledge and by making useful suggestions: Priv. Doz. Dr. Dahl (New Zealand), Prof. Dr. McLellan (England), M. Pantaleo (U.S.A.), Dr. Rating (Germany), Prof. Dr. Sanner and Prof. Dr. Rasche (Germany), Dr. Witte (Germany). They should not be held responsible for possible errors.

Prof. Dr. H. Delbrück
42369 Wuppertal, October 2007
In der Krim 39

PREFACE OF THE EUROPEAN ACADEMY
OF REHABILITATION MEDICINE

It gives us the greatest pleasure to write the preface to this book. It is the 5th published under the auspices of The European Academy of Rehabilitation Medicine by one of its members and it contributes significantly to our goal: "Making available information by experts in the field of Rehabilitation Medicine and allied disciplines; thereby enhancing the medical practice and ultimately benefiting the patients and disabled people." The previous titles in this series are: *La Plasticité de la fonction motrice*, translated in Italian language, *Assessment in Physical Medicine and Rehabilitation, Vocational Rehabilitation,* and *Les fonctions sphinctériennes.*

Cancer, in its many forms, will affect many of us, perhaps one in four. Our populations in Europe are ageing, but are often relatively healthy for a much longer period of time than previous generations. Older people may have to work longer and they will most certainly expect to remain active, however many will not have access to the quality of rehabilitation expounded in this book. The knowledge contained in this book is also incorporated into the European Boards Examination in Rehabilitation Medicine. It will be invaluable to practitioners of Oncology and other disciplines. The treatment of people with cancer, whether it is curative, arresting the disease, or palliative, is not complete until their rehabilitation has maximised their ability to engage life to the fullest.

The European Academy of Rehabilitation Medicine consists of some forty members, distinguished in the field. They come from the majority of European countries. The logo of the Academy *"Societatis vir origo ac finis"* translated "Man is both the source and goal of society" personifies its existence. We seek to improve the life of those who are disabled or newly disabled. By endeavouring to draw attention to not only its own discussions and publications, especially related to ethical matters, but also by teaching, we are continuously educating medical practitioners and the general public.

In these ways it seeks to reduce the burden of disability and enhance people's participation in the life of the community around them and the wider community.

Pr M. Anne Chamberlain,
London/Lyon, October 2006
Pr Jean-Pierre Didier,
Dijon Leeds

FIRST PART

Structural characteristics and interventions in the implementation of rehabilitation and palliation

Basics

Definition of rehabilitation and palliation

As opposed to curative aftercare (fig. 1.3), rehabilitation does not focus on a prolongation of survival but rather on an improvement of the patient's quality of life (fig. 1.1 and fig 1.2). This is also the goal of palliation. The difference between rehabilitation and palliation can been found in the fact that rehabilitation attempts to reestablish impaired functions (table 1.13), while palliation focuses on the alleviation of symptoms (table 1.15). Traditionally, once disease-modifying cancer treatment options have been exhausted, patients move to palliative care. Because of its initial ties to the modern day hospice movement, palliative medicine has been loosely defined as hospice care, terminal care, and end-of-life care.

The World Health Organisation (WHO), in a 1990 report on the topic, defined palliative care as "the active total care of patients whose disease is not responsive to curative treatment". This definition stresses the terminal nature of the disease. However, the term can also be used more generally to refer to anything that alleviates symptoms, even if there is also hope of a cure by other means; thus, a more recent WHO statement (WHO 2006) calls palliative care "an approach that improves the quality of life of patients and their families facing the problems associated with life-threatening illness." In some cases, palliative treatments may be used to alleviate the side effects of curative treatments, such as relieving the nausea associated with chemotherapy.

Rehabilitation and palliation are not mutually exclusive. Rehabilitation does not require the patient to be free of tumour. Rehabilitative measures are sensible even in the terminal phase of the illness. In this phase the focus of rehabilitation is merely shifted. Rehabilitation in terminally ill patients aims to promote capacities that are still intact. The patient's self-esteem and physical and mental integrity are to be preserved, as long as possible, by rehabilitative measures. Terminally ill patients are painfully reminded daily of the abilities that they have lost. Their functional capacities can be actively supported through various rehabilitation measures even in the final months of their lives.

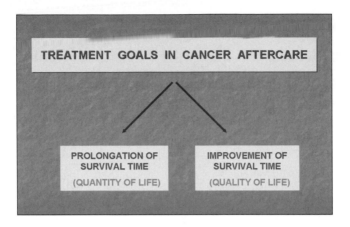

Fig. 1.1 - After being treated for cancer there must be an after care or follow up. The goal is to lengthen survival time and to improve quality of life as well.

Synonymous terms of rehabilitation in Europe

In practice the term of "oncological rehabilitation" is named very differently in various countries. What is considered to be oncological rehabilitation in one country would not be included in rehabilitation in another country (table 1.1).

Table 1.1 - Synonymous terms of rehabilitation in Europe.

France: soins de suite ou de réadaptation, médecine physique et de réadaptation, rééducation fonctionnelle, réinsertion, réadaptation, reconvalescence
Italy: riabilitazione, medecina fisica e riabilitativa
The Netherlands: revalidatie
Sweden: rehabilitering
Slovakia: rekonditionierung, health spa, fyziatria, balneologia & liecebná rehabiliácia
Great Britain: aftercare, support, rehabilitation
Germany: rehabilitation, Nachsorge, Kur

The International Classification of Function, Disabilities and Health (ICF)

The concept behind the practical implementation of rehabilitation is based on the ICF (International Classification of Function, Disabilities, and Health). As opposed to the ICD (International Classification of Diseases), which is generally accepted within curative medicine, this classification system includes not only the biological effects of illnesses but also the psychosocial aspects. Forms of assistance with participation in social life are an essential component of the ICF: In addition to the ICIDH classification system (WHO, 2001; Barat *et al.*, 2004), which was previously common within the field of rehabilitation, the ICF places less emphasis on deficits and gives more attention to resources. Assistance with participation is thus an integral component of the ICF (table 1.2). Social support is an important element to reduce and compensate for the disadvantages that result from tumour illnesses and their therapies. Assistance with daily life includes support with the organization of everyday activities (table 3.1).

The ICF is a classification of human functioning and disability. It groups health and health-related domains that describe physical functions and structures, activities, and participation. Activity is defined as the execution of a task or action by an individual. Participation consists of involvement in a particular life situation. Limitations of activity are defined as difficulties that an individual may have in performing the actual activity. Participation restrictions are made up of problems that an individual may experience in life situations (Barat and Franchignoni, 2004).

Table 1.2 - Activities and participation (performance capacity).

- Acquiring and applying knowledge.
- General tasks and demands.
- Communication.
- Mobility.
- Self-care.
- Domestic life.
- Interpersonal interaction and relationships.

The domains are classified by physical, individual, and social perspectives. Since an individual's functioning and disability occurs within a given context, the ICF also includes a list of environmental factors. For example "functioning" is a global term that encompasses all physical functions, activities, and participation. Similarly, "disability" serves as a global term for all impairments, activity limitations, and restrictions in participation. The ICF also lists environmental factors that interact with all of these constructs. It thus enables the user to record useful profiles of the individual functionning ability, disability, and health in various domains. Two persons with the same illness can have different levels of functioning ability, and two persons with the same level of functioning ability do not necessarily have the same health condition. By categorizing their abilities it enhances data quality for medical purposes. Use of the ICF should not bypass regular diagnostic procedures. In other areas of use, the ICF may be used alone. The ICF provides a classification of human functioning and disability. It systematically groups health and health-related domains. Within each component, domains are further grouped according to their common characteristics (such as their origin, type, or similarity) and are ordered in a meaningful way. The classification is organized according to a set of principles. These principles relate to the degree of interrelation between the levels and the hierarchy of the classification (sets of levels). However, some categories in the ICF are arranged in a non-hierarchical manner, with no ordering, but rather as equal members of a branch (WHO, 2001). Future enhancements in the ICF should address the following issues in table 1.3.

Table 1.3 - Future issues for ICF.

– Goals must be developed individually for each patient
– Its success is dependent on numerous factors.
– The prognosis of the illness is required.
– The cooperation of the patient is necessary.
– The cooperation of the therapist is necessary.
– The patient's motivation and trust in the process are necessary.
– It demands creativity.

Goals of rehabilitation

The term "rehabilitation" refers to a process aimed at enabling persons with disabilities to achieve and maintain their optimal physical, sensory, intellectual, psychiatric and/or social functional levels, thus providing them with the tools to adapt their lives towards a higher level of independence.

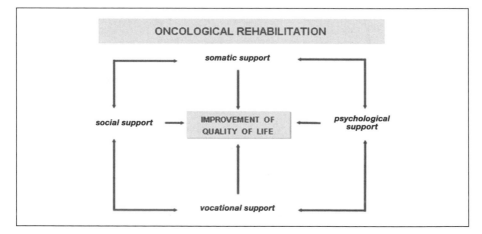

Fig. 1.2 - Measures to influence quality of life (rehabilitation).

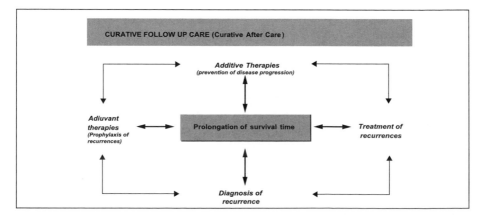

Fig. 1.3 - Measures to influence survival in the after care of cancer patients (medical aftercare).

Table 1.4 - Rehabilitation goals of cancer patients according to the stages of the disease.

– *Preventive rehabilitation therapy* is started early after the diagnosis of cancer is made, that is, before or immediately after cancer therapy
– *Restorative rehabilitation therapy* is directed at the comprehensive restoration of maximum function for patients who have a residual physical impairment and disability.
– *Supportive rehabilitation therapy* attempts to increase the self-care skills and mobility of the cancer patient with growing cancer and progressive impairment and disability by the application of quick, effective methods. Supportive rehabilitation therapy also includes physical exercises to prevent the effects of immobilization, such as joint impairments, muscle atrophy, weakness, and pressure scores.
– *Palliative rehabilitation therapy* aims to increase or maintain the comfort and function of patients with terminal cancer by improving their well-being, giving pain relief, avoiding joint impairments and pressure sores, and to provide at least partial self-sufficiency.

The main goals of maintenance rehabilitation in chronic conditions are improvement in affected body functions and an increase in activities. They should enable the patient to return to work and avoid early retirement. Methods used include physical therapies, training, diet, psychological interventions and health education, social and vocational support.

The overall aim of rehabilitation is to enable people with disabilities to lead the life that they would wish, given any inevitable restrictions imposed on their activities by impairments resulting from illness or injury (table 1.5). In practice, this is often best achieved by a combination of treatments to overcome or work around their impairments and remove or reduce the barriers to participation in the patients environment. Such a process will optimize both activity and participation.

Table 1.5 - Frequent impaired functions in tumour patients that require rehabilitative intervention.

– Impairments of physical / psychological / social / professional capacities.
– Impairments of interpersonal relationships.
– Impairments of mobility.
– Impairments of nutrition.
– Impairments of cognition.
– Impairments of coping.
– Impairments of financial independence.
– Impairments of orientation.
– Impairments of activities (such as attending school, working and earning money, housekeeping, recreational activities).

Interventions in rehabilitation

Assessment

Since cancer patients often avoid discussing their problems, especially their psychosocial problems, an active assessment prior to therapy planning takes on particular importance. Both somatic and psychosocial competencies and resources must be determined (tables 1.6, 1.7). The diagnostic instruments available for such an assessment consist of the determination of the medical history, discussions with family members, questionnaires, and explorations to determine the patient's activities of daily living (transferring, continence, dressing, bathing, grooming, eating, etc.) and instrumental activities of daily living (shopping, using transportation, providing for one's meals, money management, ability to take medications, etc.) (table 3.1). An analysis of the workplace environment and an inquiry into potential resources are recommended, since they are important for evaluation and quality control (3).

Table 1.6 - Functional assessments in rehabilitation.

– Clinical functional examination (e.g. muscle training, range of motion, coordination).
– Standardized/clinical tests (e.g. timed up and go).
– Cardiovascular function tests, oxygen saturation, graded exercise test, physiological cost of energy.
– Electro-physiologic testing (electromyography, nerve conduction studies and evoked potentials).
– Biochemical and pathological testing.
– Pulmonary function tests.
– Technical tests (gait and movement analyses).
– Ratings, scales, various scales, instruments and indices and questionnaires.
– Pain testing.
– Mobility and reaching/dexterity.
– Sensation and special senses.
– Swallowing and nutritional status.
– Sexuality.
– Continence.
– Tissue viability (skin problems and pressure scores).
– Bowel/bladder functioning.
– Communication (speech, language and non-verbal).
– Mood, behavior, personality.
– Coping.
– Neuropsychological testing (perception, memory, executive functions, attention and others).

Table 1.7 - Activity and participation assessments.

– History/anamnesis, check-lists and questionnaires.
– Relevant environmental factors (social situation, family, community, occupation and employer, functional and other assets, etc.).
– Care needs.
– Equipment needs (e.g. wheelchairs, irrigation equipment, etc.).
– Environmental adaptations (e.g. accommodation).

The degree of functioning deficits ultimately determines the remaining quality of life and the patients' ability to continue with their lives independently.

Shortly after admittance to inpatient or outpatient rehabilitation program an initial team conference is held at which the patient's medical, functional, psychological, social, vocational, and recreational status, as well as the rehabilitation potential and prognosis are presented and discussed. More specific rehabilitation goals are set, needs for equipment and personal assistance are assessed. Team rehabilitation conferences are held several times to discuss the patient's progress and plans for discharge.

Rehabilitation is a multi-professional activity, which depends upon good communication between staff and the individual skills of the professionals involved (fig. 1.4). For it to work, the team must have clear rehabilitation objectives for the patient, in which the patient and his/her significant others should be full participants.

Many tools can be used to evaluate global and specific functional capacity as well as the rehabilitation process (table 1.8). Some cross the individual ICF components. For instance, the functional Independence Measure (FIM) (table 3.8) and the Barthel-Index (table 3.7) incorporate aspects of body functions and activities as well as relevant co-morbidities and the extent of external support needed. The choice of measures will depend on the phase and aims of the rehabilitation process and the functional capacity of the individual.

Diagnostics and assessment in rehabilitation comprise all dimensions of body functions and structures, activities and participation issues relevant for the rehabilitation process. Additional relevant contextual factors are assessed. Clinical evaluation and measurement of functional restrictions and functional potential with respect to the rehabilitation process constitute a major part of diagnostics.

Assessment in elderly cancer patients. The role of concomitant illnesses. Function tests in elderly patients

The clinical assessment of the older person must address questions of life expectancy, risk of functional decline and need of assistance, tolerance to stress, rehabilitation, and management of reversible conditions, such as depression, malnutrition, and polypharmacy, that may compromise survival, function, and quality of life if left untreated (Balducci, 2003).

Table 1.8 - Methods to assess patient's activities.

– Standardized activities of single functions performed by the patient (e.g. walking test, grip test or handling of instruments, performance in standardized occupational settings). These tests can be evaluated qualitatively or quantitatively.

– Assessments of more complex activities, such as the activities of daily living (washing, sitting, etc.). These assessments may be performed by rehabilitation professionals or may be as self rated using standardized questionnaires.

– Participation is mainly analyzed in the interview with the patient through standardized questionnaires. Socio-economic parameters (e.g. days of sick leave) are used in order to evaluate social or occupational participation.

– The relevant contextual factors with respect to the social and physical environment are evaluated by interview or standardized ICF based checklists. For the diagnosis of personal factors, e.g. coping strategies of the patient's standardized questionnaires are available.

When developing a rehabilitative treatment plan for elderly cancer patients, it is essential to consider the functional deficits caused by age-related changes, the remaining compensation mechanisms, and the patient's expectations (Harlacher and Füsgen, 2000). A poor correlation of the Karnofsky and ECOG scores (table 3.4 and 3.5) with the function scores used in the rehabilitation setting is particularly seen in older patients (Extermann *et al.*, 1998).

Function tests that describe the degree of *deficits in social care* are considerably more concrete and much more important for the goals of rehabilitation. They include the Test for Activities of Daily Life (transferring, continence, dressing, bathing, grooming, eating, etc.) (Barthel Index, table 3.7), the Functional Independence Index (FIM, table 3.8) and the Test for Instrumental Activities of Daily Life (IADL Test) (shopping, using transportation, providing for one's meals, money management, ability to take medications, etc.). These tests primarily examine and document the patient's skills with regard to the ability to lead an independent life (Mahorney and Barthel, 1965; Kempen *et al.*, 1990; Suurmejer *et al.*, 1994; Barat and Fanchignoni, 2004; van Weert, 2004).

Numerous instruments are available for the assessment of *co-morbidity*. The Charlson Co-morbidity Test (Charlson *et al.*, 1987) is the best known of these.

Cognitive dysfunction increases with age. Medicinal therapy doubles the risk that the patient may develop *cognitive problems*, which may be seen for example in learning and memory problems. The Mini Mental State Evaluation Test (MMSE) and the Clock Completion Test (CCT) (Ferruci *et al.*, 1996) are used to measure cognitive disorders.

Depression is often underestimated in elderly patients. The distressing situation of being confronted with a malignant illness and its considerable emotional consequences often makes it difficult to distinguish between depression and the development of dementia. Specialized tests can be helpful in making this determination (Bach *et al.*, 1995).

Immobility, disturbances of balance, and the resulting increase in the risk of falling and fractures pose frequent difficulties in advanced age. Simple yet valid instruments are available for the assessment of the individual risk of falling (Tinetti, 1990).

The use of simple checklists to assess oral problems can also be recommended in elderly patients, since caloric and/or protein related malnutrition is often present (Morley, 1995).

Table 1.9 - Rehabilitative assessment in elderly oncological patients as a supplement to the measurement of the activities of daily living (ADL).

– **Ability to help oneself:** ADL (based on Mahoney and Barthel) and IADL

– **Cognition:** Folstein Mini Mental Status, Clock Completion Test (based on Ferruccil)

– **Emotional conditions/Depression:** Geriatric Depression Scale (test based on Bach)

– **Co-morbidity:** Number of co-morbid conditions and co-morbidity indices

– **Mobility:** Test based on Tinetti, Timed Up & Go, hand grip

– **Nutrition:** Mini Nutritional Assessment (MNA)

– **Polypharmacy:** Number and types of drugs being taken concomitantly

– **Decubitus:** Norton Scale

– **Geriatric syndromes:** Delirium, dementia, depression, falls, incontinence, spontaneous bone fractures, neglect and abuse, failure to thrive

– **Social situation:** Structured anamnesis, extended Barthel Index

Rehabilitation plan

Before the start of rehabilitation a rehabilitative assessment with rehabilitation planning and goal definition should take place (table 1.10). A medical intervention should not be offered unless measurable benefits will result. Certain minimum information about disease status (table 1.11) is a precondition. Without this preparation, there is a risk of failure of the rehabilitation measures.

Patients participate fully and actively in its development along with the other members of the patient-centered team (fig. 1.3). The plan must be regularly reviewed and updated by the rehabilitation team and forms the basis of team members' regular communication on patients' progress during rehabilitation.

Table 1.10 - Information to be asked and fixed in the rehabilitation plan.

– Diagnosis (activity, extent of the cancer disease)

– Presenting problems

– Complaints of the patient

– The individual's goals

– The professionals' goal

– Evaluation criteria

Table 1.11 - Minimum information required before initiating rehabilitative measures in cancer patients.

– Extent of tumour (e.g. pTNM before primary treatment and in the case of progression)?
– Curative or palliative therapy approach (e.g. R0, R1 or R2 resection of the tumour)?
– In the case of tumour progression information about the site and extent of the tumour foci (e.g. localisation of metastases)?
– Operative procedure (e.g. continence-preserving or creation of a stoma)?
– Has hormone-, chemo- or radiation therapy taken place? (e.g. which cytostatic agents, which hormones and at what dosages were given? What were the results?)
– Which radiotherapies have been performed? What dosages were prescribed and what were the results?
– Chemotherapy (which cytostatics, dosage, what were the results)?
– Psychosocial information regarding the family structure (statements pertaining to degree of patient information, any problems with coping or compliance, amount of support given by family members, social and occupational problems, etc.)

Rehabilitative therapies

With rehabilitation and palliation it is not the influencing of the illness, but rather the reduction of disabilities due to the tumours and therapy and improvement of quality of life which constitute the aims of therapeutic procedures. It is the intention to alleviate the negative effects of the cancer disease and therapy, not only physically, but also psychologically, socially, and vocationally. It is not influencing the illness, but rather the improvement of activities in daily life for the rest of life which constitute the aims of rehabilitative and palliative procedures (table 1.12).

Table 1.12 - Interventions in the rehabilitation of cancer patients.

– **Physical therapies** ("rehabilitation to prevent disability"): e.g. improvement of physical strength, mobility, nutritional status, physical fitness by pain therapies, supportive therapies, stoma care, prosthetic care, lymphatic drainage, health training

– **Psychological support** ("rehabilitation to prevent withdrawal and depression"): e.g. helps to cope with illness, to combat fatigue, to promote compliance, to relief and cope pain, to reduce stress, to improve self-help training, assistance with fear/depression, relaxation training, to deal with family members, health training

– **Social support** ("rehabilitation to preserve social life and autonomy"): e.g. measures for the reduction of nursing requirement, assistance in finding social aids, organization of helps to facilitate daily activities, information on hospice programs/palliative wards, counselling for family members, dealing with family members, promotion of self-help groups, health training

– **Vocational helps** ("rehabilitation to prevent unnecessary early retirement"): e.g. improvement of vocational fitness, assessment of harmful occupational substances to avoid in workplace, assistance in returning to work

– **Participation helps** ("rehabilitation to optimize social participation"): e.g. information, counselling, promotion of self-help groups

Table 1.13 - Frequent restorative and supportive therapies used in the rehabilitation of cancer patients.

– **Therapies aiming at restoration or improvement of body structures and/or function, e.g. improvement of physical performance** (pain therapy, nutritional therapies, inflammation therapy, lymph therapies, regulation of muscle tone, dysphagia management, disability equipment and assistive technology such as prosthetics, speech and language therapies, orthotics, technical supports and aids)
– **Adjuvant and additive cancer therapies for relief of symptoms and at the same time being necessary to prevent progression of the cancer disease** (chemo-hormono-biological therapies)
– **Physical treatments to improve physical well-being** (massage therapies, kinesiotherapies and exercise therapies, electrotherapies, ultrasound, heat and cold applications, phototherapy, hydrotherapy, diathermy, biofeedback therapy, pelvic floor exercises)
– **Therapies to improve psychological well-being** (psycho pharmacotherapy, treatment of depression, anxiety and of fatigue, neuropsychological interventions, behavior therapies, coping therapies, occupational therapies, art therapies, ergotherapies, improvement of cognition)
– **Therapies to improve participation** (health training, self help therapies, vocational and social counselling, family counselling)

Evaluation and outcome

Evaluation and outcome measurements of the rehabilitative therapies should constitute an important part of rehabilitation work. The spectrum of previous endeavors to improve the quality of life of cancer patients and to use the degree of quality of life for evaluation is very large. There are numerous recommendations for self-rating scales (table 1.14) and assessment scales for the evaluation of rehabilitative measures. Activities of daily life are of great importance in this context.

The evaluation of rehabilitative and palliative measures in tumour patients is directed not at survival time, but rather at quality of life criteria. This involves primarily subjective parameters such as improvement of pain, appetite, weight, mobility, overcoming fears, etc. and not such parameters as are found in association with primary therapy (response, remission and length of remission). The effectiveness of rehabilitation interventions is judged by the patient's degree of functional independence.

Basically, improvement in quality of life is attained when there is less nursing care. ("rehabilitation to combat the need of care"), when the patient can be vocationally reintegrated ("rehabilitation to combat early retirement"), when he/she feels secure ("rehabilitation to combat resignation and depression") and when the patient's physical handicaps and functional limitations are at a minimum ("rehabilitation to combat disability").

Quality of life questionnaires of the European Organization for Research and Treatment of Cancer such as EORTC QLQ C-30 and the functional assessment of cancer therapy (Fact) (Barat and Franchignoni, 2004) are internationally validated questionnaires and have been used on multiple studies. They can be used in rehabilitation as well. They are composed of multi-item scales and yes/no questions assessing physical, role functioning, cognitive, emotional, and social effects. The EORTC QLQ C-30 also includes symptom measures and a global health and QL scale

The outcome of measures for rehabilitation is dependent on numerous influential factors. Even well validated and widely used methods for the measurement of quality of life demonstrate heterogeneity across different settings and cultures, such as the Functional Independence Measure or the Barthel Index (Mahoney and Barthel, 1965), the Quality of Life Questionnaire QLQ-C36 or C30 (Aaronson *et al.*, 1993), the US equivalent to this scale, the Functional Assessment of Cancer Therapy questionnaire (FACT-G) (Bonomi *et al.*, 1996), the Rotterdam Symptom and Check List (RSCL), the Functional Assessment of Cancer Therapy-Anaemia (FACT-An), the Symptom Distress Scale (SDS), the Medical Outcome Study Short Form 36 (SF-36), the Hospital Anxiety and Depression Scale (HADS), the Functional Living Index-Cancer (FLI-C), and the Daily Diary Card (DDC). These scales ask a similar set of generic questions that consist of several subscales for specific quality of life domains, including physical well-being, and social, physical, emotional, and cognitive functioning.

Effectiveness parameters in the rehabilitation and palliation of pancreatic carcinoma patients may serve as an example for the complexity of outcome measurements in rehabilitation (table 1.14).

Different outcome scales in *palliative care of cancer patients* have been developed (Aspinal *et al.*, 2002; Bausewein *et al.*, 2005). The scales cover physical and psychological symptoms, spiritual considerations, practical concerns, emotional concerns of the patient and family, and psychosocial needs of the patient and family. The Palliative Care Outcome Scale (POS) is a multi-dimensional instrument covering these physical, psychosocial, spiritual, organizational, and practical concerns.

Table 1.14 - Possible therapeutic aims and their effectiveness parameters in the rehabilitation and palliation, e.g. of pancreatic carcinoma patients.

Reduction of disorders resulting from surgery/chemotherapy/radiation therapy	WHO Toxicity scale, CTC classification, assessment of organ function. Questionnaires : FLIC, SIRO
Pain relief	Pain diary, reduction of analgesic drugs, pain sensitivity scales. Questionnaires: PDI, EORTC QLQ- C30, SE36, SDS, RSCL
Improvement of nutritional status	Weighing, determination of total protein, albumin concentration, biometric impedance analysis, FACT-CT
Improvement of metabolic status in diabetics	Blood sugar daily profiles, HbA1, diabetes journal
Clarification and alleviation of malassimilation/maldigestion symptoms	Stool fats/stool weight

Table 1.14 - (suite).

Improvement of physical fitness	Ergometry, Karnofsky index, WHO and EORTC performance status, walking distances, muscle force (hand held dynamometry), exercise capacity (symptom limited bicycle ergometry, vigorimeter, QLQ-C30. Questionnaires: FACT-Ct, FACT-G, FACT-An, SIP, SF-36, Nottingham Health profile
Family member counselling	Questionnaires
Information on illness, follow-up care, signs of recurrence, therapy in case of recurrence, behavior-influencing illness	Questionnaires, tests
Reduction of anxiety, depression	Rating scales. Questionnaires: STAI, Poms, BDI, BSI, HADS-D, PAF
Coping with illness	Questionnaires: FKV, FKV-LIS, BEFO, TSK, FIBECK
Clarification and improvement of vocational fitness, return to work	Resumption of vocation, length of time of inability to work
Reduction of necessity of nursing care	Questionnaires: Barthel index, FIM, ADL
Relief of physical and psychological symptoms in the palliative situation	Questionnaire: POS

Structural characteristics

Inpatient rehabilitation – outpatient rehabilitation

Rehabilitation can be performed in both inpatient and outpatient settings. Outpatient clinic service is for patients who are ambulatory but do have symptoms that can be treated at home. In nearly all countries, such outpatient rehabilitation measures are given priority, except for Germany where almost all rehabilitation measures are predominantly performed within inpatient programs in special cancer rehabilitation hospitals. In most other countries the inpatient rehabilitation units are located in cancer hospitals with an in-house physician on call and the various medical and surgical consultation services available at all times. Residence in a rehabilitation clinic generally begins directly following the hospital stay.

Most German cancer rehabilitation hospitals are located in a nice surrounding. One of the pros for these inpatient rehabilitation measures is the experience that rehabilitation is greatly helped by an appropriate environment, in which the patient's fears and anxieties may be relatively limited. Patients can share their experiences with one another in this environment and are given social care around the clock. This setting is intended to provide the basis for further social care. These rehabilitation clinics have specially trained personnel (fig. 1.4).

Hospice/ Home care services

The palliative and supportive services of a hospice program provide physical, psychosocial, and spiritual care for patients with terminal cancer diagnoses and their families (table 1.15).

Table 1.15 - Characteristics of hospice and palliation wards.

– Multidisciplinary hospice services are available to dying patients and their families and include home-based hospice, inpatient hospice, residential hospice or respite care. Services provided include medical, nursing, psychosocial, spiritual, and bereavement. Services may be provided by hospice program staff, volunteers, or through a written agreement with an individual, institution, or agency.

– The hospice program assures continuity of care through assessment of the patient and family needs, development and review of the care plan, and management of care needs until discharge or until death and the bereavement period.

– Hospice services are available 24 hours a day, 7 days a week.

– Homemaker and home health aide services are available.

– Acute and chronic cancer pain management is available to all patients.

– Hospice services are provided with sufficient nursing personnel to meet the level of care required by hospice patients.

– Respite care is available to family and other caregivers.

– The hospice program meets appropriate licensing and accreditation requirements.

– Policies and procedures are established for all hospice components including: Admission and discharge criteria, bereavement care, and psychosocial, medical and nursing care management.

Palliation (relief of symptoms, table 1.16) should always be an important part of patient care. In the advanced cancer patient, it may be the only care when curative care is no longer the goal (Lagman and Walsh, 2005).

Hospices and palliative units may be incorporated with home health agencies or hospitals.

Table 1.16 - Frequent symptoms in the advanced stage of cancer that require palliative intervention (meta-analysis of 10 studies, based on Zech, Grond *et al.*, 1994).

– Pain (70%)
– Dry mouth (68%)
– Anorexia (61%)
– Weakness (47%)
– Constipation (45%)
– Difficulty breathing (42%)
– Nausea, vomiting (36%)
– Insomnia (34%)
– Sweating (25%)

– Problems swallowing (23%)
– Urinary symptoms (21%)
– Neuropsychiatric symptoms: disorders of consciousness, cramps, dizziness, restlessness (20%)
– Skin problems: itching, allergic reactions, infections, decubitus ulcers (16%)
– Dyspepsia (11%)
– Diarrhea (70%)

The rehabilitation team for cancer patients

Rehabilitation is a complex discipline that involves the interaction of numerous treatment providers, each with a particular area of training (fig. 1.4). Communication among members of the rehabilitation team, a most critical component, is facilitated through informal meetings during which specific concerns are shared and discussed.

The value of teamwork in this setting is that the output of the team is greater than the sum of the individual professional inputs. The teamwork approach scores high because they can share their expertise and workload. There are fairly blurred margins between the roles of the team members, successful team's thrive on everyone contributing despite professional boundaries.

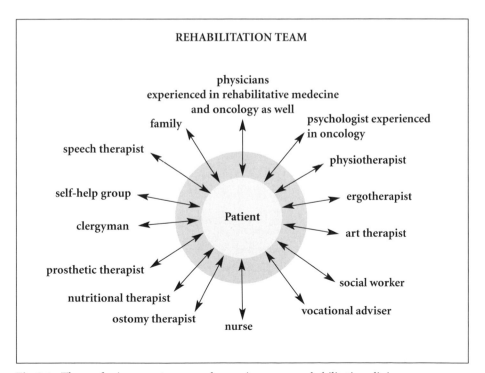

Fig. 1.4 - The professions most commonly seen in a cancer rehabilitation clinic.

The role and necessary qualifications of the cancer rehabilitation team members

The professional qualification of the personnel involved in rehabilitation and palliation varies greatly. While specialist nurses in England (such as breast cancer nurses, PEG nurses, special nurses for artificial nutrition, colorectal nurses, stoma care nurses, rehabilitation nurses, community nurses, lung cancer nurses, health supervisors) have a very high degree of professional qualification and psychosocial competence and their own education and training programs, these advanced training programs don't exist in most other countries.

The role and competences of a physician working in rehabilitation oncology

The team should be led by an oncologist having special knowledge in medical rehabilitation. He is the team's primary link with other treating physicians. He introduces the patient and family to the goals of the cancer rehabilitation team and meets regularly with the team, as well as with the patient and family, to direct and coordinate their efforts, while taking into account the patient's progress and changing needs.

Table 1.17 - The role and necessary competences of a physician working in rehabilitation oncology.

– Competences in clinical oncology
– Knowledge of reversible, irreversible late chemotherapy side effects
– Knowledge of reversible, irreversible late radiation side effects
– Knowledge of reversible and irreversible immunotherapy side effects
– Knowledge of reversible, irreversible hormone therapy side effects
– Knowledge of reversible, irreversible complication of surgery
– Knowledge to handle chemo and hormone therapy
– Knowledge of cancer therapy indications
– Knowledge of alternative and complementary therapies
– Knowledge to coordinate rehabilitative activities of the rehabilitation team
– Knowledge of social system and legislation on disablement
– Basic knowledge of economic (and financial) aspects of rehabilitation
– Knowledge, experience and application of medical and physical treatments (including physical modalities, natural factors and others evaluation and measurement of outcome)
– Knowledge of vocational restrictions
– Knowledge of carcinogenic occupational noxious agents
– Knowledge of vocational legislation
– Prevention and management of complications
– Prognostication of disease/condition and rehabilitation outcomes
– Knowledge of rehabilitation technology (orthotics, prosthetics, technical aids and others)
– Knowledge of pain therapy procedures
– Knowledge of psycho-oncological therapeutic indications
– Teamwork with psycho-oncologist
– Teaching skills (e.g. patients, team members, self help groups)
– Competences in health training
– Team dynamics and leadership skills

The role and competences of a nurse working in rehabilitation oncology

The complex needs of patients with cancer and their families require specialized oncology nursing knowledge and skills to achieve optimal rehabilitation outcomes.

The rehabilitative nurse is a nurse who has specialty training in rehabilitative aspects of nursing care. Particular emphasis is placed on bowel and bladder management in the patient with neurogenic disorders of waste elimination and on wound management. The rehabilitation nurse may be involved with wound, continence problems, ostomy care and with the training of the patient or family in the management of catheters, ostomy equipment, and surgical dressings. The enterostomal therapist (ET nurse) plays a major role in helping the cancer patient with an ostomy (i.e. colostomy, ileostomy or urostomy) to understand the principles of ostomy care, to learn the different aspects of ostomy management, and to adjust to the altered self-image (table 1.18b). Specialist Breast nurses (SBNS) make an important contribution to improved outcomes for women, by providing information and support and promoting continuity of care (Yates *et al.*, 2007). Nurse Practitioners/Advanced Practice Nurses in England are highly qualified and play an important role in rehabilitation and palliation of cancer patients.

Table 1.18a - The role and necessary competences of the nurse in rehabilitation oncology.

- To serve primarily as easily accessible resource to the nursing staff giving care to the cancer patient, as well as to the patient and the family
- To evaluate the patient's specific nursing needs
- To plan the patient's care
- To help to obtain nursing supplies
- To educate other nurses, the patient, and his or her family about nursing techniques
- To facilitate patient and family self-management
- To monitor discharge plans and assist in the discharge process
- To maintain close contact with patients and families
- To educate patients and families on how to manage their symptoms at home

Table 1.18b - The role and necessary competences of the wound and ostomy nurse in rehabilitation oncology (Enterostoma therapist).

- Assessment and management of acute and chronic wounds, including surgical wounds, pressure ulcers, arterial and venous lower leg ulcers and diabetic foot ulcers
- Recommendations for treatment modalities and wound care products
- Patient and family education related to care of wounds
- Preoperative counselling and stoma localisation
- Assessment of stomal functioning, pouching system and stomal and peristomal skin status
- Recommendations related to ostomy management and care, peristomal care and prevention of stomal and peristomal complications
- Recommendation and use of appropriate skin care products that can promote healing and provide protection
- Patient and family education related to self-care, lifestyle modifications and activities of daily living
- Supportive care and counselling
- Assistance with dietary, sexual and lifestyle issues
- Initiation and recommendation of home health care, and other referrals when deemed appropriate

– Referrals to other health care providers when appropriate
– Adherence to medication and treatment regimens
– Recommendation and use of specific types of containment devices
– Post discharge care and counselling

The role and competences of psychologists working in rehabilitation oncology

Psycho-oncology is concerned with the psychological, social, behavioral, and ethical aspects of cancer. This subspeciality addresses the two major psychological dimensions of cancer: The psychological responses of patients to cancer at all stages of the disease, and that of their families and caretakers; and the psychological, behavioral and social factors that may influence the disease process. Psycho-oncology is an area of multi-disciplinary interest and has boundaries with the major specialities in oncology: The clinical disciplines (surgery, medicine, pediatrics, radiotherapy), epidemiology, immunology, endocrinology, biology, pathology, bioethics, palliative care, rehabilitation medicine, clinical trials research and decision making, as well as psychiatry and psychology.

Psychologists play a crucial role in the cancer rehabilitation team. Virtually all cancer patients must address issues of death and dying and many need the support of someone trained in this area. Patients may have difficulties dealing with changes in their body image. Clinical neuropsychologists may be involved with the evaluation of cognitive impairment.

Table 1.19 - The role and necessary competences of the psycho-oncologist in rehabilitational oncology.

– To assess the patient's cognition and behavior, including intelligence, personality (i.e. emotional, behavioral, and character patterns, personal history, motivation, reaction to illness, and coping skills)
– To assist the patient and the family in coping, as well as to counsel and consult with the rehabilitation team members in managing the emotional reactions

The role and competences of physical therapists working in rehabilitation oncology

Physical therapists often institute and supervise an exercise program to improve mobility, strength, and stamina. In elderly patients they are primarily concerned with improving mobility, with a major emphasis on safe independence (e.g. minimizing the risk of falling). If involved early in the course of treatment, they can instruct the patient and the family in a basic exercise program to prevent muscle atrophy or contractures and maintain fitness. Typically, physical therapists provide assessments of ROM, manual muscle testing, and gait. They use orthotics and other adaptive devices to correct specific neuromuscular impairments.

The prosthetist-orthotist is involved with the fitting and fabrication and artificial limbs. In cases of limb-sparing procedures, the orthtist often needs to fabricate devices that substitute for weak muscle groups or unstable joints.

Table 1.20 - The role and necessary competences of the physical therapist in rehabilitation oncology.

- To teach the patient to perform specific exercises to strengthen muscles, to increase stamina, and to maintain or improve joint range of motion and trunk flexibility
- To improve balance and coordination
- To improve functional skills: Transfers into and out of bed, wheelchair locomotion, and ambulation with or without assistive devices
- To apply physical modalities to reduce pain, such as superficial and deep heat, cold, transcutaneous electrostimulation (TENS), and massage
- Physical exercise with the patient, such as muscle-strengthenig exercises (isometric, isotonic or isokinetic)

The role and competences of dietists working in rehabilitation oncology

The nutrition professional manages nutrition. He provides dietary guidelines about reducing nutritional deficiencies due to the cancer and/or treatments through program materials and services to the community. The nutritional needs of patients are unique to each individual.

A registered nutritionist is available to work with patients and their families, especially those identified at risk for having nutritional problems or special needs.

Nutritional status can be adversely affected by the disease process, including treatments such as chemotherapy, surgery, immunotherapy, and radiation therapy. The nutrition professional works in conjunction with patients, families, and members of the multidisciplinary team to help maintain optimal nutritional status throughout the course of disease, treatments, remission, and/or recurrence.

The nutrition professional has been trained and is experienced in the specialized nutritional needs of patients with cancer and in minimizing the progress of cancer and (therapy-induced) functional deficiencies through dietary counselling. Staffing of nutrition professionals is adequate to meet the needs of cancer patients and their families. The nutrition professional provides training to medical and nursing staff to ensure necessary assessment and referral of patients.

Table 1.21 - The role and necessary competences of the nutritionist in rehabilitation oncology.

- Identifies common nutritional problems the patient may encounter during the course of his/her disease and treatment
- Evaluate the patient's nutritional condition, assess the additional metabolic demands the cancer places on the body
- Performs an initial nutritional assessment and follow-up nutritional planning as needed with the patient and family
- Formulates an individualized nutrition care plan based on assessment findings
- Counsels the patient and family on basic nutritional needs

– Recommend the optimal diet with respect to specific clinical condition, caloric intake, food ingredients of choice, optimal consistency for easy swallowing, and the individual's tastes Judge total food intake by closely monitoring the patient's weight and counting calories and, if nutrition is inadequate, recommend interventions to facilitate adequate intake in the presence of poor appetite and swallowing disorders
– Assesses the patient's and/or family's ability to understand and comply with nutritional education and instruction
– Teach the patient and the family general and specific dietary principles
– Consult with the clinical staff on the optimal parenteral nutrition when the need for that arises

The role and competences of the social worker working in rehabilitation oncology

Social workers provide counseling and support. They provide important input into the rehabilitation process for the cancer patient, evaluating the complete home environment and determining the availability, willingness, and strengths of family members who can assist with care and support of the patient. They ensure that the rehabilitation process is continuing and coordinated beyond the hospital inpatient phase. The social worker is usually the principal liaison with the patient and family and helps to establish open channels with the rest of the team. The social worker may help the family regarding its financial resources and provide information on available services.

Table 1.22 - Role and necessary competences of the social worker in rehabilitation oncology.

– Discharge planning, facilitating a smooth transition from the hospital to the community
– Ensure continuity of care
– Secure appropriate follow-up services after discharge
– Secure financial resources, including health insurance coverage, and social security and disability compensation
– Obtain authorization and payment for necessary devices and home help
– Arrange need for transportation, attendant, or nursing care, home modifications, and other appropriate post-hospital services

Recreational therapist

Table 1.23 - The role and necessary competences of the recreational therapist in rehabilitational oncology.

– To offer activities to meet the different needs and interests of disabled individuals both in and out of the hospital, such as art therapy, music therapy, attending art shows and sport events, going to theaters
– Facilitate the institutional discharge for the physically disabled person and re-integration into community life

Pastoral care

Spiritual and psychological issues are confronted by cancer patients and their families, staff members, and the community at large; therefore, effective pastoral care is an integral part of relating to such issues. Virtually all cancer patients must address issues of death and dying: Many need the support of someone trained in this area. Spiritual guidance can help the patient appreciate his or her life prior to the cancer illness, and also to find new ways of living in the current situation.

Hospice chaplains are often assisted by largely untrained volunteers, visiting homes, hospital wards, and retirement centers, depending on the needs of their subjects. To the patient who may not see anyone unrelated to their medical condition (i.e. doctors and nurses), visits from hospice chaplains, which frequently involve prayer and simple conversation, can provide a welcome relief from routine and isolation. These visits are usually one-on-one, in person or on the phone, and generally occur weekly or more often. Because of the amount of individual contact, caretakers and patients often form lasting friendships.

Table 1.24 - The role and necessary competences of pastoral care in rehabilitational oncology.

– Pastoral care is supervised by a qualified professional chaplain with appropriate education (college and accredited theological school) and clinical training (units of clinical pastoral education are preferred).
– Spiritual needs may be identified and referred to a professional chaplain by all members of the oncology team.
– Spiritual assessment by a professional chaplain is incorporated into basic patient assessment.
– A clearly defined and functional referral system is established and maintained.
– Pastoral care involves sacramental, liturgical, and counselling services in keeping with the beliefs of patients and their families.
– Spiritual guidance in decision making related to patient care and biomedical ethics is available to patients and their families as well as caregivers.
– Ongoing multidisciplinary staff education and support is provided.
– Pastoral care recognizes diversities of faith, culture, and race. Pastoral care staff communicates with and supports clergy in the community.
– Pastoral care is available to staff members through individual counselling and group sessions.

Quality assurance

The generally accepted oncological guidelines give very little or no attention to the social effects of the illness and its therapy or to aspects of participation and activity. Most oncological guidelines and the evaluation of most therapy studies in cancer patients concern themselves with response rates, remission rates, the duration of the remission period, and survival time; all factors that are of secondary importance in rehabilitation which is concerned primarily with the effects of the illness on somatic, social, and mental integrity.

Only Germany has guidelines that exclusively concern oncological rehabilitation. However, these too are only applicable to inpatient rehabilitation, since outpatient rehabilitation is still in the process of being developed in Germany (Delbrück, 1998; Bundesarbeitsgemeinschaft für Rehabilitation, 2003).

The medical discharge report in the inpatient rehabilitation setting fulfills an important task in the quality assurance of social and professional rehabilitation measures in Germany. It fulfills three primary tasks. As a "classical medical report", it documents the status of the patient at the beginning and end of the medical interaction and describes the course of rehabilitation and the tasks that were performed. Furthermore, it has the function of a medical review for the pension funds and insurance companies by assessing the effects of the illness and/or its therapy on the patient's capacity within his or her professional life and within further psychosocial care. Finally, it serves as verification of the kind and extent of the rehabilitative services provided as well as their degree of quality.

Bibliography

1. Aaronson NK, Ahmedzai S et al. (1993) The European Organization for Research and Treatment of Cancer QLQ-C30: A quality of life instrument for use in international clinical trials in oncology. J Natl Cancer Inst 85, 5: 365-76
2. Balducci L (2003) Management of cancer pain in geriatric patients. J Support Oncol 1: 175-91
3. Barat M, Franchignoni F (edit) (2004) Assesssment in physical medicine and rehabilitation. Maugeri Foundation books. PI-ME Press Pavia
4. Bonomi AE, Cella DF et al. (1996) Multilingual translation of the functional assessment of cancer therapy (FACT) quality of life measurement system. Qual Life Res 5, 3: 309-20
5. Bundesarbeitsgemeinschaft für Rehabilitation (2003) Rahmenempfehlungen zur ambulanten onkologischen Rehabilitation. Bundesarbeitsgemeinschaft für Rehabilitation Frankfurt
6. Delbrück H, Haupt E (edit) (1998) Rehabilitationsmedizin. Ambulant – teilstationär – stationär. 2. Auflage Urban & Schwarzenberg München
7. Deutsche Krebsgesellschaft (1997) Standards und Qualitätskriterien in der onkologischen Rehabilitation. W Zuckschwerdt Verlag München
8. Ferrucci L, Cecchi F et al. (1996) Does the clock drawing test predict cognitive decline in older persons independent of the mini-mental state examination? J Am Geriatr Soc 44: 1326-31
9. Harlacher R, Füsgen I (2000) Geriatric assessment in the elderly cancer patient. J Cancer Res Clin Oncol 126: 369-74
10. Kempen G, Suurmeijer T (1990) The development of a hierarchical polychotomous ADL-IADL scale for non-institutionalized elderly. Gerontologist 30: 497-502
11. Lagman R, Walsh D (2005) Integration of palliative medicine into comprehensive cancer care. Semin Oncol 32: 134-8
12. Mahoney FI, Barthel DW (1965) Functional evaluation: The Barthel index. MD State Med J 14: 61-5
13. Morley J, Silver A Nutritional issues in nursing home care. Ann Intern Med 123: 850-9

14. Torosian M, Biddle VR (2005) Spirituality and healing. Semin Oncol 32: 232-6
15. Van Weert E, Hoekstra-Weebers JE, Grol BM *et al.* (2004) Physical functioning and quality of life after cancer rehabilitation. Int J Rehabil Res 27: 1, 27-35
16. Weaver A, Flannelly K (2004) The role of Religion/Spirituality for cancer patients and their caregivers. Southern Medical Journal 97, 12: 1210-4
17. Weis J, Bartsch HH, Erbacher G (1996) Rehabilitation needs and outcome of inpatient rehabilitation program for cancer patients. Psycho-oncology 5: 3-5
18. World Health Organization (1980) International classification of Impairments, Disabilities, and Handicaps. WHO, Geneva
19. World Health Organization (2001) International classification of functioning, disabilities and health. www.WHO.int/classification/ICF
20. World Health Organization. Retrieved on March 07, 2006
21. Yates P, Evans P, Moon A (2007) Competency standards and educational requirements for specialist breast nurses in Australia. Collegian 14, 1: 11-5
22. Zech D, Grond S, Lynch J *et al.* (1995) Validation of world health organization guidelines for cancer pain relief: a 10-year prospective study. Pain 63: 65-76

Psychological support and self-help groups in cancer rehabilitation and palliation

Need for psychological support

The cancer aftercare phase is accompanied by considerable psychosocial problems (table 2.1). Coping with cancer poses enormous mental strain. Additional strain can be caused by the effects of the therapy, which are sometimes more severe than those of the cancer itself. Fear and depression are frequent. Feelings of sadness, helplessness, and aggression can arise. Researchers in the USA estimate that at least one third of all cancer patients develops psychosomatic symptoms requiring psychotherapy.

Table 2.1 - The most significant psychosocial stressors in the aftercare phase.

- Emotional problems (fear, depression, aggression, suicidal tendencies, hopelessness and pessimism, loss of meaning, problems with self-esteem and identity).
- Partnership or family problems (communication and relationship problems, changes in role functions, sexuality).
- Vocational problems (restrictions and changes in the professional career, early retirement, etc.).
- Social problems (isolation, insecurity in interacting with friends and acquaintances, changes in recreational behaviour, etc.).
- Compliance problems (avoidance of stressful diagnostic and therapeutic measures).

Perceptions that mental factors alone, such as stress, depression, the loss of a loved one, or a patient's personality, may play an etiological role in the development of cancer belong to popular myths that lack any scientific foundation. Psychotherapy has equally as little influence on the tumour itself as rehabilitation measures have on the progression of the tumour illness.

Although more recent studies do not confirm earlier claims that psychosocially treated patients have a longer survival time, they do show that psycho-oncologically treated patients experience an improvement in mood (depression/melancholy, tension/fear, anger/hostility, and confusion/dismay) and a reduction of perceived pain, in short, an improvement in their quality of life (Goodwin *et al.*, 2001).

Measures for psychological assistance are always of a supportive nature and never curative. They must never be performed independently of other measures of somatic, social, and professional support (fig. 1.2). Insufficiently treated somatic symptoms and functional deficiencies are an obstacle for successful psycho-oncological care.

Structural characteristics and qualifications of professional assistance

Special attention, conversations, a "pat on the shoulder", or social activities alone seldom suffice as methods of aftercare for cancer patients. Rather, it is necessary to actively address the given mental problems – if necessary, with professional assistance. Professional psychosocial support is particularly important within the framework of integrated aftercare. In some countries such as Germany, special psycho-oncological training is available for clinical psychologists who are specifically involved with the mental problems of cancer patients (www.dapo-ev.de/wpo.html). Psychologists with such training are primarily active in cancer rehabilitation clinics and tumour centers, and less so in private practices. The personnel structure of a cancer rehabilitation clinic in Germany includes at least one psycho-oncologist for every 100 patients (*deutsche Krebsgesellschaft*, 1997). In other countries, such as in Sweden, it is the social workers or, as it is the case in the U.K., the nursing staff (breast cancer nurses, stoma care nurses) who have specific psychotherapeutic training and provide the majority of the psychological care for cancer patients. These nurses are also predominantly active in an outpatient setting (Delbrück, 2004).

The role and competences of psychologists working in rehabilitation oncology

Psychologists play a crucial role in the cancer rehabilitation team (fig. 1.4). Virtually all cancer patients must address issues of death and dying and many need the support of someone trained in this area. Patients may have difficulties dealing with changes in their body image. Clinical neuropsychologists may be involved with the evaluation of cognitive impairment.

Table 2.2 - The role and necessary competences of the psycho-oncologist in rehabilitational oncology.

- To assess the patient's cognition and behaviour, including intelligence, personality (i.e. emotional, behavioural, and character patterns, personal history, motivation, reaction to illness, and coping skills)
- Person centred therapy
- To assist the patient and the family in coping, as well as to counsel and consult with the rehabilitation team members in managing the emotional reactions

Psychological tasks within the rehabilitation team

Specific psychological intervention measures based on cognitive-behavioural, person-centred therapy, and hypnotherapy treatment concepts can be very helpful. This psychosocial healthcare approach encompasses not only the provision of care for affected patients and their families but also the supervision of the medical personnel (table 2.3). The supervision should ideally be performed by psychologists from outside of the rehabilitation team, whereas the psychological staff of the rehabilitation team can provide psychological care for and training of the personnel.

Table 2.3 - Psychological tasks within oncological rehabilitation.

– Support to cope with the illness
– Instruction in relaxation methods
– One-on-one psychotherapeutic sessions
– Involvement in training workshops/health training
– Crisis intervention
– Support for families

Psychosocial support includes one-on-one psychological therapy sessions as well as topic-oriented group support, such as life goals, sexuality, relationships, reduction of fear, depression, and feelings of helplessness and hopelessness, teaching coping skills, teaching strategies for stress management and the promotion of active participation and involvement in the treatment or rehabilitation, improvement of communication between patient, partner, and family, and medical/non-medical personnel. It also includes the instruction of various relaxation techniques (such as autogenic training, progressive muscle relaxation, imaginative and hypnotherapeutic procedures), and art therapies (such as music therapy, art therapy, dance therapy) (table 2.4).

Table 2.4 - Complementary therapies to combat tension, anxiety, depression, fears.

– Attitude therapy (includes techniques aimed at keeping problems such as pain at a distance). The objective is to accept the pain and put the pain issue into perspective.
– Biofeedback (controls body functions such as heart rate, blood pressure, and muscle tension).
– Distraction (takes off worries or discomforts. Talking with friends or relatives, watching TV, listening to the radio, reading, going to the movies, doing needlework or puzzles, building models, or painting are all ways to distract. Music or creative art therapies, dance therapies can be very helpful.) Include various methods of focusing thought.
– Hypnotherapeutic procedures (modifies perception of pain so that the latter is no longer perceived as distressful; helps to reduce discomfort and anxiety; help to lower the pain threshold).
– Imaginative procedures (takes away tension).
– Counter activity (overrides pain; similar to distraction strategies, art therapy, music therapy and occupational therapy are typical examples of counter-activity).
– Massage therapy (achieves muscular relaxation).
– Meditation and prayer (is especially helpful when mind and body are stressed from cancer treatment).

– Muscle tension and release (normalizes the circulation, produces slower, more effective respiration, reduces oxygen consumption, lowers the heart rate, lowers the blood pressure, relaxes the musculoskeletal system and keeps pain away).
– Progressive muscle relaxation (achieves relaxation subsequent to muscular contraction).
– Physical exercise (lessens pain, strengthens weak muscles, restores balance, and decreases depression and fatigue.
– Rhythmic breathing (achieves relaxation).
– Visualization (works similar to imagery).
– Yoga, humour, journaling, reiki, pet therapy.

If somatic causes are determined, the psychologist's role takes on an accompanying function. He or she should develop strategies with the patient that can be used to cope with the symptoms and improve quality of life.

Interventions

Fear

The mere diagnosis of cancer leads to fear, completely independent of the severity of the illness and any therapeutic intervention (table 2.5). Many patients suffer from fear and depression long after the conclusion of a successful primary therapy (Bottomley, 1998; Montazeri et al., 2001).

Table 2.5 - Fears in cancer patients.

– Fear of a progression of the illness
– Fear of helplessness, fear of death
– Fear of the side-effects of the therapy
– Fear of pain
– Fear of an agonizing death
– Fear of a deterioration of the partner relationship
– Fear of altered relationships
– Fear of becoming unemployable
– Fear of not being able to provide for the family
– Fear of social isolation
– Fear of being a burden to others
– Fear of being dependent on nursing care

Important fundamentals of therapeutic intervention measures for fear include conversations in a stress-free, calm environment, taking one's time, listening, and conveying a sense of trust. This must be required of the entire rehabilitation team, not only of the psychologists. If the fear is connected with medical, social, or professional problems, then explanations, information, and counselling can aid in achieving a lessening of the fear. If the fear is accompanied by pain, adequate measures to alleviate the pain must first be undertaken before psychotherapy is possible. An adequate therapy of the fears and depression is a prerequisite for other somatic rehabilitation measures (e.g. occupational rehabilitation).

Anxiety disorders can develop into clinically significant panic disorders. Panic disorders are often based on irrational fears and a misinterpretation of physical perceptions or hyperventilation. Cancer fears are usually real fears. Patients should learn to live with the uncertainty and insecurity of the further course of the illness (even in cases with a good prognosis). Relaxation methods and cognitive therapies are helpful, that is, methods of confronting and dealing with one's own fears. Sufficient information about underlying somatic factors and the course of therapy is necessary.

Medicinal support may be considered, but it cannot replace cognitive therapy. Benzodiazepines should be preferred to other substances due to their tolerability, their low number of side-effects, and the breadth of their therapeutic effects. Short-term substances, such as lorazepam, midazolam, and oxazepam, have proven their effectiveness. If fear symptoms emerge again before the next dose is to be taken, the medicinal therapy should be transferred to benzodiazepines (such as diazepam or clonazepam) due to their long-acting effects.

Neuroleptic drugs also have strong anxiolytic qualities. Haloperidol, which is often used in cases of simultaneous confusion or hallucination, should be particularly mentioned in this context. Tricyclic antidepressants are primarily considered when fear emerges in conjunction with depression. However, these drugs may not become effective for up to two weeks. Should a discontinuation of anxiolytic drugs be considered following a longer period of their use, then the discontinuation should occur gradually over the course of two to three days in order to prevent withdrawal symptoms.

States of delirium (confusion, disorientation, and hallucinations) predominantly emerge in the terminal phase of the illness. Treatable medicinal or illness-related causes (such as hypercalcemia) should always be ruled out prior to the introduction of symptom-oriented therapy. Within symptom-oriented therapy the use of neuroleptics (such as haloperidol) is appropriate in cases of delirium, and benzodiazepines (such as lorazepam and midazolam) are well suited for states of anxiety or agitation and motoric restlessness.

Depression

Depression occurs very frequently. It is important for the ensuing therapy to first perform a differential diagnostic assessment in order to discriminate between feelings of sadness, despondence, listlessness, and fatigue and a full, clinical depression (Hahn *et al.*, 2004).

Mental impairments such as depressions can also be caused by somatic, social, or professional factors (fig. 2.1) Should sudden changes in mood occur, the possibility of cerebral metastasization or hypercalcemic syndrome should be considered. Hormone therapies and hormone withdrawal may also accompany mental alterations. Somatic causes must therefore be ruled out before psychological care is implemented. Interdisciplinarity is necessary in both assessment and therapy.

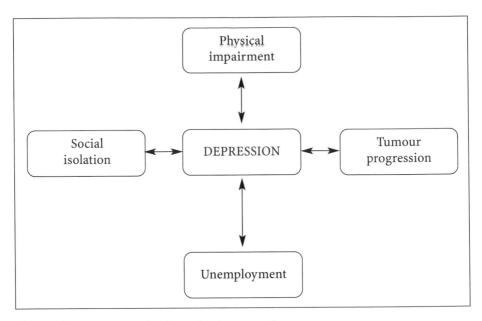

Fig. 2.1 - Frequent reasons for depression in cancer aftercare

The focus of therapy is personal and psychosocial care. Fears and depression should not be automatically treated with antidepressants, but rather treated with supportive and clarifying conversations. The specific implementation of psycho-oncological measures can make the use of psychotropic drugs unnecessary for many cancer patients.

The choice of antidepressant in cancer patients with depression requires consideration of psychological and behavioural symptoms, adverse effect profile, route of metabolism, drug half- life, and drug-drug interactions. Among the safest and most effective drugs are venlafaxine, sertraline, buproprion, citalopram, and escitalopram, as they have few drug interactions through inhibition of P450 enzymes. If a medicinal therapy is necessary, the first choice are often tricyclic antidepressants. Their doses should be increased step by step from 75mg to 150mg to achieve an antidepressive effect. It is important to heed that in contrast to the sedative effect the entry of the antidepressive effect may last up to 2 weeks. However, their usefulness is limited in the late stage of a tumour illness. The side effects, such as sedation and dry mouth, may then be potentially dominant and limit the benefit of the drugs.

Diminished self-esteem

The course of cancer is often accompanied by the patient's loss of self-esteem. There are many potential reasons for this. One may be the patient's isolation from his or her environment and friends. Not only do the people in the patient's environment pull back, but the patient himself or herself may also withdraw. The experience with the intimidating, overwhelming medical system can also create a feeling of helplessness and of being at the mercy of the medical specialists, with a reduction in the patient's feeling of self-worth. Other factors that may lead to a reduction of self-esteem are the uncertain outcome of the illness, the fear of test results, and the fear of therapies that the patient may not understand.

One of the tasks of psychotherapy in rehabilitation can be to prevent this.

Coping

Many patients want information about coping strategies (Stewart *et al.*, 2000). There is not a standardised approach to coping with the disease; every patient reacts in a different way (Manuel *et al.*, 2007). Some, often those with a firm religious belief, may do very well without any professional psychological help (Lauver *et al.*, 2007).

There are various reaction phases over the course of a cancer illness (table 2.6). The beginning and endpoints of these phases generally have no clear demarcation. They may occasionally be skipped or occur in parallel, and they can accompany differing phases of the illness (Kübler Ross, 1984; Muthney, 1996). Support from a clinical psychologist can be recommended in all of these phases.

Table 2.6 - Reaction phases in cancer patients and behavioural recommendations for rehabilitation (based on Muthney, 1996).

Phase	Patient's behaviour	Recommended behaviour for the caregiver
Denial	Denial, isolation	Cautious explanation, prevention of isolation
Shock	Anger, aggression	Understanding – no confrontation, support – no antagonizing or dispassion – no emotional accusations
Reaction	Trying to come to terms, vowing to succeed	Development of an alliance in treating the illness, promotion of positive thinking
Depression	Sadness, exaggerated attempts at amusement	Emphasis of positive aspects, but allowing the patient to experience his or her sadness
Reorientation and coping	Compliance, acceptance of dying	Accompaniment

There are various forms of coping. It still remains open as to which forms of coping should be considered effective, and which coping behaviours indicate a need for psychological intervention (Cunningham, 1995) (table 2.6). Suggestions that certain forms of coping, such as a "fighting spirit", or even "denial", may have an effect conducive to survival (Greer *et al.*, 1989) are to be viewed critically (Buddeberg *et al.*, 1991). Although they may contribute to better coping with the problems in individual cases, they are not suitable for all cancer patients. The same is the case for coping concepts that view the cancer as a challenge, as something to be fought and overcome. Even if there is evidence that active, problem-oriented coping strategies are accompanied by a better mental state, this cannot be considered an overall truth for all cancer patients.

It is important that patients develop the largest possible repertoire of different coping strategies. In certain circumstances, this can be aided by conversational exchange in support groups. The goal of psychotherapeutic assistance should always be an improvement of the patient's sense of well-being achieved by reinforcing the patient's confidence in his own coping-skills and extending the skills being available.

Social support, individual or group cognitive behavioural treatments and other psycho-educational interventions, education and discussion groups, ergo- and art therapy (tables 2.4 and 2.7) can have a positive influence on coping with the illness (Kash *et al.*, 2005).

Self-help groups (support groups) are also a possible source of emotional support and therefore can contribute to quality of life of patients with cancer. Knowing that others had similar symptoms and reactions, and that those experiences are normal, is very important for self-help group participants.

The risk of dysfunctional coping caused by improper behaviour on the part of members of the therapeutic team or the family is often neglected. Both the medical personnel and the family should be asked to remain supportive. They too should be advised to participate in psychological supervision in certain circumstances.

Anxiety, restlessness

Causes of anxiety disorders can be very complex (Love 2002; Norton *et al.*, 2004). Anxiety and fear of follow-up diagnostic tests, fear of progression or recurrence, fear of the uncertain future, and also family, economic and social problems, are frequent (Black, 2004).

In cases of disease progression anxiety, depression and fears are often linked to pain. Increased attention, conversations, "taps on the shoulder", and social activities on their own are often not sufficient to solve psychological problems. It may be necessary to involve a psycho-oncologist.

Fears and depression, as well as restlessness and pain can be reduced through complementary therapies (table 2.4) (Luebbert *et al.*, 2001).

Therapies such as ergotherapy allow for the non-verbal expression of emotions (table 2.7) (Devlin, 2006; Haun, 2001; Rose *et al.*, 2004; Dibbel-Hope, 2000; Stanton *et al.*, 2002; Deane *et al.*, 2000) and contribute to relaxation and, at least temporarily, to an improvement of the patient's quality of life. In classical group settings (music therapy, dance therapy, expressive/creative, art and occupational therapies) (fig. 2.2, 2.3, 2.4), the ergotherapists responsible for the groups should help locate problem patients, who should then be offered one-on-one sessions with a clinical psychologist.

Art work has been shown to be particularly helpful where individuals are unable to express their feelings. This may be owing to cognitive impairment, expressive or receptive dysphasia, or because the person does not have the vocabulary to express his/her feelings clearly (Devlin, 2006).

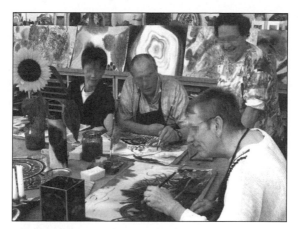

Figs 2.2 - Art therapy in a German rehabilitation centre as a complementary therapy for cancer patients.

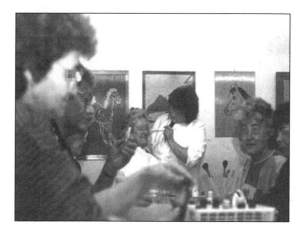

Figs 2.3 - Distraction by cosmetics in a German cancer rehabilitation centre as a complementary therapy to combat tension, anxiety, depression, fears of breast cancer patients

In addition to classical psychological rehabilitation, the geographical location of an oncological rehabilitation clinic can contribute to mental relaxation. It cannot be denied that inpatient rehabilitation in a beautiful environment has a positive influence on the mood of many patients, and the distance from household problems can be a sensible aid for coping with the illness. However, critics of the inpatient rehabilitation setting, which is very prominent in Germany, now charge that too much value has been given to this distance and relaxation in the past. Instead, they demand that a greater emphasis be placed on dealing with the illness in closer proximity to the patient's residence and family (Delbrück, 1998).

Table 2.7 - Characteristics of ergotherapy in cancer rehabilitation.

– Ergotherapy is a component of psycho-oncological care.
– Ergotherapy for cancer patients has more creative aspects than merely occupying the patient
  or providing physical-rehabilitative tasks, or even employment-oriented rehabilitative goals.
– The focus is placed on group work (therapeutic painting, therapeutic sculpting with clay,
  walks on therapy trails, cosmetics classes, etc.).
– The patients should learn to communicate with one another.
– The patients should learn to occupy themselves with new topics, in order to achieve a distance
  to their illness that aids them in better comprehending their difficulties and dealing with them
  more rationally.

Medications for anxiety include the benzodiazepines and the antidepressants. Lorazepam is often the first choice in managing anxiety. As with depression, physical causes for the anxiety must be explored at the same time that anxiolytes are provided. Adequate sleep medication can also reduce daytime anxiety.

Sexuality

Sexual counselling is an important task in aftercare that is occasionally carried out by psychologists. Disturbances in sexual experience and behaviour often emerge as an accompanying problem or subsequent problem in many cancer illnesses. For the affected patients, these disorders often mean a significant loss in their quality of life, their self-esteem, and their satisfaction within their partnership. Psychotherapy can help women cope with difficult changes in their physical appearance and sexual functioning (Anilo, 2000; Avis, 2004).

It can be assumed that only a small percentage of patients will bring up their sexual problems on their own. Most patients wait for questions from their physician or psychologist. The topic of sexuality, and in particular of "sexual incompetence", is accompanied by considerable inhibitions. Fears and feelings of guilt play a central role. These can be reduced through discussion. Under certain circumstances, it is advisable to include the partner in such a discussion, or to offer the partner individual counselling.

Hormone and chemotherapy impair ovarian and testicular function. They have a major impact on sexual function. Much of the loss of desire for sex in women with ovarian failure is linked to dyspareunia from vaginal atrophy. Hormonal changes influence libido and sexual behaviour (Ferell et al., 2003; Schover, 2005). Disturbances in sexual experience and behaviour often emerge as an accompanying problem which may mean a significant loss in quality of life, self-esteem and satisfaction within their partnership.

Fatigue syndrome

Cancer-related fatigue is defined as sustained, agonizing, physical and mental exhaustion that can emerge even years after the conclusion of treatment. In contrast to normal exhaustion, cancer-related fatigue does not improve with rest, adequate nutrition, and sleep (Weis and Bartsch, 2000; Watson, 2004). The triad of tiredness, inefficiency, and depression that is typical for fatigue syndrome has somatic, functional, and mental aspects. The genesis is multifactorial (Flechtner and Bottomley, 2003) (table 2.8). There seems to be no significant correlation between disease burden and fatigue.

Table 2.8 - Possible etiologic factors of fatigue.

– Fatigue is a frequent manifestation of anaemia in patients with cancer. However, many patients who are not anaemic, also report high degrees of debilitating fatigue.
– Chemotherapy and radiotherapy.
– Immune therapies and targeted therapies. Fatigue is a common side effect of interferon, interleukin and TNF therapy.
– Loss of nutrients as a result of anorexia, nausea, vomiting or hyper-metabolism.
– Emaciation.
– Tumour burden and tumour spreading. (There is no significant correlation between disease burden and fatigue).
– Cytokines. During tumour activity, a disrupted balance of endogenous cytokine levels and their natural antagonists can occasionally influence cancer-related fatigue, which is why a reduction of fatigue symptoms can be expected to accompany successful tumour therapy.
– Fatigue symptoms are more frequent in certain kinds of tumour illnesses, such as in malignant lymphomas. In other tumours, such as gastro-intestinal tumours, fatigue symptoms are more seldom. Patients with a combined chemo, radio, and hormone therapy display the highest degree of fatigue.

When assessing cancer-related fatigue, the health-care provider needs to include both subjective and objective data (table 2.9). As in all aspects of subjective experience, an objective measurement of fatigue symptoms is difficult. The methods available for the measurement of fatigue are predominantly based on self-rating scales. There are a number of questionnaires that aid in determining physical well-being, mental condition, and conditions in the social environment. These questionnaires then allow feedback on the extent of the fatigue syndrome (Cella, 1997; Schwartz, 2002).

Table 2.9 - To determine the cause and best treatment for fatigue, the person's fatigue pattern must be determined, and all of the factors causing the fatigue must be identified.

– Fatigue pattern, including how and when it started, how long it has lasted, and its severity, plus any factors that make fatigue worse or better.
– Type and degree of disease and of treatment-related symptoms and/or side effects.
– Treatment history.
– Current medications.
– Sleep and/or rest patterns and relaxation habits.
– Eating habits and appetite or weight changes.
– Effects of fatigue on activities of daily living and lifestyle.
– Psychological profile, including an evaluation for depression.
– Complete physical examination that includes evaluation of walking patterns, posture, and joint movements.
– How well the patient is able to follow the recommended treatment.
– Job performance.
– Financial resources.
– Other factors (for example, anemia, breathing problems, decreased muscle strength).

Underlying factors that contribute to fatigue should be evaluated and treated when possible. Contributing factors include anemia, depression, anxiety, pain, dehydration, nutritional deficiencies, sedating medications, and therapies that may have poorly tolerated side effects (table 2.8). Patients should tell their doctors when they are experiencing fatigue and ask for information about fatigue related to underlying causes and treatment side effects.

All therapeutic measures attempt to determine relevant causes or interrelated effects in order to allow a therapeutic approach to fatigue syndrome. However, every form of treatment should involve a psychosomatic approach. If anemia is the cause, transfusions of erythrocyte concentrates or a physiological increase of hemoglobin with erythropoietin can lead to improvement. However, the effects are marginal if hemoglobin values are greater than 12g/dl. A balanced and vitamin-rich diet is important, since fatigue symptoms are occasionally caused by improper and unbalanced nourishment. Some centers successfully use megestrol acetate for the treatment of both emaciation and fatigue symptoms. Psychostimulants (such as methylphenidate) are sometimes effective.

Many studies indicate the positive effects of physical activity (fig. 2.4). Bicycle ergometer training, walking, weight training, aerobic exercises, and athletic activity are shown to have not only a positive effect on physical fitness and psychological well-being, but also on fatigue symptoms (Oldevoll, 2004). A gradual increase in the training intensity is recommended, starting with 15 to 30 minutes three to five days a week. It is important to clarify to both the patient and to family that physical inactivity, which may be intended as rest, will be more likely to promote symptoms of fatigue than to alleviate them (Watson, 2004).

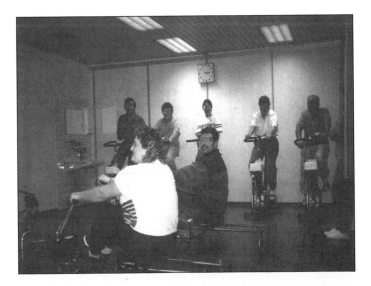

Figure 2.4 - Bicycle ergometer training may be overriding tensions, anxiety and fatigue

Many patients experience a feeling of relief when informed about the somatic causes of fatigue syndrome. They are often distraught because they believe they are suffering from depression with mental causes. When it is explained to them that the symptoms can emerge in conjunction with, for example, chemotherapy, they are very relieved and motivated to begin with physical training.

Table 2.10 - Non- pharmacological interventions in fatigue.

– Education and support groups. With appropriate educational grounding, patients can prepare for side-effects and adopt managemenet strategies.

– Exercise. The theory supporting exercise as a treatment for fatigue proposes that the combined toxic effects of cancer treatment and the decreased degree of physical activity during treatment cause a reduction in the capacity for physical performance.

– Rest and sleep. Patients with cancer report significant disruptions in sleep. The essential issue may be sleep quality rather than quantity.

– Energy conservation and activity management. Decreasing activity to save energy could contribute to deconditioning and decreased activity tolerance

– Stress reduction and stress management. Cancer-related fatigue could be a response to stress, or the emotional state of a patient could affect the way he or she perceives and reports fatigue. Although a strong correlation exists between emotional distress and fatigue, the precise relation is not clearly understood.

– Ergotherapy for cancer patients has more creative aspects than merely occupying the patient or providing physical-rehabilitative tasks, or even employment-oriented rehabilitative goals. The focus is placed on group work (therapeutic painting, therapeutic sculpting with clay, walks on therapy trails, cosmetics classes, etc.).

– Tailored behavioural interventions.

Clarification of the progression of the illness

Explaining to the patient what he or she should expect in the progression of the illness is one of the physician's tasks. It requires a particular sensitivity. Physicians must not be allowed to delegate this task to nursing staff or the psychologist. Family members must not be used as mediators for information between the physician and the patient.

General attitudes concerning the provision of information to the patient have changed fundamentally in recent years. Providing the patient with information is mandatory today for at least legal reasons. Without informed consent, medical treatment is considered personal injury. But apart from legal requirements, there are also psychological reasons for providing the patient with information. Information and explanation can reduce the patient's fear (Keller, 2001). Knowledge about the severity of the illness can free some patients from feelings of obligation to people in their environment. These feelings may otherwise embed the patients in the activities of daily life, detracting from the time and relaxation they require in order to cope with their own situation.

The manner in which the patient is informed of factors surrounding in his or her illness is very important (table 2.11). The conversation should take place in a comfortable setting (the physician's office, a single room). It is wise to tell the patient ahead of time that this is to be an informative conversation, and to check to see if the patient would like to include family or other people close to him or her in this conversation. The patient must provide prior consent before further persons are involved in the discussion.

Table 2.11 - Conditions for the briefings for informed consent.

– Not in the presence of other patients
– Not in the hallway of the ward or unit
– Not "in passing" or "in a hurry"
– Without interruption by telephone calls or pagers
– Not on the telephone
– Not in the evening

The patient must not be informed of a life-threatening situation without the simultaneous offer of aid and support. Informing the patient of the aspects of the illness must involve more than just the simple conveyance of facts. The physician should inform the patient of the severity and consequences of the findings in this conversation, but particulars regarding time factors related to the prognosis should not be given at this time, especially since illnesses may often progress in an unforeseeable manner. In cases of an unfavourable prognosis, the positive aspects should also always be mentioned (such as references to the advancements in palliative therapy, improvements in pain relief, that situations such as suffocation in lung cancer patients or starvation in patients with gastro-intestinal cancer are an absolute exception nowadays). The inability for the patient to bear the prospects of their future carries with it the risk that the patient will look to scientifically unfounded sources for support. This is reason enough to avoid speaking with the patient about the future.

It can be wise to offer the patient a therapy option that is oriented toward the cancer itself, even if the chances of success are low. However, the prerequisites for this are that this therapy is tolerable, that the patient actually desires therapy, and that the physician emphasizes the palliative character of this therapy.

The cognitive capabilities of the patient are often limited, and he or she may not be completely able to absorb and process extensive information. It is thus important to continually signalize a readiness to talk to the patient, to listen, and to be sure of what the patient has understood and which significance these conversations have for the patient. The patient's desire to repress thoughts about the situation, either temporarily or over sustained periods of time, should be respected.

It is undisputed that the patient must always be provided with comprehensive information when treatment options are offered, even in cases of an unfavourable prognosis. When treatment options are not available in conjunction with an unfavourable prognosis, the situation becomes more difficult.

If there are several accepted treatment methods available, the physician must explain each of the alternatives and their risks to the patient, even if the physician does not consider all of the given methods equally effective. As a basic principle, the physician must inform the patient of the risks and consequences of the measures mentioned.

Spirituality

Spirituality, faith, and religion can have a tremendous impact on physical and mental well-being. (Torosian and Biddle, 2005). Research has shown that religiosity and spirituality significantly contribute to the psychosocial adjustment to cancer and its treatments. Religion offers hope to those suffering from cancer, and it has been found to have a positive effect on cancer patients' quality of life. Numerous studies have shown that religion and spirituality also provide effective coping mechanisms for patients as well as for family members. Research indicates that cancer patients who rely on spiritual and religious beliefs to cope with their illness are more likely to use an active coping style, in which they accept their illness and try to deal with it in a positive and purposeful way (Holland, 1999; Weaver and Flannelly, 2004; Lauver *et al.*, 2007).

The recognition of imminent death means an intensification of loneliness and powerlessness for the cancer patient. Thoughts about the meaning of life and the forthcoming separation take on particular significance. Many dying patients desire and need spiritual and religious support in the face of their imminent death. However, spiritual guidance should not be limited to the task of supporting and preparing the patient in the path towards death. Instead, it also serves the purpose of supporting and influencing the patient's ability to experience his or her remaining life. Spiritual guidance can help the patient appreciate his or her life prior to the cancer illness, and also to find new ways of living in the current situation.

For many patients, their faith is a great help in their confrontation with dying, since for them death does not represent an end but rather a transition. This situation can have very different specific traits depending on the given religion. But what they all have in common is the belief that death is merely a passageway. Activities such as praying together, spiritual guidance, eating together, blessing the patient, and many other undertakings can help the patient to experience his or her final days and hours in a valuable manner.

Spiritual counsellors are employed in many German tumour centers and in most German cancer rehabilitation clinics. Physicians are wise to take advantage of these counsellors and integrate spiritual guidance into the treatment team and the rehabilitation and palliation concepts. In some situations, conversations with a spiritual counsellor are more helpful than medical authority, psychological support, antidepressants or tranquilizers, and anxiolytic medication. Charges that spiritual guidance in clinics merely attempts to "compel the patient to convert at the last minute" are not justified.

Support by families

Family members should be involved in aftercare as a basic principle, unless the patient desires otherwise. Sympathy, visits, and help from friends and family are very important both during the acute phase of the illness and afterwards. However, family members will sometimes be afraid that cancer is contagious, and that they too may become ill. They must be relieved of this fear. One of the means by which this is possible is participation in educational cancer training.

Observations of crisis management behaviour show that people in acute crises are particularly grateful for help from friends due to their own mental strain and disorientation. Emotional support from family is irreplaceable. This often brings the people in the patient's environment to their own maximal capacity for stress, creating a need for support and professional psychological care among friends and family.

Even if it is difficult for family, friends, and acquaintances to witness the suffering in the clinic without being able to provide any direct assistance, they should still make time for visits. Even if they believe that they can't find the right words or say the right things in conversation with the patient, they should still try to talk with the patient. "Just listening" is often enough, and their presence alone is meaningful for the patient.

Support for family members

Cancer not only places strain on the patient but also has direct effects on the partner and entire family (Keller, 1995). Research surveys show that emotional stress, depression and anxiety are almost as common among patients' partners as among patients themselves (Bishop et al., 2007). It is helpful if carers can be seen alone from time to time, perhaps by the family doctor, asked how they are coping and invited to talk over any emotional distress.

Distress affects the families of older tumour patients as well as the families of children suffering from cancer; the focus is merely shifted. Tremendous communication problems often arise. Previously existing tensions and conflicts can emerge in the form of aggressions or feelings of guilt. This can place great stress on the patient and can negatively affect the patient's ability to cope with the illness. Psychological support for both the patient and family members, provided by the physician, the spiritual counsellor, or a psycho-oncologist, can be helpful in these cases.

Cancer can cause considerable distress especially for the healthy partners of older cancer patients, which is experienced in addition to the impairments resulting from age-related changes in their own lives. They lose the security provided by continuity in their relationship prior to the cancer. Plans for a "peaceful retirement" are shattered, prospects for their life in old age must be reconsidered and redeveloped. The physical exertion involved in caring for the patient as well as the financial costs of old and new burdens pose substantial problems for the family. The transition in role allocation from "being provided for" to "being the provider" places high demands on the family's ability to adapt to the new situation. In addition to conflicts between the family members' own needs, the desire for autonomy and obligations to the ill parent, conflicts also often arise between caring for the patient and fulfilling responsibilities in the adult child's own family or professional career. The partners of older cancer patients particularly experience emotional distress, while the adult children of cancer patients more frequently describe their stress as the result of confusion in roles. This particularly applies to middle-aged daughters, who fulfill the responsibilities of several roles simultaneously, who more commonly experience stress and fear, and who are less able to fall back on support from their social environment.

Support options for families are internationally very limited with regard to financing by insurance companies or other cost carriers. In Germany, these options are restricted to "family health care" within pediatric oncological rehabilitation clinics, in which children suffering from cancer are cared for together with their parents for a period of three to six weeks. Most German cancer rehabilitation clinics offer the spouse/partner the option of residing in the clinic with the patient for the cost of room and board.

It is desirable for the patient's partner to participate in educational cancer training. Informing patients and their families that physical inactivity can hinder the treatment of fatigue should be one of the problems focused upon in group therapy sessions. A number of German cancer rehabilitation clinics that have a basis on therapy close to the patient's residence explicitly integrate psychosocial care into both their inpatient and their outpatient/semi-outpatient treatment concepts. Spiritual guidance is given emphasis in such cases, especially since it provides the opportunity for further care by placing the patient in contact with the local religious congregations. Self-help groups for family members have also been established. In some regions of Germany there are special centers and organizations (Alpha) that promote the support of family members of the terminally ill.

Desire for information – Motivation – Activation

Education and information are important aids in overcoming illness. This involves the patient's understanding of what is happening to his/her body and why a certain form of therapy has been chosen. Many patients want information pertaining to the disease, treatment, and self-care issues. Many patients express they would like to participate in a counselling programme to discuss psychological issues caused by suffering from breast cancer (Liang *et al.*, 2002; Lauver *et al.*, 2007).

The goals of patient education (also known as "health training", "health education", and "health promotion") include reducing fear and depression, bringing about potentially sensible changes in lifestyle, and above all promoting self-help skills. "The patient should be activated from being treated to being active" (Bourbonniere *et al.*, 2004; Zibecchi *et al.*, 2003).

The educational sessions should take place in small groups whenever possible. These groups should be made up of patients with the same illness or problems so that they can exchange their experiences and perceptions (table 2.12). In Germany, these groups are often moderated by psychologists in conjunction with other members of the rehabilitation team (fig. 1.4). In Anglo-American and Scandinavian countries, the nursing staff or social workers predominantly assume this task. It has proven to be advantageous when patients who have recently been discharged from the hospital following an also recent operation are brought together with other cancer patients, whose treatment is already several years back. The "more experienced" patients function as positive models encouraging the recently diagnosed patients. Family members should also be allowed to participate in the group sessions.

The information and tips provided in the educational sessions should also be given to the patients and their family members in written form.

Table 2.12 - Topics for group education programs for cancer patients.

- Diagnostic and therapeutic options of traditional medicine
- Causes of cancer
- Heredity of cancer
- Psyche and cancer
- Fear and courage to live
- Tasks of aftercare
- What can the patient do to prevent the illness/impairment from progressing? (salutogenesis)
- Increased autonomy
- What can medical science do to prevent the illness/impairment from progressing?
- Symptoms of a relapse
- Modes of behaviour during the course of an illness
- Options for coping with fear
- Options for pain relief
- Relaxation and guided imagery
- Side effects of therapy
- Healthy nourishment
- Effects of the illness/therapy on the career
- Effects of the illness/therapy on recreational activity
- Significance of alternative therapies
- Social rights and support
- Rehabilitation options

Assessment and evaluation

Assessment (initial psychological diagnosis) is primarily concerned with the determination of a need for psychological intervention. Standardized questionnaires are primarily used for this measurement (Endicott *et al.*, 1976; Bergner, 1981; Folkman and Lazarus, 1988; Wiersam, 1990). The same questionnaires are generally used to assess the progress of the therapy and to evaluate the measures that are performed. The Hospital Anxiety and Depression Scale (HADS), the Spiegelberger State-Trait Anxiety Inventory (STAI) are frequently used to assess the parameters of "fear", "depression" and "anxiety" (Bjelland *et al.*, 2002; Marteau *et al.*, 1992).

The analysis and relevance of the assessment of mental problems based on a questionnaire is disputed. The reproducibility of the responses is often difficult, and subjective fluctuation within the patients is difficult to objectify. Mental distress is subject to strong interactions of somatically caused disorders. On the other hand, assessments made by people other than the patient often don't represent the patient's actual mental state. Thus, others sometimes assess the mental problems of patients with severe symptoms to be worse than the affected patient would rate them.

Many of the questionnaires that are recommended in the assessment of need for psychosocial care and the evaluation of psycho-oncological support measures are intended for the research setting and are thus hardly useable in routine practice. Others are more representative of the attempts at transparency and monitoring of psycho-oncological work that are desired by the cost carriers than they are of an endeavour to meet the legitimate psychological requirements of diagnosis and therapy. Procuring evidence of effectiveness and evaluating psychosocial intervention in cancer patients are extraordinarily difficult undertakings (Weis and Dormann, 2005).

Self-help groups

Providing contact addresses of self-help groups is helpful. Participation in support groups can be an important source of emotional and informational support for patients. There are various motives for becoming and remaining member of a patient association. Motives for membership reflect both benefits for the individuals and the welfare of others. Many patients say they wanted to use the association's information and activities. These comments are very common in members of a breast cancer association (Carlsson et al., 2005).

A support group may help to cope with the practical and emotional aspects of the disease. Talking with other patients may help ease feelings of isolation. Self-help groups have the effect of motivating the patient and contribute to a reduction of fear and depression (Montazeri, 2001; Keller, 2000).

Self-help groups organize talks with others affected by the same illness and provide information on certain difficulties that are specific to a given impairment or illness. They also offer knowledge on the chances for success of various treatment and rehabilitation options as well as on the adequate use of cancer resources.

In addition of psychological support, self-help groups often provide their members with specific knowledge about medications and resources as well as social laws. Self-help groups play an important role with regard to the aims of follow-up.

There are various motives for becoming and remaining a member of a patient association. Motives for membership reflect both benefits for the individuals and the welfare of others. The topic of "cancer patients' needs and experiences" is very common among members of breast cancer associations, whereas "making use of the association's information and activities" is more common among members of prostate cancer associations (Lyons, 2001; Carlsson et al., 2005).

Motivation and assistance in achieving self-help skills hold a very high value in oncological rehabilitation. In addition to psychological support, self-help groups often provide their members with specific knowledge about medications and resources as well as social laws. Moreover, they have the effect of motivating the patient and contribute to a reduction of fear and depression (Montazeri, 2001; Keller, 2000).

The concept behind self-help groups is based on the idea that mutual experience and situations offer a person strength. The participants discover they are not alone in their experiences and emotions, and other patients experience the same problems. These common experiences and feelings are intended to strengthen the patient's feeling of self-worth. The patients are to adopt an active attitude towards themselves, their illness, and their environment. The members of self-help groups have first-hand knowledge of the illness and its resulting medical, mental, social, and professional problems ("experts in their field"). Thus they are often more successful than professional healthcare providers at winning the trust of the other patients and offering them support with their physical emotional, and social problems. Self-help groups help to absorb some of the patient's mental distress. Even close family members, relatives, or friends – and of course even physicians and psychologists – have limits to how much they can offer in this regard. Through activities of many different kinds, self-help groups show the patient that a meaningful and fulfilling life is possible even after cancer. Members who have overcome their illness in a positive way serve as a positive role model for newly ill patients. Cancer patients can better overcome the isolation caused by the illness in this way. Enormous reassurance and support is received by the interaction of individuals with the same conditions, when they have the chance to discuss their feelings and how they deal with family, friends, fellow-workers, and society at large.

The first formal, organized ostomy support group in the world began at the Mount Sinai Hospital in 1950. Since then the tasks and concepts of self-help groups have changed over time in many European countries. While treatment deficits, such as in stoma treatment, once led to the establishment of cancer patient groups, today these groups are more and more frequently formed for psychosocial reasons, as well as for the gain of political influence. The nationwide patient organizations in Western Europe have tremendous influence on the health policies of their countries. They call for improved structures, such as the installation of hospices or improved early diagnostics. Thanks to their extensive, Europe-wide contacts, they aid in the foundation of patient organizations in other countries, especially in the Eastern European countries. In these countries, self-help groups still assume treatment responsibilities, such as the psychological care of breast cancer patients or stoma treatment in Slovakia (Witte, 2003).

Internet chat groups and telephone support groups fulfill similar needs. They connect patients who are homebound, isolated, or otherwise unable or unwilling to travel to meet together (Colon, 1996).

Membership in a self-help group is not suitable for all cancer patients. Not every self-help group can be recommended, especially since the groups often have a very particular, individual focus. Participation in self-help groups is to be discouraged when the group interferes with the patients' trust in their physician or in the medical system, or when they advise participation in alternative or supplementary therapy forms that have been scientifically shown to be ineffective or even potentially harmful.

As a basic principle, however, physicians should consider self-help groups to be partners and not rivals in the medical and psychosocial rehabilitation of their patients. Experience shows that patients from these groups turn to non-traditional medical disciplines when they are not taken seriously enough or sufficiently advised by traditionally oriented physicians.

Self-help groups for cancer patients exist in most countries. Regional self-help groups are frequently short-lived, especially since their activities are often dependent on the initiative and capacities of individual cancer patients. In this respect, the address lists must be continually updated. The national cancer societies generally have address lists that are regularly updated.

Bibliography

- Ahlberg K, Ekman T, Gaston-Johansson F *et al.* (2003) Assessment and management of cancer-related fatigue in adults. Lancet 362 (9384): 640-50
- Anilo LM (2000) Sexual life after breast cancer. Journal of Sex & Marital Therapy 26, 3: 241-8
- Aspinal F, Hughes R, Higginson I *et al.* (2002) A user's guide to the palliative care outcome scale. Palliative care & policy publications. Kings College, London
- Avis N, Crawford S, Manuel J (2004) Psychosocial problems among younger women with breast cancer. Psycho-oncology 13, 5: 295-308
- Bausewein C, Fegg M, Radbruch L *et al.* (2005) Validation and clinical application of the german version of the palliative care outcome. J Pain Symptom Manage 30: 51-62
- Bjelland I, Dahl AA, Haug TT *et al.* (2002) The validity of the Hospital Anxiety and Depression Scale. An updated literature review. J Psychosom Res 52, 2: 69-77
- Bottomley A (1998) Anxiety and the adult cancer patient. Eur J Canc Care 7: 217-24
- Bourbonniere M, Kagan SH (2004) Nursing intervention and older adults who have cancer: Specific science and evidence based practice. Nurs Clin North Am 39: 529-43
- Buddeberg C, Wolf C, Sieber M *et al.* (1991) Coping strategies and course of disease of breast cancer patients. Psychother. Psychosom 55: 151-7
- Carlsson C, Baigi A, Killander D *et al.* (2005) Motives for becoming and remaining member of patient associations: A study of 1,810 Swedish individuals with cancer associations. Support Care Cancer 20
- Colon Y (1996) Telephone support groups: A nontraditional approach to reading underserved cancer patients. Cancer Pract 4, 3: 156-9
- Cella D (1997) The functional assessment of cancer therapy anaemia (FACT-An) scale: A new tool for the assessment of outcomes in cancer anemia and fatigue. Semin Hematol 34 (suppl 2): 13-9
- Cunningham A (1995) Group psychological therapy for cancer patients: A brief discussion of indications for its use, and the range of interventions available. Supportive Care Cancer 3: 244-7
- Delbrück H, Haupt E (edit) (1998) Rehabilitationsmedizin. Ambulant – teilstationär – stationär. 2. Auflage Urban & Schwarzenberg München
- Deutsche Krebsgesellschaft (1997) Standards und Qualitätskriterien in der onkologischen Rehabilitation. W. Zuckschwerdt Verlag München
- Deane K, Fitch M, Carman M (2000) An innovative art therapy program for cancer patients. Can Oncol Nurs J 10: 147
- Delbrück H, Witte M (2004) Vergleich onkologischer Rehabilitationsmaßnahmen und-strukturen in Ländern der Europäischen Gemeinschaft. Nordrhein-Westfälischer Forschungsverband Rehabilitationswissenschaften Wuppertal
- Devlin B (2006) The art of healing and knowing in cancer and palliative care. Int J Pallative Nurseing, 12, 1: 16-9
- Dibbell-Hope S (2000) The use of dance/movement therapy in psychological adaptation to breast cancer. Arts in Psychotherapy 27: 51-68
- Endicott J, Spitzer RL, Fleiss JL *et al.* (1976) The sickness rating scale: A procedure for measuring overall severity of psychiatric disturbances. Archives of General Psychiatrie 33: 766- 71

- Flechtner H, Bottomley A (2003) Fatigue and quality of life: Lessons from the real world. Oncologist 8 Suppl 1: 5-9
- Folkman S, Lazarus RS (1988) Manual for the ways of coping questionnaire (WOC). Palo Alto, Consulting
- Goodwin PJ, Leszcz M, Ennis M et al. (2001) The effect of group psychosocial supprt on survival in metastastatic breast cancer. N Engl J Med 345: 1719
- Greer S, Moorey S, Watson M (1989) Patients adjustment to cancer (MAC) Scale vs clinical ratings. J Psychosomatic Research 33: 373-7
- Kübler-Ross E (1980) Interviews mit Sterbenden. Gütersloher Verlagshaus
- Hahn C, Dunn R, Halper E (2004) Routine Screening for Depression in Radiation Oncology Patients. Am J clin Oncol 27, 5: 497-9
- Haun M, Mainous RO, Looney SW (2001) Effect of music on anxiety of women awaiting breast biopsy. Behav Med 27: 127-32
- Holland JC, Passik S, Kash KM et al. (1999) The role of religious and spiritual beliefs in coping with malignant melanoma. Psychooncology 8: 14-26
- Kash K, Mago R, Kunkel EJ (2005) Psychosocial oncology: supportive care for the cancer patient. Semin Oncol 32: 211c-8
- Keller M, Sellschopp A, Beutel M (1995) Spouses between distressand support. IN: Cooper C, Baider L, Caplan de Nour A (edit) (1995) Cancer and the family. Wiley. Chichester
- Keller M (2001) Effekte psychosozialer Interventionen auf Lebensqualität und Krankheitsverlauf von Krebspatientinnen. Onkologe 7: 133-42
- Lauver DR, Connally-Nelson K, Vanig P (2007) Stressors and coping strategies among female cancer survivors after treatments. Cancer Nurs 30, 2: 101-11
- Luborsky L (1962) clinicians judgements of mental health. Archives of general psychiatry 7: 407-17
- Luebbert K, Dahme B, Hasenbring M (2001) The effectiveness of relaxation training in reducing treatment-related symptoms and improving emotional adjustment in acute non-surgical cancer treatment: A meta-analysis review. Psycho-oncology 10: 490-502
- Lyons A (2001) Ileostomy and colostomy support groups The Mount Sinai J Med 68, 2: 110-3
- Manuel J, Burkwell S, Crawford S et al (2007) Younger women perspectives of coping with breast cancer. Cancer Nurs 30, 2: 85-94
- Marteau T, Bekker H (1992) The development of a six – item short-form of the state scale of the Spiegelberger Stait-Trait inventory. Br J Clin Psychol 31, 3: 301-6
- Montazeri A, Jarvandi S, Haghighat S et al. (2001) Anxiety and depression in breast cancer patients before and after participation in a cancer support. Patient Educ Couns 45, 3: 195-8
- Muthny F (1996) Wege der Krankheitsverarbeitung von Krebspatienten und Möglichkeiten von Hilfen. Hefte zur Krebsnachsorge. Hartmann Bund, Bad Neuenahr
- Oldervoll L, Kaasa S, Hjermstadt M et al. (2004) Physical exercise results in the improved subjective well-being of a few or is effective rehabilitation for all cancer patients? Europ J cancer 40: 950-62.
- Rose JP, Brandt K, Weis J (2004) Music therapy in oncology. Psychother Psychosom Med Psychol 54: 457-70
- Schwartz AH (2002) Validity of cancer-related fatigue instruments. Pharmacotherapy 22 (11): 1433-41

– Stanton AL, Danoff-Burg S, Sworowski LA *et al.* (2002) Randomized, controlled trial of written emotional expression and benefit finding in breast cancer patients. J Clin Oncol 20: 4160-8
– Torosian M, Biddle VR (2005) Spirituality and healing. Semin Oncol 32: 232-6
– Watson M, Denton S, Baum M *et al.* (1988) Counselling breast cancer patients: A specialist nurse service. Couns Psychol Q 1: 25-34
– Watson M, Haviland JS, Greer S *et al.* (1999) Influence of psychological response on survival in breast cancer: A population-based cohort study. Lancet 354: 1331-6
– Watson T, Mock V (2004) Exercise as an intervention for cancer-related fatigue. Phys Ther 84: 736-43
– Weaver A, Flannelly K (2004) The role of religion/spirituality for cancer patients and their caregivers. Southern Medical Journal 97, 12: 1210-14
– Weis J, Bartsch HH, Erbacher G (1996) Rehabilitation needs and outcome of inpatient rehabilitation program for cancer patients. Psycho-oncology 5: 3-5
– Weis J, Domann U (2006) Interventionen in der Rehabilitation von Mammakarzinompatientinnen. Eine methodenkritische Übersicht zum Forschungsstand. Rehabilitation (in press)
– World Health Organization (2001) International classification of functioning, disabilities and health. www.WHO.int/classification/ICF
– Wiersma D, Dejong A, Kraaikamp HJM *et al.* (1990) The Groningen Social disabilities schedule. Manual and questionnaires 2nd version. University of Groningen, Department of social psychiatrie, World Health Organisation
– Zech D, Grond S, Lynch J *et al.* (1995) Validation of wrld health organization guidelines for cancer pain relief: A 10-year prospective study. Pain 63: 65-76
– Zibecc L, Greendale GA, Ganz PA (2006) Continuing education: Comprehensive menopausal assessment: An approach to managing vasomotor and urogenital symptoms in breast cancer survivors. Oncol Nurs Forum 30: 393-407

Social support in cancer rehabilitation and palliation

Definition and goals of social support

Social support and assistance with daily life are important elements of the endeavor to reduce and compensate for the disadvantages that result from tumour illnesses and therapies. Social measures to avoid impairments of activities and performance should be given priority because an essential factor affecting quality of life is independence. Activities of daily living dependency is associated with lower quality of life ratings in cancer patients (Cheville, 2005) (tables 1.9, 3.1, 3.2, 3.3).

Oncology social workers help patients and their families regarding practical concerns that accompany the diagnosis, treatment and after care of cancer.

Table 3.1 - Goals of social support in rehabilitation and palliation.

– To develop maximum skills in activities of daily living (ADL) allowed by the disability
– To avoid impairments of activities and performance
– To prevent and to reduce nursing care
– To guarantee social compensations for handicaps
– To give social counselling
– To provide nursing care

Table 3.2 - Functioning disorders in tumour patients as a result of the tumour or the therapy.

– Mobility disorders (walking, climbing stairs, running)
– Disorders of physical capacity (work capacity, endurance, housekeeping, self-care)
– Disturbances in the environment (family, career, recreation)
– Disturbances in activities of daily life (ADL) (eating and drinking, bathing, getting dressed/undressed, physical hygiene, housekeeping, shopping, preparing meals, use of the toilet, etc.)

Table 3.3 - Activities of Daily Living (Lawton and Brody, 1969).

– Eating and drinking
– Bathing and grooming
– Getting dressed/undressed
– Managing bladder and bowel functions
– Physical hygiene
– Caring for health and fitness
– Toileting
– Moving in bed
– Changing position
– Walking
– Housekeeping
– Shopping
– Preparing meals
– Using transportation
– Money management
– Ability to take medications

Due to the fact that the onset of cancer frequently occurs by older persons, many cancer patients have an increased need for social assistance, independent of the progression of the illness and any functioning disorders that may result from therapy (Harlacher and Füsgen, 2000).

Interventions in social care

Assessment of needs for social support

The planning and organization of social care is an important element in rehabilitation and palliation. Questions of a patient's needs for nursing care must be resolved, who can provide inpatient and outpatient support, where this can be provided, and whether the need for care can be prevented or at least reduced through rehabilitation measures.

The best known and most frequently used parameters for the measurement of functional status and capacity within the field of oncology are the Karnofsky Index (table 3.4), the capacity scales of the Eastern Cooperative Oncology Group (ECOG-Performance status, table 3.5), and the WHO Performance Status (table 3.6) (Extermann, 1988). These indices are primarily used in curatively oriented therapy studies. They aid in determining the prognosis and in developing therapy planning. They do not meet the bio-psychological requirements and goals of oncological rehabilitation and palliation.

Table 3.4 - Karnofsky performance status scale definitions rating (%) criteria.

Able to carry on normal activity and to work; no special care needed.	100	Normal, no complaints; no evidence of disease.
	90	Able to carry on normal activity; minor signs or symptoms of disease.
	80	Normal activity with effort; some signs or symptoms of disease.
Unable to work; able to live at home and care for most personal needs; varying amount of assistance needed.	70	Cares for self; unable to carry on normal activity or to do active work.
	60	Requires occasional assistance, but is able to care for most of his personal needs.
	50	Requires considerable assistance and frequent medical care.
Unable to care for self; requires equivalent of institutional or hospital care; disease may be progressing rapidly.	40	Disabled; requires special care and assistance.
	30	Severely disabled; hospital admission is indicated although death not imminent.
	20	Very sick; hospital admission necessary; active supportive treatment necessary.
	10	Moribund; fatal processes progressing rapidly.
	0	Dead

Table 3.5 - ECOG Performance Status.

Grade	ECOG
0	Fully active, able to carry on all pre-disease performance without restriction.
1	Restricted in physically strenuous activity but ambulatory and able to carry out work of a light or sedentary nature, e.g., light house work, office work.
2	Ambulatory and capable of all self-care but unable to carry out any work activities. Up and about more than 50% of waking hours.
3	Capable of only limited self-care, confined to bed or chair more than 50% of waking hours.
4	Completely disabled. Cannot carry on any self-care. Totally confined to bed or chair.
5	Dead.

Table 3.6 - Categories of WHO Performance Status.

– Scale 0: Patient is fully active and more or less as he was before the illness.

– Scale 1: Patient cannot carry out heavy physical work, but can do anything else.

– Scale 2: Patient can look after himsself, but is not well enough to work .

– Scale 3: Patient is in bed or sitting in a chair for more than half the day; he needs some help in looking after himself.

– Scale 4: Patient is in bed or a chair all the time and needs a lot of looking after.

A standardized assessment of functional status is the only approach that allows a comparison of results and forms the basis for monitoring progress. It should be based on procedures that have been proven to be valid, sensitive and reliable. Good indices for the assessment of social needs in rehabilitation and palliation are the Barthel Index (Mahoney and Barthel, 1965) and the Functional Independence measurement (FIM).

The Barthel Index (table 3.7) consists of ten items with a possible score of 100 points. The index is an ordinal scale consisting of ten activities of daily living. The Barthel Index can be derived from asking the patient, the patient's friends and relatives as well as from direct observation. The Barthel Index is at its best when recorded over periods of time by a single individual, a measure of improvement of a patient. It is an assessment that enables health professionals to determine the degree of disability in a particular individual. Generally speaking, a score of 14 indicates some disability, usually compatible with the level of support found in a residential home, a score of 10 compatible with discharge home provided there is maximum support and a care giver in attendance.

The *Functional Independence Measurement* (FIM) (table 3.8) is an 18-item measure that evaluates the following: self-care, sphincter control, mobility, locomotion, communication, and social cognition. The items on the FIM are scored on a seven point ordinal scale ranging from 1 to 7. The range of the scores on the FIM is a minimum of 18, which indicates the low level of functioning, to a maximum of 126, which indicates very high level of functioning. The FIM is a structured interview that is administered during the first few days of admission to the hospital. It is administered periodically through the hospital stay and once again at the time of discharge. The FIM is useful in measuring rehabilitation outcomes with individuals with disabilities. FIM is one such instrument that has been used with various disability groups to assess functionality.

Table 3.7 - The Barthel Index.

1. Bowel status	0 point - Incontinent (or needs to be given enema)
	1 point - Occasional accident (once a week)
(Question 1 of 10)	2 points - Fully Continent
2. Bladder status	0 point - Incontinent or catheterized and unable to manage
	1 point - Occasional accident (max once per 24 hours)
(Question 2 of 10)	2 points - Continent (for more than seven days)
3. Grooming	0 point - Needs help with personal care: face/hair/teeth/shaving
(Question 3 of 10)	1 point - Independent (implements provided)
4. Toilet Use	0 point - Dependent
	1 point - Needs some help but can do something alone
(Question 4 of 10)	2 points - Independent (on and off/wiping/dressing)
5. Feeding	0 point - Unable
	1 point - Needs help in cutting/spreading buffer, etc.
(Question 5 of 10)	2 points - Independent (food provided within reach)
6. Transfer	0 point - Unable (as no sitting balance)
	1 point - Major help (physical/one or two people)
	2 points - Can sit minor help (verbal or physical)
(Question 6 of 10)	3 points - Independent
7. Mobility	0 point - Immobile
	1 point - Wheelchair-independent (including corners, etc.)
	2 points - Walks with help of one person (verbal or physical)
(Question 7 of 10)	3 points - Independant
8. Dressing	0 point - Dependent
	1 point - Needs help but can do about half unaided
(Question 8 of 10)	2 points - Independent (including buttons/zips/laces, etc.)
9. Stairs	0 point - Unable
	1 point - Nedds help (verbal/physical/carrying aid)
(Question 9 of 10)	2 points - Independent up and down
10. Bathing	0 point - Dependent
(Question 10 of 10)	1 point - Independent bathing or showering

Table 3.8 - The Functional Independence measurement (FIM).

Patient's functional status	Scoring
Completely dependent	1
Requires maximal assistance	2
Requires moderate assistance	3
Requires minimal assistance	4
Requires supervision	5
Relatively independent	6
Completely independent	7

The patient's score varies from 18 points (the patient is completely dependent) to 126 points (the patient is completely independent).

The following is the detailed questionnaire:

Evaluation 1: Self-care
– Item 1. Food
– Item 2. Care of appearance
– Item 3. Hygiene
– Item 4. Dressing upper body
– Item 5. Dressing lower body

Evaluation 2: Sphincter control
– Item 6. Control of bladder
– Item 7. Control of bowel movements

Evaluation 3: Mobility
– Item 8. Bed, chair, wheel chair
– Item 9. To go to the toilets
– Item 10. Bath-tub, shower

Evaluation 4: Locomotion
– Item 11. Go, wheel chair
– Item 12. Staircases

Evaluation 5: Communication
– Item 13. Auditive comprehension
– Item 14. Verbal expression

Evaluation 6: Social adjustment/cooperation
– Item 15. Capacity to interact and to socially communicate
– Item 16. Resolution of the problems
– Item 17. Memory

Total scoring: from 18 to 126 points

Compensations for handicaps

One of the tasks in rehabilitation is to inform the patient and his family about governmental and non governmental helps, voluntary organizations and about support groups.

Cancer imposes heavy economic burdens on both patients and their families. For many people, a portion of medical expenses is paid by their health insurance plan. For individuals who do not have health insurance or who need financial assistance to cover health care costs, resources are available, including government-sponsored programs and services supported by voluntary organizations. There are numerous non profit organizations providing financial and social help.

Many countries provide legal concessions and privileges for the severely handicapped. These privileges span from tax breaks and employment protection to financial relief and other financial services. The extent of such aid varies from country to country depending on the influence of political and social factors (table 3.9).

Table 3.9 - Legally defined privileges for cancer patients in Germany (Delbrück, 1998).

– Increased dismissal protection at the workplace.
– Support in maintaining or obtaining a handicapped accessible workplace, for example technical aids or labor expense subsidies for the employer.
– Option of early retirement or retirement pay.
– Exemption from overtime (at the wish of the employee).
– Entitlement to an additional five days of vacation leave each year.
– Preferential processing of documents and official matters in civil service offices.
– Tax breaks.
– Special concessions for the use of public transportation, public swimming facilities, museums, etc.
– Additional tax exemptions in conjunction with applications for housing subsidies.
– State subsidized housing in compliance with certain requirements (such as in consideration of the annual income).
– Frequently, reduced membership fees for organizations and associations.
– Depending on additional criteria, cost relief is also offered for radio and television taxes, motor vehicle registration fees, travel fare exemption, reduction of admission charges.
– In cases of extreme impairment in operating motor vehicles (as with severe breathing impairments following pneumonectomies in bronchial carcinomas, or with seizures in cases of brain tumours), patients can use public transportation at a low cost within a radius of 50km; special parking concessions, a motor vehicle registration reduction of 50%, and a motor vehicle insurance reduction of 25% are also available.
– Persons who are excluded from meeting in public (such as transplant patients with immunosuppression, contagious tuberculosis, or with an unpleasant odor in cases of an insufficiently maintained preternatural anus, frequent expectoration or coughing in cases of laryngeal or bronchial carcinomas) are exempt from radio and television taxes and are given a reduction in their base telephone fees.
– For persons permanently dependent on support from others (such as paraplegics, amputees, the blind and severely visually impaired, the severely hearing impaired, people who suffer from seizures, severely mentally impaired persons), the transportation in public transportation systems is provided free of charge for an accompanying assistant, fare reductions of 50% are provided to the disabled person, and transportation of an accompanying assistant is free of charge on German domestic flights.

The special concessions are intended to compensate for the disadvantages that result from the illness and its treatment. However, they are also intended to strengthen the autonomy and self-help options of the disabled, to facilitate the disabled persons' participation in daily life and in the community, to increase productivity, and finally, to reduce healthcare costs.

In Germany, all cancer patients are entitled to a legal certificate stating that they are severely disabled if they apply for one, independent of the dimension and extent of the disability and their prognosis. This certificate makes them eligible for special advantages (table 3.9) that are specially oriented towards aspects of their professional life, such as increased employment protection. However, not all cancer patients apply for these certificates (which must be renewed at least once every five years), since they can also lead to various disadvantages. Such disadvantages effect particularly young patients and patients intensely active in their career, although the legal "advantages" were originally intended especially for them. Official status as "severely disabled" can lead to difficulties in selecting a career, changing a profession, or in advancing within a given profession, since many employers have false presumptions concerning the professional capacity of cancer patients and may be afraid of having more difficulty dismissing them. Young patients who have successfully overcome lymphomas, leukemia, or testicular cancer, for example, are often advised against applying for disabled status.

Participation

Assistance with participation in social life is an integral component of all rehabilitation work in disabled people. It is based on principles defined by the International Classification of Function, Disabilities, and Health (ICF) (Barat M, Franchignoni F, 2004; World Health Organization, 2001).

An essential factor affecting quality of life is independence. All measures that help to avoid or to reduce the dependence of cancer patients play a key role in rehabilitation and palliation (table 3.3, 3.10).

Table 3.10 - Targets being given priority in palliative oncology.

– Avoiding impairments of activities and performance
– Recognizing and supporting independence and competence
– Delaying or avoiding the need for care and the resulting dependence
– Enabling the patient to remain at home or in his or her familiar environment

Family counselling

Family members must be informed early of possible nursing-care problems that can arise within homecare so that they can procure appropriate assistance. They should be provided with addresses of healthcare organizations that offer such assistance.

The involvement of family members in nursing care is essential to maintain continuity in the patient's healthcare and social support, particularly as the patient nears the end of his or her life. Family care givers often assume this role under sudden and extreme circumstances, with minimal preparation and unbalanced guidance and support from the healthcare system. The primary nursing care setting for cancer patients has shifted from the hospital to the home as a result of several factors, including the increased use of outpatient services for cancer treatment, shortened hospital stays, longer survival times, and the trend for care givers to accommodate patients' desire to be cared for at home as long as possible. Caring for a family member with cancer poses significant challenges, with considerable psychological and physical consequences for the care giver (Glajchen, 2004).

Homecare for terminally ill patients is unimaginable without intensive support from the family. Aside from the fact that patients sometimes have no family available, this support is often insufficient when caring for highly symptomatic tumour patients. In many countries, state and semi-state organizations, charity groups, funding organizations, or self-help groups thus offer assistance with the homecare of cancer patients who are dependent on individual healthcare.

Social counselling

Assistance in social care is available in most countries. This aid is offered to both patients and families in different forms in different countries. In France nearly all hospitals employ social workers *(assistance sociale)* who have high reputations and who are responsible for securing post-stationary social care. In some countries, such as Germany, special state sponsored and semi-state sponsored cancer counselling centers are available to the public. In other countries, charity institutions, self-help organizations, and support groups assume the social and legal aspects of outpatient patient care (such as the organization *Lutte contre le cancer* in France) (Delbrück, 2004).

The social services of most clinics, as wells as the health insurance organizations and the information and counselling services of the national cancer organizations and self-help groups, maintain address lists that they can give to the patient, the family, or the physician responsible for further outpatient care.

With the explosion of the Internet, many cancer centers and hospitals, news networks, pharmaceutical companies have websides on which various topics are featured. Many of these websites are dedicated to cancer therapy in general and focus on specific topics in various formats. Occasionally patients can become overwhelmed with all of the information. That is why it is important for patients to use the information obtained as part of the shared decision-making process with their physicians regarding their treatment.

Table 3.11 - Services provided by cancer counselling centers in Germany (Delbrück, 1998).

– Procuring information about questions concerning medical care, nursing care, social-legal issues, and practical issues
– Support in coping with the illness and the disability
– Psychosocial counselling in the form of individual sessions as well as family or group settings
– Therapeutic support – either psychotherapy or family therapy
– Provision of practical and economical services
– Visitation services
– Gymnastic offers, autogenic training, relaxation and breathing exercises
– Creative therapy offers
– Initiation of rehabilitation measures and access to health care centers
– Mediation of contact to other patients affected by the same cancer, self-help groups
– Organization of work groups and collective events
– Coordination of existing cancer aftercare services
– Support for self-help groups
– Public relations work

Due to the forthright efforts of cancer patients, there are now many organizations and list serves (e-mailing lists) that cancer survivors can turn to for help before, during, and after cancer treatment. There are several organizations that provide invaluable services to cancer patients and have been in existence for a very long time. Most notably are the services offered by the national cancer societies. Most organizations not only provide written material for cancer patients but also have helplines for patients to call. The creation of interactive online support is becoming a reality. Non profit organizations provide information, education, support, and counselling for patients and their families.

The limited ability to obtain credit poses a particularly large problem for cancer patients who would like to arrange an independent existence and require financial coverage in order to do so, such as in the form of life insurance.

Most life insurance providers only accommodate potentially curatively treated cancer patients who show no signs of tumour activity. In general, they accept the clinical findings that were obtained in the framework of the aftercare examinations when concluding the contract.

Moreover, life insurance companies make a distinction between various risk classes, based primarily on life expectancy (prognosis). These risk classes result in different waiting periods. This means that if the patient desires to take advantage of insurance claims in the event of illness related damages, the insurance sum is only paid out following a specific waiting period, the length of which is dependent on the prognostic criteria.

Even when the carcinoma is in an early stage and exhibits a good prognosis, the life insurance companies require a postponement of payment for two years beginning at the inception of therapy. Even after this time period has passed, additional risk fees amounting to between 1 and 2 percent of the insurance sum are imposed. In other cases, such as when the cancer has spread to a higher degree, when the risk of relapse is high, and in cases of a poor prognosis, the insurance companies generally decline life insurance.

Structural characteristics

Qualification and competences of personnel

In some countries, physicians assume the responsibility for initiating social assistance, while in other countries the nursing staff, social workers, or charity organizations and support groups take up this role. The social worker and the vocational counselor (tables 3.12, 3.13) have many important roles in the rehabilitation of the cancer patient.

Great Britain has the system of "specialist cancer nurses" (e.g. breast cancer nurses, stoma nurses, lung cancer nurses, community nurses), who are available to cancer patients for counselling and coordination from the beginning of their illness to the end. These specialist cancer nurses are both vital in providing information about the disease and its treatments, as well as in providing counselling and support for patients and their families. Their role is crucial in guiding the patient through the complexities of the multi-disciplinary treatment team and in accessing support from other services, such as social workers, community follow-up, and physiotherapy. Patients and care-givers feel assured that the nurse is an approachable point of contact at any stage of their illness (Delbrück, 2004).

Table 3.12 - Role and necessary competences of the social worker in rehabilitation oncology.

– Discharge planning, facilitating a smooth transition from the hospital to the community
– Individual social counselling and initiation of social support
– Ensure continuity of care
– Procurement of support for families, support from the patient's environment (self-help groups, charity organizations, etc.)
– Secure appropriate follow-up services after discharge
– Secure financial resources, including health insurance coverage, and social security and disability compensation
– Obtain authorization and payment for necessary devices and home help
– Arrangement need for transportation, attendant, or nursing care, home modifications, and other appropriate post-hospital services
– Contact to business and civil services
– Counselling and initiation of career support services
– Counselling for retirement issues
– Nursing care (e.g. homecare, assistance with housekeeping, etc.)
– Initiation of rehabilitation measures
– Access to palliative care or hospice care

Table 3.13 - Role and necessary competences of vocational counselor in rehabilitation oncology.

– Detailed evaluation, counselling, testing, career exploration, educational planning
– Visits to work or school sites and consult with employers and teachers to facilitate the transition from disability to productivity as a worker or student
– Make the initial referral to offices of vocational rehabilitation and maintain a close cooperative and effective relationship with the offices of vocational representatives

Evaluation, quality assurance

To assess and monitor function accurately, the performance in different activities of self-care, mobility, and communication must be numerically rated according to the patient's level of independence: completely independent; independent with devices; requires assistance (supervision, "spotting", reminding, physical help); or completely dependent.

Several evaluation scales for social measurements in handicapped patients exist. Some are simple and easy to use but provide incomplete information, whereas others are detailed but time consuming, as they address a whole range of quality of life factors which include mobility, self-care, employment, income, education, family activities, living arrangements, and transportation. The functional evaluation scale that is currently gaining the widest acceptance by rehabilitation professionals is the Functional Independence Measurement (FIM) (table 3.8).

Bibliography

- Balducci L (2003) Management of cancer pain in geriatric patients. J Support Oncol 1: 175-91
- Barat M, Franchignoni F (edit) (2004) Assesssment in physical medicine and rehabilitation. Maugeri Foundation books. PI-ME Press Pavia
- Bishop M, Beaumont J, Hahn E (2007) Late effects of cancer on spouses or partners compared with survivors and survivor-matched controls. J Clin Oncol 25, 11: 1403-11
- Bonomi AE, Cella DF et al. (1996) Multilingual translation of the functional assessment of cancer therapy (FACT) quality of life measurement system. Qual Life Res 5, 3: 309-20
- Bundesarbeitsgemeinschaft für Rehabilitation (2003) Rahmenempfehlungen zur ambulanten onkologischen Rehabilitation. Bundesarbeitsgemeinschaft für Rehabilitation Frankfurt
- Cella D (1997) The functional assessment of cancer therapy anaemia (FACT-An) scale: A new tool for the assessment of outcomes in cancer anemia and fatigue. Semin Hematol 34 (suppl 2): 13-9
- Cheville A (2005) Cancer rehabilitation. Semin Oncol 32: 219-24
- Charlson M, Pompei P et al. (1987) A new method for classifying prognostic comorbidity in longitudinal studies. J Chronic Dis 40: 373-83
- Dejong A, Giel R, Sloof C et al. (1985) Social disability and outcome in schizophrenic patients. Br J Psychiatr 147: 621-36
- Delbrück H, Haupt E (edit) (1998) Rehabilitationsmedizin. Ambulant – teilstationär – stationär. 2. Auflage Urban & Schwarzenberg München
- Delbrück H, Witte M (2004) Vergleich onkologischer Rehabilitationsmaßnahmen undstrukturen in Ländern der Europäischen Gemeinschaft. Nordrhein-Westfälischer Forschungsverband Rehabilitationswissenschaften Wuppertal
- Extermann M, Overcash J et al. (1998) Comorbidity and functional staus are independent in older cancer patients. J Clin Oncol 4: 1582-7
- Ferrucci L, Cecchi F et al. (1996) Does the clock drawing test predict cognitive decline in older persons independent of the mini-mental state examination? J Am Geriatr Soc 44: 1326-31
- Glajchen M (2004) The emerging role and needs of family care givers in cancer care. J Support Oncol 2: 145-55
- Harlacher R, Füsgen I (2000) Geriatric assessment in the elderly cancer patient. J Cancer Res Clin Oncol 126: 369-74
- Kempen GIJM, Suurmeijer TPBM (1990) The development of a hierarchical polychotomous ADL-IADL scale for non-institutionalized elderly. Gerontologist 30: 497-502
- Lawton M, Brody E (1969) Assessment of older people: Self maimtaining and instrumental acrivities of daily living. Gerontologist 9: 179-86
- Mahoney F, Barthel DW (1965) Functional evaluation. The Barthel Index. Md State Med J 14: 61-6
- Tinetti M (1990) A simple procedure for general screening for functional disability in elderly patients. Ann Intern Med 112: 699-706
- United Nations (1994) The standard rules on equalization of opportunities for patients with disabilities

- World Health Organization (2001) International classification of functioning, disabilities and health. www.WHO.int/classification/ICF
- Wright B, Linacre JM (1993) Performance profiles of the functional independence measure. Am J Phys Med Rehabil 72: 84-9

Vocational integration in cancer rehabilitation[1]

Delbrück H

Tasks and goals

In cancer rehabilitation, influencing the illness is less of an issue than the reduction of subsequent problems caused by tumours and therapies. Negative effects on patients' professional lives are additional elements in rehabilitation apart from somatic, psychological and social problems (Gobelet, 2005). Assistance designed to promote vocational integration is thus part and parcel of the tasks involved in oncological rehabilitation (Delbrück, 1998; Delbrück, 2003). Vocational inactivity not only means financial and existential disadvantages for those concerned as well as for society, but also involves a risk of social isolation and a reduction in self-esteem. In short, it leads to a reduction in the quality of life (Maunsell *et al.*, 1999).

Epidemiology

The prevalence of cancer patients living in Western Europe who are capable of gainful employment can only be estimated – in contrast to mortality. Among civil servants in Germany, the percentage of cancer patients under the age of 60 is put at 30%. Additionally, the percentage frequency of people taking early retirement following cancer can only be estimated. In Germany, neoplasia (8%) is in fourth place as a cause for early retirement in civil servants following mental illnesses (47%), musculoskeletal diseases (15.4%) and cardiovascular diseases (11%) (Lederer *et al.*, 2003).

Cancer is a collective term for a very heterogeneous group of malignant diseases with differing prognoses and differing therapeutic requirements. Special cancer diseases occur with different degrees of frequency in infancy and adolescence, in adulthood and in old age.

Cancer diagnoses most frequently involving a need for vocational rehabilitation in the past 20 years include malignant haematological and lymphatic system diseases, testicular tumours and sarcomas, which have very good lifetime prognoses thanks to the introduction of more recent chemotherapy. As a result of the temporal shifts of certain

[1] This article, up-dated, has been already published in C. Gobelet, F. Franchignoni, Vocational Rehabilitation *(2006): 209-23.*
© Springer-Verlag Paris.

tumour diseases and thanks to improved precautionary diagnostics, rehabilitation doctors are, however, currently faced to an increasing degree by the vocational problems suffered by patients with gynaecological, gastro-intestinal and pulmonary tumours. Whereas, today, improved therapy strategies and possibilities result in certain tumour diseases either being cured more frequently than before or being converted to a chronic stage, this is often at the cost of considerable side-effects that also affect patients' vocational abilities.

What cannot be disputed is the fact that there have been considerable changes in the prevalence of cancer diseases among patients in employment as well as in vocational issues in the last 20 years. Changes in environmental influences are less responsible for this than improvements in early diagnostics and the improvement in treatment possibilities. In future, it can be assumed that there will be a further increase in the prevalence of cancer patients in gainful employment and thus an increase in the need for vocational rehabilitation.

Due to changing attitudes to work, not to mention the job situation, the need for vocational rehabilitation, the willingness to undergo rehabilitation as well as the likelihood of the success of vocational rehabilitation assistance for cancer patients have changed, not only quantitatively, but also qualitatively.

Tasks involved in the vocational rehabilitation of cancer patients

The following tasks are of major importance. They are commented on in detail below:
– Assessment, i.e. identification of any vocational limitations. Statement on the negative as well as the positive performance prospects of the person undergoing rehabilitation (sociomedical opinion);
– Measures designed to improve general physical and mental performance;
– Measures designed to safeguard and to maintain workplaces;
– Introduction of measures for vocational reintegration;
– Assessment, evaluation and quality assurance of vocational rehabilitation measures.

Assessment of any vocational limitations. Statement on the negative as well as the positive performance prospects of the person undergoing rehabilitation (sociomedical opinion)

The assessment, the identification of a need for rehabilitation, primarily refers to the identification of dysfunctions and restrictions associated with vocational activities. It describes both the "actual status" as well as the "nominal status" of the performance required to carry out vocational activities. It represents the basis for rehabilitation planning, rehabilitation therapies and evaluation.

Vocational limitations can be conditional;
– on the cancer disease itself;
– on the vocational environment;
– on the effects of therapy.

A summary of the assessment with a description of the negative and positive performance status of the person concerned is given in the sociomedical statement

Table 4.1 - Assessment at the start of the vocational rehabilitation of a cancer patient.

– Does the patient have a job?
– Does the patient carry out a skilled trade? Did he or she pursue this most recently or was it a semi-skilled activity?
– Is the patient expected to be able to resume the vocational activity most recently pursued at some time in the future?
– What problems might arise on resumption of work? Can problems be expected when carrying out work?
– Is any form of job reallocation meaningful?
– Is a gradual resumption of work possible or meaningful?
– Does some form of vocational reorientation appear meaningful?
– How does the patient view his or her vocational future?
– Should an invalidity pension be considered?
– Should a temporary invalidity pension be considered?
– Are any vocational-rehabilitation related aids meaningful, possible and promising?
– Have any vocational-rehabilitation related aids been introduced? (Severely-disabled pass, company physician, workplace transfer, pension application?)

Cancer and limited ability to work

Incurable cancer for which there is no treatment generally involves an incapacity to work. However, there are numerous exceptions. For many cancer patients, work represents the only opportunity for self-affirmation and contact with their surroundings. For psychological considerations alone, an incurable tumour should basically not be equated with vocational inactivity. Patients afflicted with chronic cancer can work to a limited degree if the vocational activity pursued is not accompanied by discomfort and a drop in performance.

In a palliative situation, there is an obligation to enable the dying person to live until he dies, at his own maximum potential, performing to the limit of his physical and mental capacity with control and independence whenever possible (Cheville, 2001). This can also include aids to assist in the continuation of his or her work. Apart from this possible human obligation to promote the resumption of vocational activities, an R1 resection (indication of residual tumors) or incomplete remission following chemo- or radiotherapy should not necessarily be equated with working incapacity and the granting of a pension even after an extensive metastisation and despite widely held opinions. Some tumours cause no discomfort or have no effect on people's capacity to work for many years; there may be no requirement for any therapy for many years; some therapies cause so little strain and partial remissions can be so stable that the vocational performance of those concerned is barely affected despite an obvious tumour problem. (Table 4.2). These patients are frequently capable of work for a long time despite tumour activity. In the case of these patients, however, vocational rehabilitation aids are restricted to aids designed to maintain workplaces.

Table 4.2 - Cancer disorders that frequently do not involve any discomfort.

- Chronic myeloid leukaemia in the chronic phase
- Chronic lymphatic leukaemia in the stages Rai 0-II (Binet A)
- Indolent non-Hodgkin's lymphoma of low malignancy
- Early-stage prostate carcinoma
- Early-stage thyroid carcinoma
- Localised carcinoids
- MALT lymphomas of the stomach (low malignance)
- Renal carcinoma without any impairment of kidney functions
- Early-stage bladder carcinoma

Restrictions on working capacity in the case of potentially curably treated cancer patients

In the case of a potentially curative therapy (R0 situation), all macroscopically and microscopically visible tumour tissue could be removed, residual tumour tissue can no longer be traced with imaging detection procedures (sonography, computer tomography, NMR and PET) and the tumour markers are in the standard range. If there are any indications of residual tumours, this is called an R1 or even an R2 resection. In the case of palliative therapies, we are frequently dealing with patients according to R1 and R2 therapies respectively.

Incapacity to work is generally encountered during tumour therapy and in the subsequent recovery phase. Dependent on the type of treatment and dependent on individual disposition (WHO, ECOG and/or Karnofsky index), the recovery phase can differ in duration. The times for working incapacity given in table 4.3 are average values that may be subject to considerable deviations in individual cases.

In the case of adolescent patients with good prognoses, working motivation and compliance, consideration can be given to measures both designed to retain workplaces as well as promote jobs - including those involving a vocational reorientation.

Table 4.3 - Average duration of working incapacity following potentially curative treatment and uncomplicated progress (without the help of chemotherapy and/or radiotherapy).

Tumour diseases	Treatment	Months of working incapacity
Stomach carcinoma	Gastrectomy	6-8
	Partial stomach resection	3
Colon carcinoma	Hemicolectomy	3
Rectal carcinoma	Rectal resection	4
	Rectal amputation	6
Bronchial carcinoma	Pneumonectomy	6
	Lobectomy/bilobectomy	3
Prostate carcinoma	Radical prostatectomy	5
Renal carcinoma	Nephrectomy	2
Bladder carcinoma	Partial resection	2
	Cystectomy with orthotopic neo-bladder	6
	Cystectomy with ileal conduit	4-6
Breast carcinoma	Tumorectomy	2
	Breast amputation with axillary lymph node resection	3

Vocational environment and restrictions in working capacity

Doctors involved in rehabilitation investigate the vocational environment of cancer patients for any physical and mental stress, for employers' and colleagues' attitudes to cancer diseases not to mention for the possible level of exposure to carcinogenic materials at work. Even if most of the carcinogenic substances concerned with problems listed in table 4.4 and table 4.5 have a long induction period, cancer patients should discontinue any activities in which they are exposed to carcinogenic substances. It is presumed that potentially carcinogenic substances have a stronger carcinogenic effect in the case of "cured" cancer patients than is the case of healthy people. A workplace transfer or even a vocational reorientation may be necessary.

Table 4.4 - Vocational activities with frequent exposure to asbestos.

– Shipbuilding activities
– Construction industry activities
– Asbestos mine activities
– Fuel-trade activities

Table 4.5 - Professional groups exposed to respirable quartz dusts.

Ore and uranium ore miners
- Tunnelers
- Casting fettlers
- Sandblasters
- Furnace bricklayers and moulders in the metalworking industry
- Personnel in fine-china companies
- Personnel in dental laboratories

Effects of cancer therapies and restrictions of working incapacity

A difference must be made between:
- The acute or reversible effects of tumour therapy;
- The long-term or irreversible effects of tumour therapy.

The acute or reversible effects of tumour therapy

Early and reversible post-operative problems include physical weakness, problems with wound healing, anaemia from bleeding, scar weaknesses, reversible problems caused by chemotherapy (e.g. tiredness, nausea, diarrhoea, anaemia, fatigue), reversible side-effects of radiation (e.g. radiation sickness, enteritides). Work is impossible during these acute side-effects. In this phase, rehabilitation therapies predominantly consist of toughening measures and measures designed to strengthen functions so that those affected are fit to resume their original jobs as early as possible. Given physical as well as mental invigoration, a full restoration of working capacity can usually be expected after the acute side-effects have receded.

The long-term or irreversible effects of tumour therapy

This includes consequential disorders, some of which appear many years after the conclusion of treatment. As a result, they are also called late sequelae.

Irreversible disorders include syndromes after the removal of organs (e.g. after gastrectomies conducted on stomach carcinoma patients, with intestinal carcinoma patients with short bowel and/or artificial anus, with bronchial carcinoma patients after pneumonectomies, with bladder carcinoma patients after cystectomies, etc.). These also include undesirable side-effects after radiation therapy (e.g. lymph oedema, pulmonary fibrosis, cardiovascular disorders, etc.) or after chemotherapy (e.g. blood count problems, bone marrow and pulmonary fibrosis, etc.). The effects of irreversible late sequelae can only be relieved and/or compensated for. These patients need rehabilitation measures that go beyond physical and mental invigoration.

Some disorders such as coronary heart disease in the case of lymphoma patients after mediastinal irradiation or cardiac insufficiency in the case of patients with leukaemia or mamma carcinoma treated with anthracycline only appear very late on. These anticipated disorders following therapy must be prevented or at least reduced.

To reduce vocational handicaps, preventive measures are required. Vocational advisory services are very important, in particular for adolescents who have been cured. For example, leukaemia patients treated with meningeal-irradiation should avoid vocational activities that require a high degree of concentration and fast reactions. Following chemotherapy involving anthracycline or mediastinal irradiation, no jobs involving physically strenuous activities should subsequently be attempted due to cardiac risks.

The tables 4.6-4.10 list the possible vocational restrictions to which cancer patients with irreversible late disorders may be subject.

Table 4.6 - Workloads that cured patients with malignant lymphatic and leukaemia diseases should avoid.

Restrictions	Reason for the restrictions
No physically strenuous activities	Frequency of chemotherapy and radiation therapy side-effects on the circulation (e.g. anthracycline, mediastinal irradiation)
No activities in surroundings involving a risk of infection	Frequent immune deficiency syndrome due to illness and therapy
No activities requiring particular concentration and attentiveness	Only after meningeal irradiation
No activities with particular physical and mental stress	Frequent lapses in concentration, effects on the immune system?

Table 4.7 - Workloads that cured stomach carcinoma patients should avoid after a total gastrectomy (R0).

Restrictions	Reason for the restriction
Jobs connected with frequent bending	Danger of gastro-oesophageal reflux
Physically tough jobs, no lifting or carrying heavy loads	When underweight, danger of gastro-oesophageal reflux
Jobs that presuppose a good head for heights (e.g. roofers)	Dumping symptoms with pains caused by hypoglycaemia
Jobs that require continuous attention	Dumping symptoms with pains caused by hypoglycaemia
Activities in the first six post-operative months	Fairly slow adaptation to the modified stomach-bowel passage
Activities involving unpleasant odours or acrid fumes	Provocation of vomiting, nausea and diarrhoea
Absolutely no night work or shift work	Lower stress threshold
Jobs in which more frequent breaks unusual for the business are possible	More frequent intake of small meals necessary
Unsuitable as a full-time truck driver	More frequent breaks unusual for the job, mental and physical stress, risk of a dumping syndrome with lapses in concentration

Table 4.8 - Workloads that cured rectal carcinoma patients should avoid after an abdomino-perineal rectal resection (R0).

— Severe physical workloads (this includes lifting, working above head-height, jobs connected with severe vibrations and in which more than 5kg have to be frequently lifted)
— Unfavourable working posture (e.g. squatting or lying)
— Extreme climatic situations (e.g. working in the heat)
— Unfavourable working hours (shift and night work)
— Unfavourable working breaks (in order to be able to eat meals regularly and in peace, regular breaks of adequate length are required)
— Rhythmic jobs (it must be possible to take individual breaks in the case of irregular evacuation of the bowels without interfering with colleagues' work flow)

Table 4.9 - Workloads that cured bronchial carcinoma patients should avoid after a pneumonectomy (R0).

— Heavy physical loads (these include lifting, working above head-height)
— Jobs connected with strong vibrations
— Unfavourable working posture (e.g. doing jobs when squatting or lying)
— Activities connected with extreme or frequently fluctuating temperatures
— Unfavourable working hours (shift and night work)
— Rhythmic jobs: An individual break has to be able to be taken without interrupting fellow workers' workflow
— Piece-work
— Activities in dusty professions, with serious air pollution, dry air or powerful and irritating odours
— Activities in chemical laboratories

Table 4.10 - Workloads that cured breast carcinoma patients with manifest lymph oedem (R0) should avoid.

— Work done by clerks, workmen and cleaners
— Activities carried out under unfavourable heat radiation or lengthy exposure to the rays of the sun
— Activities accompanied by an excessive load on the affected arm
— Activities involving a possible risk of injuring the affected arm
— Easy, monotonous activities with the affected arm lasting several hours
— Activities in which restrictive clothing is required or shoulder straps have to be placed on the shoulder of the affected side
— Activities in a water bath or thermal bath higher than 33°C

Sociomedical opinion

A rehabilitation oncologist is required to assess a negative and positive performance status. He must form an opinion on the current ability of the person undergoing rehabilitation with regard to the specific, existing workplace; what prospective working capacity with regard to vocational alternatives exists, just how his or her ability to perform it in the trade learnt, in semi-skilled jobs or on the general labour market and how the chances of success of any vocational rehabilitation measures can be estimated (table 4.11).

For the assessment of the vocational performance of potentially cured patients, the same principles apply as those for the assessment of patients with acute or chronic benign diseases and disabilities. Theoretically, a more or less poor prognosis has no influence on a sociomedical assessment (Pannen, 1997; Verband Deutscher Rentenversicherungsträger, 1995); in practice, however, it influences at least the type and the scope of any rehabilitation measures that may possibly be introduced. Consequently, in the case of young patients with small-cell bronchial carcinoma in an R0-situation or patients with acute myeloid leukaemia in complete remission, one would be satisfied purely with job-retaining measures due to the poor long-term prognosis evidenced by experience and dispense with vocational reorientation.

Table 4.11 - Criteria involved in the sociomedical assessment among cancer patients.

– Comparison of requirements and working capacity
– Description of particular vocational stresses
– Information on the possible duration of work
– Description of positive "activity profiles"
– Description of negative "activity profiles"
– Recommendations for job-promoting measures
– Patient's self-assessment on his or her vocational ability

Measures designed to improve general physical and mental performance

Measures designed to improve vocational ability to work under pressure. Increase in general physical and mental capacity

Physically strengthening as well as mentally stabilising measures designed to promote motivation for work are frequently required. A range of different in- and outpatient methods are available for this purpose.

In Germany, every cancer patient old enough to be in gainful employment has a statutory claim to in- and outpatient rehabilitation measures that have been specially designed to meet their requirements (Tiedt, 1998). They extend from general, illness-unrelated physically strengthening and mentally stabilising measures to illness-related, individually adapted rehabilitation therapies. The aim of regimens designed to invigorate or promote recovery is to facilitate the resumption of work (Pannen, 1997). In Germany, these toughening rehabilitation measures are therefore not financed by medical insurance companies, but by pension funds. It is in their interest for contributors to their schemes to resume their professional activities as speedily as possible. They should remain in their jobs as long as possible instead of depriving the pension fund of benefits and pensions. Outpatient sports and swimming courses designed to maintain vocational abilities as long as possible are promoted. With regard to promotion, these out- and inpatient measures are conditional on their being carried out by a qualified rehabilitation team. Apart from medical oncological skills, sociomedical experience and expertise are essential in an oncological rehabilitation team (fig. 4.1) (table 3.13). It is often necessary to address a cancer patient's specifically vocational problems. His or her remaining capacity must be assessed and recorded and vocational rehabilitation measures introduced and documented (table 4.6-4.10).

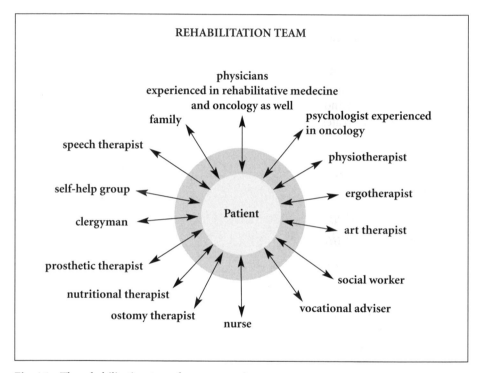

Fig. 4.1 - The rehabilitation team for cancer patients.

Up to now, Germany is the only country in Europe in which pension schemes conduct these rehabilitation measures specially designed for cancer patients, the aim being to promote vocational reintegration. Roughly one-third of all gainfully employed cancer patients in Germany take advantage of the opportunity of this kind of rehabilitation measure. In all other countries of the European Community, it tends to be medical or social reasons that lead to the introduction of in- or outpatient rehabilitation in the case of cancer patients.

Tumour patients frequently suffer from resignation, fears and depression. These influence patients' vocational willingness to work and, alongside a lack of motivation, are a substantial reason for frequent early pensions. Some authors consider that fatigue symptoms are the most frequent reason for the unsuccessful vocational reintegration of cured cancer patients (Curt, 2001; Spelten et al., 2003). Help in coping with the disease, the reduction of fears, depression, helplessness and hopelessness as well as the boosting of compliance and motivation are important. These are the main tasks of a psycho-oncologist. He or she has a vital position in the rehabilitation team for cancer patients (fig. 4.1), in particular where vocational rehabilitation is concerned. The purpose of intensive psychological care is to influence a patient's resigned attitude and to promote his or her desire to perform.

Self-help groups fulfil an important role in terms of motivation for self-assistance, help towards self-help and in dealing with tendencies to retreat from society. They exert an activating influence on those concerned and thus contribute towards a willingness to resume work.

Training and medical advisory services are prerequisites for an active and independent approach. For example, some patients are unaware of the numerous vocational protective measures and benefits that are granted in many countries to chronically handicapped employees in the pursuit of their profession as well as to employers when hiring those affected. What cannot be disputed is that well-informed cancer patients have greater opportunities for social and vocational reintegration than uninformed patients.

Here, too, self-help groups make an important contribution in the fields of advisory and information services.

Measures designed to improve resistance to vocational pressure and to increase specific physical and mental performance

In the case of stomach carcinoma patients, it largely consists of training sessions to prevent and reduce postgastrectomy symptoms, in particular, postprandial discomfort. Good nutritional advice can help to reduce the numerous vocational restrictions resulting from gastrectomy when carrying out one's job. The appearance of postprandial dumping problems prevents, among other things, the pursuit of jobs that require a head for heights (e.g. roofers) or jobs that require permanent attentiveness (e.g. bus drivers, production line workers or pieceworkers). A workplace transfer is necessary in these cases and in physically demanding activities.

In the case of bronchial carcinoma patients, the restrictions imposed by lung function prevent or restrict all physically demanding activities. By means of breathing exercises, inhalations, accompanying therapies involving medicaments and anti-obstructive physical therapy measures, it is possible to improve patients' ability to handle physical demands. Workplace transfers are frequently required.

In the case of rectal carcinoma patients with an artificial anus, it is a mastery of irrigation that makes patients independent of dealing with pouches, which reduces the adverse effect of noises and thus opens up to them so many vocational activities that would otherwise be impossible. Non-irrigating colostomy wearers are frequently unable to conduct any activities involving customer contact. However, almost all activities are possible for irrigating rectal carcinoma patients.

The restoration of the ability to communicate using speech is a cardinal task of rehabilitation after laryngectomy in the case of patients suffering from laryngal carcinoma. It is a basic prerequisite for the resumption of work in many professions. Vocational rehabilitation planning is a multidisciplinary task for these patients as the missing larynx not only affects vocal functions and sensitivity to smell and taste but also the absence of any closing of the glottis also seriously affects the normal abdominal prelum and social as well as mental problems frequently occur as a result of physical disfigurement (Cady, 2002).

Measures for the protection and maintenance of workplaces

Irrespective of the symptoms of their problems, cancer patients must fundamentally be considered severely disabled, no matter whether treated potentially curatively or palliatively. In the first years, at least, after the diagnosis of cancer, they enjoy improved protection against dismissal at their workplaces (table 4.12) and, after the conclusion of therapy, enjoy particular vocational protective measures in the first five years at least that are, however, regulated differently from country to country. In France, cancer is considered one of the *maladies de longue durée* (long-lasting diseases) that grant all civil servants and employees concerned the right to workplace retention and vocational functions for up to three years. The government even guarantees their reemployment for up to five years after the disease has been diagnosed whereby those concerned can draw a full salary for the first three years, followed by only half of this (Fédération nationale 1997).

Table 4.12 - Vocational protective measures for cancer patients in Germany (Delbrück, 2003).

– Increased protection against dismissal in the workplace; dismissal is exceptionally difficult
– Assistance in keeping or acquiring a workplace appropriate for a disabled person, e.g. technical aids or wage subsidies
– Acceleration of pension provision
– Exemption from overtime and exemption from night-shifts if so desired
– Right to five days additional holiday per year with a five-day working week

Introduction of aids and measures for vocational reintegration

Theoretically, people with cancer who are undergoing rehabilitation are not considered to be a special group in the field of occupational promotion. However, their integration in Germany is the goal, as it is with other persons undergoing rehabilitation according to the type and severity of their functional limitations (Pannen, 1997). A specific form of vocational rehabilitation designed for cancer patients does not therefore exist. Nevertheless, all benefits in the job-promotion field are open to people undergoing rehabilitation.

There are numerous forms of assistance for employees as well as for employers that are intended to facilitate vocational reintegration. Primarily, there are measures designed to keep jobs. Retraining is rarely considered and – if it is – it is only for younger patients with good lifetime forecasts. Many cured cancer patients of advanced age no longer have the mental flexibility, the stamina and the ability to adapt that are required for successful retraining. In Germany, the only retraining measures that are financed by sponsors – if at all – are for patients under the age of 40.

For the retention or acquisition of workplaces, support and assistance are granted to the employee as well as to the employer. Integration assistance amounting to between 50 and 70% of remuneration is granted for six months. In justifiable, individual cases, as much as 80% can be paid and its duration can be extended to as much as two years. Pension insurance companies are willing to participate in the financing of ergonomic working chairs, height-adjustable worktables, lifting equipment, access ramps, sanitary fittings and other aids as well as technical working aids if these measures guarantee that cancer patients will keep their workplaces.

Workplace-retaining aids and benefits that promote jobs for cancer patients in Germany include (Delbrück, 2003):
– Benefits for the maintenance or acquisition of workplaces;
– Equipment and technical aids;
– Qualification through short courses;
– Integration assistance for employers;
– Measures to pinpoint jobs and work trials;
– Vocational adjustment;
– Further training and retraining;
– Job and professional promotion;
– Supplementary benefits (interim assistance, travelling expenses, household help, work-clothes, tools, examination fees, textbooks, training allowances).

Gradual reintegration into the work process is one vocational rehabilitation measure that is frequently practised (Gobelet, 2005). Resumption of work can, for example, be done with the person concerned initially only working two to three hours every day; after a certain time, this is increased to four to six hours and then to six to eight hours until work returns to full working hours. In Germany and France, cancer patients receive their full wages from the medical insurance for the full period of this increasing workload although they are not working full shifts.

Assessment, evaluation and quality assurance. Predictors for occupational reintegration

No quality assurance is possible without assessment and without any progress documentation. Many evaluation parameters are available to examine rehabilitation targets. These not only include the start of vocational activities but also the change in risk factors, the change in obstructions and limitations, the introduction of benefits designed to promote jobs, implementation within companies, job creation, the reorganisation of workplaces to suit disabled people, training and further training in a new professional field.

The rates for the successful vocational reintegration of cancer patients given in the relevant literature vary widely from 30 to 93%. This is not simply attributable to the different quality of the rehabilitation opportunities or to differences in attitude among those affected or to financial possibilities, but it is also attributable to the different consideration given to disabled people in society. The fact that the likelihood of successful vocational reintegration is very much greater in the USA than in other countries is not merely due to improved rehabilitation for cancer patients but it is also a consequence of their having to earn a living. Financial security in the case of chronic diseases and working incapacity is very differently regulated in individual countries.

In the case of patients with head and neck carcinoma (Cady, 2002), the vocational reintegration quota is very much lower than with testicular and Hodgkin's patients. All investigations consistently showed a close correlation with the patients' age, the type of work they did as well as the type and degree of severity of their tumour disease (Maunsell *et al.*, 1999; Cady *et al.*, 2002; Spelten *et al.*, 2002; Schwiersch *et al.*, 1995). According to our own experience, which is, however, only covered to some extent by statistics, the factors mentioned in the table as well as vocational ability and the quality of the rehabilitation conducted are important (table 4.13).

Table 4.13 - Factors that can influence the introduction, implementation and the result probability of vocational rehabilitation measures in the case of cancer patients, independent of their vocational performance and the quality of the rehabilitation measures conducted as well as the type and scope of the tumour disease.

– Risk of relapse
– Lifetime forecast
– Age and gender of the patients
– Social status
– Unemployment prior to falling ill
– Level of education, earning status
– Patient's motivation and willingness to participate
– Patient's desire to be given a pension.
– Time elapsed since primary therapy
– Sponsors' expectations
– Employer's motivation and willingness to participate
– Attitude of the workforce and close colleagues
– Pressure on workforce in the company
– Previous time-limited pensioning
– General and special labour market

Whether and to what extent the intended goals are reached or not depend not only on the quality of the vocational rehabilitation measures but also on many predictors (table 4.13). Humanitarian and political labour-market reasons must also be added to these.

Apart from somatic reasons and legal reasons relating to social insurance as well as financial aspects, the decision for or against early pensioning must also give consideration to the positive psychological aspects of dealing with a disease. For many people, their profession and work mean more than just a way to meet their existential requirements. To many people, work is the only possibility for social contact and is a confirmation of their self-esteem. It represents a form of diversion, distance and suppression of the feeling of a constantly threatening Damocles' sword. It can therefore be perfectly legitimate to support cancer patients – even those with greatly reduced working capacity – in resuming their previous jobs.

The demand that the quality of vocational rehabilitation measures must be judged solely by the frequency of successful vocational reintegration must be assessed critically. The rapid introduction of a pension for those unable to pursue gainful employment in the face of an irrefutable and well-documented reduction in their ability to work can also point to good vocational rehabilitation work.

Structures and organization of vocational rehabilitation for cancer patients

The structural and process quality of vocational reintegration measures for cancer patients differs in various EC countries. In Europe, different sponsors are responsible for vocational rehabilitation. In comparison with Germany, other countries frequently do not view sociomedical assessments, the introduction and implementation of vocational rehabilitation measures to be tasks for rehabilitation medicine and most definitely not tasks for rehabilitation oncologists.

Whereas, in Germany, inpatient rehabilitation is at the focus of rehabilitation measures and statements on the ability to work, on the question of vocational forecasts, on the need for vocational rehabilitation, on the capacity for rehabilitation and on the willingness for rehabilitation on the part of those concerned are demanded and initial vocational assistance is also introduced, rehabilitation in the other EC countries is largely outpatient in nature. Rehabilitation oncologists do not consider the clarification of further vocational activity as well as the introduction and implementation of vocational assistance to be their main duties. In these countries, patients are forced to apply to the labour market authorities; a large amount of personal initiative is expected of such patients if they intend to resume work.

Unfortunately, there is no information on the important issue of whether the vocational reintegration quota is increased in Germany by its costly and time-consuming inpatient and outpatient rehabilitation measures. This deficit is attributable not only to a lack of prospective studies and to the selection of patients looked after during rehabilitation but is also a result of the rapidly growing call in recent years for the need for rehabilitation research (Koch, Weiss, 1998; Hensel *et al.*, 2002).

Bibliography

- Delbrück H, Haupt E (1998) Rehabilitationsmedizin. Urban Schwarzenberg Munich
- Delbrück H (2003) Krebsnachbetreuung. Nachsorge, Rehabilitation und Palliation. Springer Heidelberg
- Maunsell E, Brisson E, Lauzier S *et al.* (1999) Work problems after breast cancer: An exploratory qualitative study. Psycho-Oncology 8: 467-73
- Lederer P, Weltle D, Weber A (2003) Evaluation der Dienstunfähigkeit bei Beamtinnen und Beamten. Gesundheitswesen 65(1): 536-40
- Cheville A (2001) Rehabilitation of patients with advanced cancer. Cancer 92: 1039-48
- Pannen H (1997) Standards und Qualitätssicherung sozialmedizinischer Maßnahmen im Rahmen der onkologischen Rehabilitation. In Delbrück, H.(Hrsg.) Standards und Qualitätskriterien in der onkologischen Rehabilitation. W. Zuckschwerdt, Munich

- Verband Deutscher Rentenversicherungsträger (ed.) (1995) Sozialmedizinische Begutachtung in der gesetzlichen Rentenversicherung. Gustav Fischer, Stuttgart Jena New York
- Tiedt G (1998) Rechtliche Grundlagen der Rehabilitation. In Delbrück H, Haupt E (Ed.) Rehabilitationsmedizin, Urban & Schwarzenberg Munich 45-68
- Curt G (2001) Fatigue in cancer; like pain, this is a symptom that physicians can and should manage. Br Med J 322: 1560
- Spelten ER, Verbeek J, Uitterhoeve A (2003) Cancer, fatigue and the return of patients to work – a prospective cohort study. Europ J Cancer 39: 1562-7
- Cady J (2002) Laryngectomy. Beyond loss of voice – caring for the patient as a whole. Clin J Oncol Nurs 6(6): 347-51
- Fédération nationale des centres de lutte contre le cancer (1997) Prévoir demain. Guide de la réinsertion des patients traités pour les cancers. Centres de lutte contre le cancer, Paris
- Spelten ER, Sprangers M, Verbeek J (2002) Factors reported to influence the return to work of cancer survivors: A literature review. Psycho-Oncology 11: 124-31
- Heckl U (1996) Gesunde Kranke – Kranke Gesunde. Der Umgang mit einer Tumorerkrankung im beruflichen Umfeld. Europäischer Verlag der Wissenschaften, Frankfurt
- Fobair P, Hoppe R, Bloom J et al. (1986) Psychosocial problems among survivors of Hodgkin's disease. Journal of clinical Oncology 4: 805-14
- Schwiersch M, Stepien J, Schröck R (1995) Inwieweit beeinträchtigen psychosoziale Belastungen den Wiedereintritt ins Berufsleben bei Mammakarzinompatienten. In Delbrück H (Hrsg.) Der Krebskranke in der Arbeitswelt. W Zuckschwerdt, Munich
- Koch U, Weiss J (1998) Forschung in der Rehabilitationsmedizin. In Delbrück H, Haupt E. Rehabilitationsmedizin. Urban & Schwarzenberg München 150-66
- Hensel M, Egerer G, Schneeweiss A et al. (2002) Quality of life and rehabilitation in social and professional life after autologous stem cell transplantation. Annals of Oncology 13: 209-17
- Gobelet C, Franchignoni F (2005) Vocational Rehabilitation. Springer Paris

Pain management in cancer rehabilitation and palliation

It has been estimated that more than 85% of cancer patients require pain management at some point during the course of their illness. Pain may be the first symptom of disease in some cancers. In others, pain develops later on.

Pain management is one of the most thankful tasks in cancer palliation and rehabilitation. It is a challenge that places considerable demands on rehabilitation and palliation professionals.

Cancer pain is a complex biopsychosocial phenomenon (fig. 5.1). Appropriate management in rehabilitation and palliation service includes primary anti-cancer treatments, local and systemic analgesic therapies and other non-invasive techniques such as psychological and rehabilitative interventions.

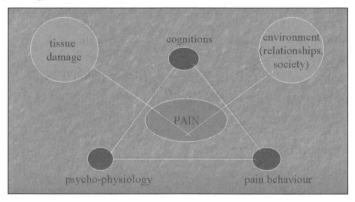

Fig. 5.1 - Pain as a biopsychosocial phenomenon.

Classification of pain and pain management strategies in cancer patients

Pain and pain management in cancer patients can be classified according to various criteria (table 5.1). These criteria and their implications for treatment are discussed in the following.

Table 5.1 - Classification of pain management strategies in cancer patients.

By cause (tumour-induced pain, iatrogenic pain, unspecific pain)
– By quality (nociceptive pain, neuropathic pain)
– By duration (acute pain, chronic pain, breakthrough pain)
– By severity (weak, moderate, strong)
– By site of origin (visceral pain, bone pain, soft tissue pain)
– By psychosocial status

Classification by cause of pain

Cancer growth

The risk of pain differs from one cancer to another. Risk factors include the disease history, histology and differentiation of cancer cells, tumour site, and probability of spread.

Various tumour cell growth mechanisms are responsible for the quality, quantity and severity of cancer pain (table 5.2). These must be assessed before starting pain management. If tumour growth is the cause, options for causal therapy (i.e., strategies impacting tumour growth) should be exhausted before initiating pain therapy. Cooperation with the patient's oncologist is essential to meet this task.

Table 5.2 - Mechanisms by which cancer induces pain.

– Cancer tissue infiltrating nerves
– Cancer tissue blocking or destroying nerves
– Peritumoural edema compressing nerves
– Cancer tissue secreting substances that irritate the nerves or lower the pain threshold
– Pathologic fractures inducing functional instability

Pain associated with tumour infiltration of nerves, plexuses, and meninges may be caused by direct tumour infiltration of the nerve, compression or metastatic fracture of bone adjacent to a nerve or nerve root. The peripheral nerve is most commonly infiltrated by tumours that invade the intercostal, paravertebral, or retroperitoneal space. Constant burning pain with dysesthesia in an area of sensory loss is the usual picture. The pain is radicular and tends to be unilateral.

Peritumoural edema

Peritumoural edema impinging on nerves differs in severity according to tumour histology, site and rapidity of growth. Measures to reduce the edema are the best analgesics in such cases.

Therapy-induced pain

(For more details, see section on Management of iatrogenic pain).

Potentially curative cancer surgery, chemotherapy and radiotherapy may be associated with chronic specific or unspecific chronic pain syndromes (table 5.3). Management of these iatrogenic pain syndromes is one of the goals of cancer rehabilitation whereas palliation is mainly concerned with cancer-induced pain syndromes.

Table 5.3 - Treatment-induced pain syndromes in cancer patients.

– Pain syndromes due to loss of organs
– Post radiation pain syndromes
– Chemotherapy-induced polyneuropathy

Pain of unknown origin

Sometimes a specific cause may be hard to identify. Small-cell cancers in particular (APUD tumours) tend to secrete paraneoplastic substances that sensitize pain receptors and may cause pain, which in most cases is diffuse and difficult to localise. Unspecific pain in these patients calls for special medication strategies.

Pain of benign origin needs other treatments than tumour-induced or iatrogenic pain (table 5.4).

Table 5.4 - Differences between cancer-induced pain and pain of benign origin.

– Cancer-induced pain tends to be chronic.
– Cancer pain is very often associated with anxiety, insomnia, loss of appetite and emotional troubles. Behavioural therapy may be necessary. Concomitant symptoms are less frequent in non-cancer pain.
– Drug treatment is the mainstay of cancer pain management; this is not the case for non-cancer pain.
– Causal therapy is more often possible for cancer-related pain management; this does not apply to non cancer pain management.
– Non-cancer pain is initially treated with non-opioid analgesics. In contrast, morphine is very often a first-line analgesic in cancer-related pain.
– Complete pain relief is the goal of treatment in palliative cancer patients. The goal in non-cancer-pain patients is to achieve pain relief, not necessarily freedom from pain. In non-cancer related pain, a compromise must be found between desirable analgesia and unwanted side effects. The principal aim is to improve function.
– Long-term side effects are less important in palliative cancer treatments than in the treatment of non-cancer-induced pain.

Classification by quality of pain

Nociceptive pain

Nociceptive pain is typically the result of a musculoskeletal or visceral injury or disease and includes somatic and visceral mechanisms. Primary afferent neurons receive nociceptive input from peripheral nociceptors. Nociceptors are activated in response to noxious stimuli, which can be thermal, chemical, or mechanical in character. Nociceptive pain usually resolves when the initial tissue damage heals, and tends to respond well to treatment with anti-inflammatory agents and opioids.

Periosteal and bone pain is a typical example of nociceptive pain. Visceral pain is in most cases nociceptive if due to cancer infiltration. Acute leukaemias and lymphomas are often complicated by nociceptive pain.

Somatic and visceral nociceptive pain syndromes are distinguished according to site of origin. Somatic pain is subdivided into superficial pain from skin or mucous membranes and deep pain from the muscles, bones or joints. Somatic pain is characterized by aching, throbbing, stabbing, and/or a sensation of pressure. Deep somatic pain tends to be dull, whereas superficial pain is initially sharp and later becomes dull. Visceral pain is characterized by gnawing, cramping, aching, sharp, and/or stabbing sensations, and its source is the internal organs.

Nociceptive pain responds well to classical analgesics such as prostaglandin synthesis inhibitors and opioids.

Most patients with cancer have a mixed pain syndrome, that is, a combination of both nociceptive and neuropathic pain, and frequently require combination drug therapy for pain management.

Neuropathic pain

Neuropathic pain may occur in cancer patients as a result of the tumour itself (e. g. infiltration of the plexus) or may be iatrogenic (following chemotherapy, surgery or radiotherapy). Typical examples include painful diabetic neuropathy, HIV/AIDS neuropathy, post-herpetic neuralgia, and cancer-induced as well as post-treatment cancer pain syndromes, such as postmastectomy syndrome, post thoracotomy syndrome and radiation and chemotherapy neuropathies (platinum, taxoids, vinca alkaloids).

Neuropathic pain occurs as a result of infiltration or compression of peripheral nerve fibres, with the pain impulse emanating from the nerve pathway rather then the nerve endings. It is characterized by hypersensitivity either in the damaged area or in the surrounding normal tissue.

Pain is usually projected to the region supplied by the affected nerve ("projected pain"). It may be difficult to localise (e.g., in polyneuropathic pain). Patients often use terms such as "burning", "numbness", "tingling", "electric", "stabbing", or "pins and needles" to describe neuropathic pain. Sensitivity disorders such as hypaesthesia, hyperalgesia, paraesthesia, dysaesthesia and allodynia are frequent. The autonomic nervous system may be affected, causing patients to report dizziness, constipation or other changes in bowel function, urinary retention, and erectile dysfunction.

Neuropathic pain in cancer patients is often treated with anticonvulsants and antidepressants. The main indication for anticonvulsants is shooting neuropathic pain. The most commonly prescribed drugs are carbamazepine and gabapentin and clonazepam and/or tricyclic antidepressants and clomipramine.

In the past, neuropathic pain was often referred to as "opioid-nonresponsive pain", but more recent studies, e.g. with oxycodone in patients suffering from painful diabetic neuropathies (Watson *et al.*, 2003) or with transdermal buprenorphine in various neuropathic pain conditions (Rodriguez-López *et al.*, 2005; Hans 2005) suggest that opioids may indeed be effective in relieving this type of pain (Paice, 2003).

Combinations with opioids and tricyclic antidepressants are often indicated. Corticoids have long been used to treat a variety of neuropathic pain states.

Classification by duration of pain

A distinction must be made between acute pain and chronic pain before deciding on the correct treatment. The type of medication will also depend on how long medication has to be given. The longer the likely period of analgesic treatment, the more important it is to take cumulative and long-term risks into account when choosing an analgesic strategy. Chronic pain and long-term pain management are major complicating factors in cancer patients.

Acute pain

Acute pain is caused by external or internal injury. It is closely correlated with the triggering stimulus and can be clearly located. Acute pain has a distinct warning and protective function, in contrast to chronic pain, which has become dissociated from the triggering event.

Table 5.5 - Basics of acute pain management.

– Single-agent therapies are allowed.
– WHO analgesic ladder step I drugs have priority.
– Opioids are given as needed and not on a time-contingent dosing schedule.
– For relief of acute pain, short-term use of a narcotic may be considered. The need for prolonged narcotic therapy should prompt a re-evaluation of the aetiology of a patient's pain.
– Cumulative and long-term side effects are less important because treatment is administered for a limited time only.

Chronic pain

Defined as pain lasting more than six months, chronic pain becomes a clinical entity in its own. Its severity has lost its warning and protective functions. It may be accompanied by depression and psychosocial problems, in turn exacerbating the pain. Insomnia and autonomic nervous system symptoms often accompany cancer pain and lower the pain threshold (fig. 5.2).

Patients become increasingly inactive, leading to social isolation and dysthymia, and potentially culminating in depression. Self-esteem is considerably shaken. Chronic pain wears the patient down, physically, psychologically and socially. Chronic pain calls for special pain management strategies including social and mental support (table 5.6).

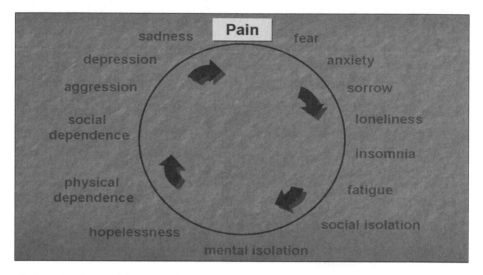

Fig. 5.2 - Psychosocial features influencing sensibility of pain receptors.

Table 5.6 - Basics of chronic pain management.

– WHO analgesic ladder step II and III drugs have priority.
– Adjuvant analgesics are often necessary (like antidepressants, anticonvulsants, corticoids).
– Opioids must be administered in sustained-release dosage forms.
– Medication is given on a time-contingent dosing schedule.
– Pain diary is necessary and medication must be adapted in response to changing conditions (breakthrough pain).
– Patients should be monitored periodically for complications.
– Chronic pain calls for more consideration of emotional and psychosocial factors.
– Cumulative and long-term side effects are very important.

Breakthrough pain

The severity of chronic pain may be consistently high or fluctuate, and may be occasionally interspersed with acute attacks of pain. These acute attacks of limited duration are called breakthrough pain. The phrases "episodic", "incidental", and "transient" pain are all consistent with breakthrough pain (BTP). Several factors promote the development of breakthrough pain (table 5.7). Three subtypes of BTP have been defined:
– incident BTP;

– idiopathic BTP;
– end-of-dose BTP.

Incident BTP describes pain occurring with activity or movement. This type of BTP is more common than idiopathic or end-of-dose BTP. **Idiopathic BTP** generally lasts longer than incident BTP and is not precipitated by a known cause. Worsening idiopathic BTP may be suggestive of advancing disease and is generally not due to analgesic tolerance. **End-of-dose BTP** occurs prior to a scheduled dose of an around-the-clock (ATC) analgesic. Characteristically, end-of-dose BTP usually has a gradual onset and longer duration than other types of BTP.

Because the cause of breakthrough pain may not be the same as that of the underlying baseline pain, it is essential that clinicians evaluate and treat it separately from baseline pain. Treatment should be tailored to the individual and the type and pattern of pain experienced. The ideal treatment for BTP would have a rapid onset of action, but a short duration to match the usual short duration of BTP. Breakthrough pain requires co-medication with rapid-action analgesics whilst continuing the patient's sustained-release medication.

In addition, nonpharmacologic measures may be useful treatments or adjuvants for BTP. In some chronic pain states, opioids may be used solely for persistent pain, and BTP is approached with nonpharmacologic strategies. Such strategies that are commonly employed include ice, heat, rest, stress management techniques (such as mindfulness meditation or self-hypnosis), and TENS.

Table 5.7 - Reasons for breakthrough pain (BTP).

– Insufficient dosage of analgesics in sustained-release formulations or end-of-dose failure (mainly observed in patients using patches). (end-of-dose-BTP)
– Physical effort. (incident BTP)
– Emotional effects (incident BTP)
– Psychosocial events, stress (incident BTP)
– No known cause (idiopathic BTP)

Classification by severity of pain

Graduation of pain severity (fig. 5.3) was the basis for the pain management recommendations published in 1986 by the WHO (World Health Organization) (fig. 5.5).

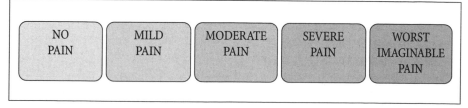

| NO PAIN | MILD PAIN | MODERATE PAIN | SEVERE PAIN | WORST IMAGINABLE PAIN |

Fig. 5.3 - Verbal rating scale (VRS)

Severity of pain is undoubtedly an important criterion when selecting a pain management strategy. The problem is that measuring severity of pain is a very subjective process. There are no satisfactory objective methods for determining severity. Physicians must therefore resort to patient self-assessment as a method for evaluating pain.

Severity is only one of several factors with implications for pain management.

Classification by site of origin

Pain may occur at various points in the **pain pathway**, starting with pain receptors in the periphery, progressing to pain transmission and ending with registration of pain in the brain. The range of treatments is correspondingly large (table 5.8).

Some tumours are likely to be associated with painful localized bone metastasis (incidences for various cancers: breast cancer 50%-80%, prostatic cancer 60%-80%, bronchial cancer 40%-70%, renal cell carcinoma 30%-50%, bladder cancer 40%-60%, thyroid gland carcinoma 40%-60%).

The pathophysiology and treatment of osseous pain differs from the pathophysiology and treatment of visceral or soft tissue pain (Sabino et al., 2005). Osteolytic and osteoblastic bone lesions each require different pain management strategies. Calcitonin can reduce the acute pain of bone lesions associated with inflammation, bisphosphonates are used to manage pain associated with osteolytic bone metastases, and bone-seeking radionuclides are mainly effective in osteoblastic bone metastasis. Hormones are good painkillers for bone metastases in hormone sensitive tumours (e.g., breast cancer and prostatic cancer) but do not work in other types of tumour-induced bone pain.

Table 5.8 - Differences in pain quality according to tumour site.

– Periosteal and/or bone pain is dull, boring, deep, but may also be sharp and lancinating. It is usually easy to locate and tends worsen during motion.
– Pain of soft tissue and muscles is often permanent and worsens under pressure, for example when the subject is sitting. The pain is usually dull, boring, continuous and diffuse in terms of location. It occurs independently of motion.
– Visceral pain is mainly due to infiltration, ulceration or compression in the gastrointestinal, respiratory or urogenital tract. Visceral pain is typically dull, deep, hard to localize, and may be colicky.

Classification by psychosocial status

Purely psychogenic pain is rare but psychosomatic complaints are a frequent component of chronic pain, resulting in a mixed presentation. Psychotherapy is recommended for patients whose pain is associated with a somatoform, anxiety, or depressive disorder. Anxiolytic drugs have anti-anxiety effects. Benzodiazepines are indicated in subjects with anxiety and/or insomnia.

In chronic pain states, somatic pain may be accompanied by other disease-related or dyspnoea, restlessness, anxiety, insomnia) (fig. 5.2) syndrome in many cases. Psychosocial problems exacerbate the pain circumstances and have a major impact, that is why "chronic pain" qualifies as a biopsychosocial entity (Kerssens *et al.*, 2002).

Pharmacotherapy on its own is usually insufficient. Pain management in these patients is about much more than analgesia.

Sequence of procedures in pain management

Table 5.9 - Basics of pain management in cancer patients.

– Assessment (history and examination, establishing the causes of pain, determining its severity)
– Planning of treatment (definition of goals. Causal therapy or symptomatic therapy? Pharmacotherapy or physical/mental therapy? Systemic or local therapy? Side effects? Compliance?)
– Conduct of therapy (treatment intervals: instant-action drugs/sustained release/dosing intervals? Dose: dose modification/duration? Single-agent or combination therapy? Comedication? Managing side effects)
– Monitoring (evaluation, quality control)

Assessment

Essentially, the assessment of pain may be performed using three strategies: pain scales, pain interviews, physical examination and behavioural observation.

Clinical examination and medical history are extremely important. They may give an indication as to which medication may work. Patients with cancer pain often have a long history of suffering, unsuccessful treatment attempts, and numerous medical consultations. A detailed case history including a psychological history is essential in order to make an exact diagnosis and avoid repeatedly unsuccessful attempts at treatment.

The clinical assessment of the older person must address questions of life expectancy, risk of functional decline and need of assistance, tolerance to stress, rehabilitation, and management of reversible conditions, such as depression, malnutrition, and polypharmacy, that may compromise survival, function, and quality of life if left untreated (Balducci, 2003).

Pain interview and questionnaire

A **pain interview** includes questions related to the severity of pain and correlation with movement and time of day. The pain interview also contains questions on the number of days pain has interfered with ADLs/IADLs, pleasurable and social activities, exercise, ability to think, appetite, sleep, energy and mood (Balducci, 2003). Other questions are designed to elicit the number and frequency of pain medications taken during the past week and how the patient rates his or her health. A good approach is to ask patients to fill out a very detailed **pain questionnaire** before they undergo a medical examination (table 5.10). In addition to detailed questions about the patient's existing pain, the pain questionnaire also asks about other diseases, therapies, medicinal drugs and social environment.

Table 5.10 - Basic questions to be answered by the patient before deciding on a pain management strategy.

– Where does the pain occur? Is the pain diffuse or on one side only? Does the pain radiate?
– How severe is the pain? Is it mild, moderate, severe or intolerable?
– How would you describe the quality of the pain? For example, is it dull, sharp, colic tingling?
– How often does the pain occur? Is it permanent or occasional? For example, once a day, once a week, once a month?
– How long does the pain last? Is it permanent or does it last for seconds, minutes, hours or days?
– When does the pain occur? Morning, noon, evening or night?
– What triggers the pain? Changes in the weather? Mental stress? Does it occur before or after meals, during exercise or at rest? Does it occur along with other symptoms, such as nausea, constipation or restlessness?
– How have you been sleeping? Do you have difficulty falling asleep or sleeping through the night? Do you get nightmares? Do you feel rested or still tired after sleeping?

Pain diary

A **pain diary** kept by the patient has proved very valuable as a means of monitoring treatment. Pain diaries are an effective way of monitoring how pain responds over time and evaluating the patient's physical and psychological status. In addition, the patient is actively motivated to comply with treatment and becomes more involved. Patients rate the severity of their pain in this diary with the aid of a pain scale.

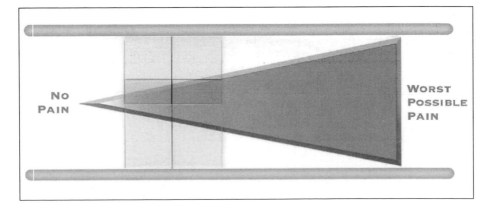

Fig. 5.4 - Visual analogue scale.

Measures to determine severity of pain

There are many factors influencing the individual pain sensitivity and the choice of pain management. In patients unable to verbalize their symptoms, behavioural observations may be used as indicators of pain (e.g. facial expressions, body movements, changes in interpersonal interactions, changes in activity patterns or routines, mental status changes).

Pain scales and assessment procedures to measure and to evaluate the effectiveness of pain management include numeric rating scales, visual analogue scales, verbal rating scales and emoticon (smiley faces) scales (fig. 5.3. and 5.4). The advantage of this method is that it gives the physician a clear idea of the patient's pain perception and gives the patient a feeling of being actively integrated in the pain management process.

As a general principle, scales that require a high level of abstract thinking, such as the visual analogs scale or the McGill pain questionnaire are unsuitable for older individuals, especially for those who are cognitively impaired or have a low educational level, because the abstractive capacity declines with age (Balducci, 2003).

Patients rate pain severity on a range from 0 – indicating no pain – to 10 –indicating maximum pain– (numeric rating scale) or pinpoint pain severity on a 10cm scale from a starting point at 0cm –no pain– up to a potential maximum score at 10cm –worst possible pain– (visual rating scale), or identify their pain status on an emoticon scale showing five different facial expressions. Pain is rated daily and treatment should be adjusted to suit the patient's pain perception score.

Table 5.11 - Relative utility of pain scales in the elderly (Balducci, 2003).

– **Numeric rating scale**	Reliable, but low completion rate Vertical positioning of numbers seems to be more suitable for older individuals
– **Verbal descriptor scale**	High completion rate Lacks a numeric component
– **Pictorial pain scale**	More suitable for adults with limited education. Evaluation of pictures showing facial expressions may be unreliable in cognitively impaired or depressed individuals
– **Visual analogue scale**	Failure rate increases with age Generally unsuitable for individuals with a low level of education
– **McGill questionnaire**	Sensitive to sensory and affective aspects of pain Not recommended for individuals who are illiterate or cognitively impaired Length may be a problem, but a short version is available

Therapeutic measures

Basically we distinguish causal (anti tumour therapies), symptomatic (therapies influencing the pain sensitivity) and co-analgesic interventions (therapies influencing the biopsychosocial environment).

Causal pain management strategies (anticancer therapies)

Inhibiting cancer growth may reduce the pain if tumour growth is the cause of pain. An oncologist should be consulted before initiating pain management and asked about anticancer therapy options to relief pain (table 5.12).

Table 5.12 - Causal pain management strategies in cancer patients.

- Surgery
- Chemotherapy
- Hormone therapy
- Radiotherapy
- Radionuclide therapy
- Bisphosphonate therapy

Surgery

Cancer surgery options are not limited to measures intended to reduce tumour size. They also encompass bypass procedures, anastomosis, and stent placement. The latter procedures are particularly likely to produce prompt and sustained freedom from pain in subjects with gastro-intestinal cancer.

Surgery may have specific and critical efficacy in the relief of pain caused by impending or evident fractures.

Chemotherapy

The analgesic effect of systemic chemotherapy depends mainly on the chemosensitivity of the primary tumour. It follows that pain in leukaemia, lymphoma, myeloma, testicular cancer, small cell lung cancer, and certain ovarian cancers responds better to chemotherapy than does the pain associated with chemoresistant cancers like melanoma and renal cancer.

Table 5.13 - Basics of chemotherapy in pain management of cancer patients.

- Pain relief correlates with cancer cell kill.
- Chemotherapy is indicated in subjects with diffuse cancer spread accompanied by pain.
- Works best in rapidly growing tumours.
- The best analgesic option is radiochemotherapy in combination with morphine.

Hormone therapy

The analgesic effect of sexual hormone therapy depends mainly on the hormone sensitivity of the primary tumour and its metastases. It follows that pain from breast cancer and prostatic cancer will respond better than pain from other cancers. Pain relief occurs just a few days after initiation of hormone therapy in subjects with these hormone sensitive cancers.

Corticosteroids are successful in joint pain and in subjects with headache and vomiting caused by brain metastases. Patients rapidly become pain-free on the first day of treatment. In subjects with rapidly growing liver metastases, corticosteroids reduce painful peritumoural inflammation and swelling. Corticoids are indicated in painful peritumoural edema but are effective for a limited period only.

Calcitonin has a direct effect on the mechanism of bone absorption and, like bisphosphonates, acts as an analgesic in the presence of bone metastasis. Calcitonin may be administered by the nasal route or subcutaneously.

Table 5.14 - Basics of hormone therapy in pain management of cancer patients.

– Sexual hormones (hormone ablation, hormones, antihormones) are most effective in treating the pain associated with hormone-dependent tumours (such as prostate cancer and breast cancer).

– Cortisones have a symptomatic analgesic effect in subjects with peritumoural edema and brain metastasis. They may be useful for causal pain management in leukaemia, lymphoma and diffuse cancer spread.

– Corticosteroids are co-administered with pharmaceutical analgesics and anti-emetics.

Percutaneous (external) radiotherapy

Radiation therapy is highly effective in palliating pain, in particular from bone metastases. Two different mechanisms apply.

The first mechanism is that of reducing tumour volume (curative radiotherapy), involving elevated cumulative therapeutic doses and fractionation (e.g, 5 x 4Gy or 10 x 3Gy). The analgesic effect of fractionated radiotherapy correlates with cancer cell kill and occurs after several days or weeks of treatment.

The second mechanism is that of symptomatic radiotherapy, requiring lower doses and only one shot (e.g., 1 x 8Gy). Pain relief is rapid. The "only" effect is reduction of peritumoural inflammatory acidosis, i.e., reduction of tumour swelling but not of actual tumour size.

Both regimens are equivalent in terms of pain and narcotic relief at three months and are tolerated with few adverse effects (Hartsell *et al.*, 2005).

Table 5.15 - Basics of radiotherapy in pain management of cancer patients.

Internal or external radiotherapy is indicated in subjects with localized tumour growth.
– Pain due to bone metastases responds very well to external radiotherapy.
– Diffuse osteoblastic tumour metastases respond very well to radionuclides.
– A low dosage (Gy) is sufficient for rapid pain relief (symptomatic analgesia). Higher doses and fractionation are necessary to kill cancer cells and stabilize pathological fractures (causal analgesia).
– Radiotherapy for rapid pain relief reduces peritumoural edema but does not affect tumour cell growth.
– Pain radiotherapy should be combined with other analgesic modalities (for example bisphosphonates in bone metastasis).

Radionuclide therapy

Systemic beta-emitting, bone-seeking radiopharmaceuticals represent a good alternative or adjuvant to external beam radiotherapy for palliation of painful osteoblastic bone metastases. Documented response rates in prostatic cancer and breast cancer patients with painful bone metastasis range from 40% to 95%. Pain relief starts within 1-4 weeks after the initiation of treatment, continues for up to 18 months, and is associated with a reduction in analgesic use in many patients (Finlay *et al.*, 2005; McEwan, 2000; Hamdy, 2001).

The most frequently used radio-isotopes in pain management are P-32-labelled phosphate, strontium-89, samarium-153, rhenium-186 and rhenium-188. Radio-isotopes have mainly been used in patients with bone metastasis from prostatic cancer because these metastases are in most cases osteoblastic (sclerotic). The majority of radio compounds accumulate where new bone is formed. Pain patients with refractory bone metastasis and a positive technetium 99m methylene diphosphonate bone scan are ideal candidates for treatment.

Toxicity is mostly haematological. Thrombocytopenia is significant and protracted. Any concomitant myelosuppressive chemotherapy should be carefully monitored. Thrombocytopenia is the main toxicity of relevance in limiting further chemotherapy. Radionuclides should not be given to patients with suspected disseminated intravascular coagulation (McEwan, 2000).

Relative contra-indications for treatment include osteolytic lesions, pending spinal cord compression or pathologic fracture, pre-existing severe myelosuppression, urinary incontinence, inability to follow radiation safety precautions, and severe renal insufficiency.

Bisphosphonates

Skeletal metastasis is frequently accompanied by increased osteoclast activity. Bisphosphonates are excellent painkillers in osteolytic metastases. They do not influence tumour cell growth but decrease the proliferation and functional activity of osteoclasts and may also be beneficial in subjects with predominantly osteoblastic metastatic processes such as skeletal metastases in prostate cancer (Hamdy, 2001). Side effects are minimal. Bisphosphonates should not be given on a long-term basis to subjects with periodontitis and dental problems because of the risk of osteonecrosis. Administration may be oral or intravenous once every four weeks (Carter and Gross, 2003).

Bisphosphonates should be initiated in subjects with asymptomatic osteolytic metastases to prevent fractures and pain. They should be administered intravenously in symptomatic subjects. Oral administration is an option for asymptomatic patients.

Symptomatic pain management strategies

Causal treatment strategies (measures to inhibit tumour growth) are not an option in many cancer patients. Symptomatic pain relief is then the only possible approach.

There are many factors influencing the individual pain sensitivity and the choice of symptomatic pain management (table 5.16). Various local or systemic pharmaceutical, physical and mental approaches may be considered depending on the sensitivity of pain receptors, pain transmission, pain perception and modulation, and depending on whether the pain is nociceptor-mediated or neuropathic, acute or chronic. Site of origin and cause are other factors to be taken into account.

Systemic pharmaceutical approach

Pharmacologic therapies for pain include non-opioids, opioids, adjuvant analgesics, disease-modifying therapies, and (in some cases) interventional techniques. A wide range of systemic pain management drugs is available with a broad spectrum of action. These agents are administered alone or in combination (table 5.16).

Table 5.16 - Systemic pharmaceuticals agents influencing pain sensitivity.

– Non-opioid analgesics
– Opioids
– Antidepressants
– Co-analgesics

Some drugs take effect at the pain origin site while others target pain transmission or pain perception and processing in the brain. The onset of action of an analgesic may be rapid or sustained. The duration of action may be short or long. Some agents reduce the sensitivity of peripheral and central pain receptors. Newer drugs aim to prevent the development of a pain memory. The side effects differ accordingly.

The World Health Organization published pain management recommendations for cancer patients in 1986 in a bid to maximise pain relief and minimise side effects. Although more than twenty years old, this WHO step system (World Health Organizatio; 1986; fig. 5.5) is still the basis for cancer pain management in the world today.

This approach consists of a three-step analgesic ladder which advocates a sequential administration of drugs according to efficacy. The progression is from low efficacy, non-opioid analgesics to weak opioids for moderate pain thence to strong opioids for severe pain, each step of the ladder being associated with adjuvant drugs and symptomatic treatment whenever necessary.

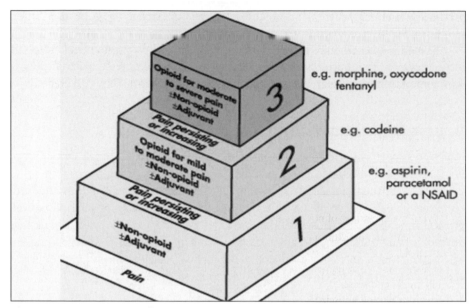

Fig. 5.5 - WHO step system for cancer pain management.

The WHO recommendations are mainly concerned with pain severity and less with pain origin, quality, duration and location. These recommendations to administer peripherally acting analgesics in subjects with pain of minor severity (step I), weak opioids in subjects with moderately severe pain (step II), and centrally acting analgesics (i.e., strong opioids) in subjects with severe pain (step III) are still correct in principle but do not take into account the progress that has been made in the field of pharmaceutical pain management during the past twenty-five years.

Non-opioid analgesics (WHO step I analgesics)

Non opioid analgesics (table 5.17) were previously termed "peripherally acting analgesics" in contrast to opioid analgesics which were termed "centrally acting analgesics". This terminology is now considered as obsolete. Non-opioid analgesics have also been found to have central effects and, conversely, opioid analgesics appear to have peripheral effects, particularly in subjects with inflammation. WHO step I analgesics include various substance classes with different modes of action.

The main mechanisms of action (table 5.18) are inhibition of peripheral prostaglandin synthesis (this applies to NSAIDs such as aspirin, ibuprofen and COX 2 inhibitors) and inhibition of central prostaglandin synthesis (paracetamol, dipyrone). Flupirtine has a special position in this group in that it does not inhibit prostaglandin synthesis.

All non-opioid analgesics have a ceiling effect the analgesic effect cannot be infinitely raised by increasing the dose. The duration of action of peripheral analgesics ranges from 2 hours (aspirin) to 4-6 hours (ibuprofen, diclofenac) to more than 24 hours (piroxicam). Half-lives differ considerably. This results in a high risk of dose dumping, particularly in elderly patients with a reduced metabolic rate. Therefore, piroxicam is not recommended for pain management in cancer patients.

Antispasmodics are first-line drugs in the management of chemotherapy-induced polyneuropathy. These drugs may reduce paroxysmal or neuropathic pain. The most commonly used antispasmodic and antiseizure drugs are gabapentin and carbamazepine.

Table 5.17 - Non-opioid analgesics (WHO step I).

– Non-steroidal anti-inflammatory drugs (NSAIDs)
– Flupirtine
– Antispasmodic agents
– Antiseizure drugs

Table 5.18 - Particularities of non-opioids.

– Ideal for acute and breakthrough pain.
– Non-steroidal anti-inflammatory drugs are good painkillers in subjects with bone metastases.
– Contra-indications for non-steroidal anti-inflammatory drugs are ulcers, clotting disorders, kidney and liver disease.
– Antidepressants and antiseizure drugs are indicated in subjects with "shooting, electric" pain (e.g., carbamazepine and gabapentin).
– Antispasmodic medication is indicated in subjects with spastic pain (dipyrone, pentazocine, N-butylscopolamine, nitro-agents).
– Tetrazepam is used as a muscle relaxant. Baclofen may be indicated for spasm control and oxazepam for restlessness and anxiety.

Opioid analgesics (weak opioid, WHO step II analgesics)

Opioids which in contrast to WHO step I analgesics are not restricted by an analgesic ceiling effect and which are therefore suitable from moderate up to very severe pain conditions, are classified as weak (WHO step II; table 5.19) and strong (WHO step III; table 5.20). They are often used in combination with non-opioids.

Table 5.19 - Weak opioid analgesics for treatment of moderate pain (WHO step II).

– Codeine
– Dextropropoxyphene
– Dihydrocodeine
– Tilidine/naloxone
– Tramadol
– Pentazocine

WHO step III strong opioids are available in a range of formulations and delivery systems. They all have a comparable spectrum of action but differ in terms of potency and severity of side effects. Some strong opioids are better for acute pain while others are more suitable for chronic cancer pain (tables 5.20 and 5.21). Various treatments routes are possible (tables 5.22 and 5.23).

Table 5.20 - Strong opioids for treatment of severe pain (WHO step III).

Morphine
– Piritamide
– Fentanyl
– Buprenorphine
– Oxycodone
– Methadone
– Hydromorphone
– Pethidine

Table 5.21 - Particularities of strong opioids (WHO step III).

– Effectiveness has mainly been demonstrated in nociceptive pain (bone and soft tissue pain, visceral pain). However, there is growing evidence for the efficacy of opioids in neuropathic pain. Apparently neuropathic pain conditions seem to be more responsive to certain opioids (e.g., tramadol, buprenorphine), than to others, probably based on the activation of different pharmacological pathways (McCormack, 1999).
– Long-term opioid therapy may be appropriate for carefully selected patients who can be monitored by their physicians and who can appropriately manage their medication. Opioids should be prescribed by only one physician (case manager).
– Whenever possible, analgesics should be given orally or in stable conditions transdermally and not injected. This provides the patient with the highest possible degree of independence and comfort, enhances quality of life and prevents side effects such as addiction and dependence.
– Sublingual tablets and transmucosal delivery systems were formerly used in subjects with dysphagia, emetic subjects and those unwilling to take tablets. Transdermal patches are the treatment of choice in these patient populations today. The main indication for sublingual tablets and transmucosal delivery systems today is breakthrough pain.
– Short-acting analgesics are the treatment of choice for acute pain states requiring immediate treatment.
– Injection or infusion ensures an immediate onset of action. Switching to subcutaneous or parenteral therapy may be necessary in the terminal phase. Subcutaneous treatment is easy to handle. Intravenous administration is an option in subjects receiving concomitant volume replacement or parenteral feeding or in subjects with a large bleeding risk.
– A different route of administration or a different opioid should be considered in subjects with intolerable side effects. Either measure may help to reduce side effects and provide more effective pain relief. When switching a patient to another opioid, differences in the effective dose must be taken into account.
– Long-acting opioids should be given on a time-contingent dosing schedule rather than as needed. This is for three reasons:
  1- To prevent the release of a neurochemical cascade and breakthrough pain;
  2- To minimize side effects such as habit formation;
  3- To reduce the total drug dose.
– Administering the agents before pain sets in increases pain relief and lowers the analgesic dose required. Chronic pain is a vicious circle that can be counteracted only by preventing pain in the first place. Constant and sufficiently high plasma levels of the analgesic drug should be maintained (e.g., by using transdermal opioid formulations).
– Strong opioids should be prescribed in sustained-release formulations. Sustained-release drugs are ideal for chronic pain.

– For breakthrough pain episodes fast acting opioids like morphine IR or transmucosal fentanyl/buprenorphine are the drugs of choice. If oral or transdermal administration is not an option, opioids may alternatively be administered sublingually, by the oral transmucosal route, rectally, by feeding tube, or parenterally.
– The patient must be actively involved in the treatment regimen, including keeping a pain diary.
– The patient should be psychologically stable.
– There should be no evidence of any (previous) dependence on opioids or other centrally acting drugs such as benzodiazepines.

Table 5.22 - Treatment routes for administering opioids.

– Oral (tablets, capsules, sustained-release and non-sustained release formulations)
– Intramuscular
– Intravenous
– Subcutaneous
– Sublingual
– Transmucosal
– Transdermal (patches)
– Epidural/intrathecal

Table 5.23 - Particularities of transdermal pain management strategies (patches).

– Indicated in subjects with chronic and stable pain conditions. Rate - controlled drug delivery.
– Long-lasting analgesic effect.
– Transdermal buprenorphine (Transtec®) up to 96 hours.
– Transdermal fentanyl (Durogesic®) up to 72 hours.
– Particularly suitable for long-term treatment.
– May be combined with non-opioids.
– May be combined with any fast-acting opioid for breakthrough pain episodes.
– Steady-state plasma levels help to minimise side effects.
– The sustained effect maximises the patient's independence with regard to administration. Increased compliance
– Transdermal therapies enhance quality of life and prevent habit formation/abuse.
– Analgesic pumps maintain steady-state levels of analgesic medication. Use of analgesic pumps has declined since the launch of transdermal analgesic patches, however. The advantage of analgesic pumps is that the analgesic reservoir only needs to be replenished approximately every four weeks while patches need to be replaced approximately every three to four days.
– Late onset of action (which applies to all sustained-release medications), i.e., it takes 12 to 24 hours to reach an analgesic effect. Accordingly, short-acting analgesics must be co-administered at the start of treatment.

Antidepressants

Antidepressants are substances with a mood-lifting effect. Some antidepressants can be used for their analgesic effect alone or in combination with other analgesics (mainly opioids). The doses used for pain management are considerably lower than those used for psychiatric treatment (Plaghki, 2004; Portenoy, 1989).

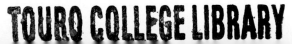

Tricyclic antidepressants are mainly indicated in neuropathic pain. Antidepressants and antiseizure medications are commonly administered for continuous burning pain and painful dysaesthesia. A treatment strategy combining opioids and antidepressants is particularly effective in subjects with plexus involvement. Antidepressants are also used with success in painful iatrogenic polyneuropathy, herpes pain and phantom pain. In addition to their antidepressant and analgesic effect, some antidepressants (amitriptyline and doxepine, for instance) also have sedative effects and may be indicated for patients with sleep disorders. Some antidepressants are associated with weight gain (e.g., amitriptyline, doxepine, maprotiline, mirtazapine) while others are used for weight loss (e. g., sibutramine, fluoxetine).

Co-analgesics

The term "coanalgesics", is often used synonymously with "adjuvant analgesics", "pain-modifying drugs", and similar descriptives. A wide variety of non-opioid medications from several pharmacologic classes have been demonstrated to reduce pain caused by various pathologic conditions or to modify the ongoing disease process in a way that specifically reduces pain. Co-analgesics do not provide direct pain relief but their mechanism of action nevertheless has an impact on pain. Co-analgesics are selected according to the pathophysiological cause of a patient's pain.

Co-analgesics may be antidepressants, anticonvulsants, alpha-2 receptor antagonists, corticosteroids, calcium metabolism regulators, centrally acting muscle relaxants, benzodiazepines or antispasmodics.

Corticosteroids are particularly useful for neuropathic, visceral, and bone pain syndromes, including plexopathies and pain associated with stretching of the liver capsule due to metastases. Corticosteroids are indicated in numerous areas of pain management. One important feature is their anti-edematous and anti-inflammatory effect, which provides rapid relief in the presence of peritumoural edema, nerve compression, joint pain, etc. Low-dose corticosteroids may have positive effects on mental status and appetite. Dexamethasone produces the least amount of mineralocorticoid effect, making it the least toxic choice. Dexamethasone is available in oral, intravenous, subcutaneous, and epidural formulations. The standard dose is 16-24mg/day and can be administered once daily due to the long half-life of this drug, but divided doses are usually used to mitigate high-dose toxic effects, such as psychosis and severe blood sugar abnormalities in diabetic patients. Doses as high as 100mg may be given with severe pain crises, similar to the doses used in acute neurologic emergencies.

Sleeplessness influences the level of pain sensitivity. Sleep quantity and quality are important in people living with cancer. If relaxation techniques and other non-medical measures are unsuccessful, pharmacotherapy is necessary (e.g., in the form of benzodiazepines).

Anxiety affects the severity of pain. Tricyclic antidepressants and/or benzodiazepines may be administered in addition to analgesics for pain relief based on anxiolysis. The mood-uplifting effect of antidepressants helps to reduce the quantity of analgesics required.

The analgesic and appetite-enhancing impact of cannabis may be impressive in the terminal stages. However, cannabis may produce disorientation, mental changes, tachycardia and other symptoms.

The pain threshold is strongly affected by lifestyle and psychosocial factors. Accordingly, psychosocial support may have a positive impact on response to pain management regimens.

Invasive approach

More than 90% of patients with cancer pain respond well to traditional and adjuvant analgesics. For those patients who experience intractable pain that is unresponsive to conventional treatment, interventional pain management techniques often provide welcome pain relief (Sloan, 2004). Interventional anaesthetic procedures for cancer pain number a variety of techniques (table 5.24). Simple, percutaneous injections of alcohol or phenol can provide much needed pain relief for patients with pancreatic, colorectal, or gynaecological cancers.

Table 5.24 - Anaesthetic interventional pain management techniques.

– **Neurolytic block:** coeliac plexus, superior hypogastric plexus, thoracic subarachnoid neurolysis, intercostal nerve, ganglion impar, lumbar sympathetic chain, stellate ganglion, other peripheral nerves (e.g. mandibular, phrenic)
– **Spinal analgesics:** epidural (external catheter vs implanted catheter or pump), intrathecal (external catheter vs implanted pump)
– **Regional local anaesthetic infusions:** brachial plexus, lumbar plexus, peripheral nerve, interpleural block, stellate ganglion
– **Other techniques:** spinal cord stimulation, vertebroplasty, lumbar epidural steroids, intracerebroventricular opioids, human chromaffin transplants

---

In neural blockade and neurolysis, pain transmission from the site of origin to the central nervous system is interrupted by severing neural conduction by surgical or chemical methods. Neuronal regeneration is possible after injection with both alcohol and phenol. Neurolytic blockade can typically be repeated in this situation.

Plexus blockade or neurolysis may produce sustained freedom from pain. Opioid administration to the cervical ganglion or stellate ganglion may be useful in subjects with neuropathic pain in the upper extremity and head. Neuropathic pain involving the lower extremity may be relieved by sympathetic blockade. Neurolytic block of the lumbar sympathetic ganglia may provide pain relief in subjects with urologic cancer. S4/S5 neurolysis may provide significant or total pain relief in subjects with strictly perianal pain such as may be associated with colorectal carcinoma.

Destruction of the **coeliac plexus** ganglia in the upper abdomen is the most common neurolytic block performed. Coeliac plexus neurolysis has often been performed in pain associated with cancer of the distal oesophagus, pancreas, stomach, and liver. Destruction of the superior hypogastric plexus in the lower abdomen has been used to provide pain relief from pelvic cancer. This lower abdominal block has effects similar to the coeliac plexus block in the upper abdomen. Neurolytic blocks have become more uncommon now that non-ablative measures are available.

Epidural anaesthesia involves the injection of analgesics near the spinal cord for reversible, temporary interruption of pain pathways. Reversible neural blockade is also used to help diagnose pain states of unknown cause. If the pain stops after anaesthesia of a particular nerve, this indicates the site of origin of the pain or the pain transmission route involved.

Both epidural and intrathecal administration of morphine have been used effectively to treat cancer pain. **Epidural intrathecal therapy** is a potential treatment alternative in subjects with opioid-sensitive pain who suffer from intolerable side effects. Excruciating pain in the thorax or abdomen, pelvis and lower extremities that does not respond to tablets, drops, infusions and injections may respond to drugs administered in the epidural space near the spinal cord. Epidural catheters may be administered under local anaesthesia in an outpatient setting. The patient or a family member can inject the analgesic into the port as needed. Small electronic pumps with analgesic reservoirs can be set to control regular epidural administration of the analgesic. If a long residence time is likely, the catheter is inserted under the skin so as to avoid interfering with personal care regimens. The catheter is attached to a port embedded under the skin.

One of the advantages of an **intrathecal catheter** –or a pump– versus epidural drug delivery is that a lower quantity of drug produces a more potent effect. Disadvantages include the need for hospitalisation for catheter implantation and the risk of infection. Uncontrolled pain states involving the head or neck may be treated by administering analgesics through an intraventricular catheter. Morphine remains the gold standard and is the only opioid approved for intrathecal use today (Sloan, 2004). Small doses of intraventricular morphine provide long lasting analgesia, and catheter systems are relatively easy to implant.

When all other pain management strategies fail, **chordotomy** may be considered. This procedure involves the severing of the pain pathways leading from the spinal cord to the brain (spinothalamic tract). Because the effect is temporary and due to the subjective discomfort involved, this procedure is performed only –if at all– in patients with a limited life expectancy. The use of destructive techniques, through surgery or anaesthetic blockade, has decreased in recent years with the advent of non-ablative measures. Invasive neurosurgery for pain relief has become less common since the launch of highly effective morphine-based sustained-release tablets and patches.

Physical approach

An important aspect of any management strategy is the use of non pharmacologic treatments. There are a variety of non pharmacologic approaches to pain that have been shown to be effective in alleviating pain for patients with advanced illness. These include physical interventions, such as positioning and active or passive mobilization (therapeutic exercise), techniques, such as TENS, massage, and heat/cold, and complementary and alternative medicine techniques, such as music, and relaxation/imagery exercises.

Physiotherapy

Physiotherapy for pain relief may be indicated in all stages of the disease. The exercises differ depending on the cause and nature of the pain involved (table 5.25). A basic distinction applies with regard to active and passive physiotherapy. Exercises to increase the subject's awareness of posture, motion patterns and breathing are designed to heighten the patient's perception of the areas where pain originates and are a basis for active processing of pain by the patient.

Table 5.25 - Components of physiotherapy in pain management for cancer patients.

– Higher awareness of motion patterns
– Relaxation of painfully tense muscles
– Anxiolysis
– Relaxation of fibrotic subcutaneous tissue
– Patient is taught behaviours calculated to relieve pain
– Patient learns relaxation techniques
– Patient learns postures designed to reduce pain

Breast resection is commonly followed by unspecific back pain that responds very well to physiotherapeutic exercises.

Breathing exercises are highly beneficial in terms of pain control for patients with lung cancer. Respiratory therapy affects both breathing technique and the breathing process, in turn helping to relieve pain (Edel and Knauth, 1999). Thoracotomised patients tend to fear pain and become tense, which increases resistance in the respiratory tract. Breathing exercises and relaxation techniques lower the breathing rate, the respiratory volume increases, and a more natural, economic and effective breathing pattern becomes possible. Anxiety, tension and pain decrease (see lung cancer section, for more details).

Patients with bone metastasis can and should avail of physiotherapy. Some physiotherapy exercises are possible even in subjects with extensive skeletal involvement. Painful positions adopted for protective reasons can be resolved by suitable physiotherapy.

Cancer patients with bone metastases tend to adopt protective or relieving postures to avoid imposing strain on the site of pain. This imposes undue strain on other muscles and causes painful areas of tension to develop. Myeloma patients in particular tend to report pain of this kind which is often misinterpreted as indicating progressive disease.

Patients who maintain a permanent relieving posture and immobility are at risk of developing painful abrasion syndromes and decalcification of bone. The risk of fracture rises. Patients were formerly advised to wear a supporting apparatus to minimise their risk of fracture. Doctors nowadays are reticent about prescribing a brace in patients with bone metastasis because the "braced" regions are particularly prone to decalcification, in turn increasing the risk of fracture.

Manual therapy (chiropractice)

Chiropractic pain management is commonly used to treat back pain caused by degenerative phenomena. Manual treatment of this kind should be administered to cancer patients only if tumour growth-related causes have been ruled out by imaging and lab tests.

Massage and warm baths

Massage exerts mechanical tractive and compressive forces that can resolve painful tension, correct false posture that causes pain, and halt pathological processes.

Massage produces rebound vasodilation, thereby increasing the oxygen supply to the tissues and accelerating the removal and breakdown of pain mediators.

The mentally soothing and relaxing effects of massage act on the limbic system to lower the sensitivity to pain. The same applies to warm baths. Fatigue, distress, nausea and anxiety scores are significantly reduced (Deng et al., 2004). Adding aromatic oil to massage oil enhances the effects of the massage. There is good evidence that aromatherapy with massage and massage alone may be helpful for anxiety reduction for short periods. Patients with high levels of psychological distress respond best to these therapies (Soden et al., 2004).

Underwater pressure massage combines the mechanical effects of massage with the lifting and warming effects of hydrotherapy.

Massage has no effect on pain caused by tumour growth. Massage should be applied judiciously. Contra-indications must be observed (table 5.26).

Table 5.26 - Contra-indications for baths and massage.

– Baths are not suitable for subjects with severe heart failure, high blood pressure or acute inflammation.
– Opioid-containing transdermal patches should not come into direct contact with heat (thermal lamp, fango mud packs, etc.) because of the risk of releasing an elevated quantity of morphine into the skin.
– Massages should be avoided in subjects with dermatosis, phlebitis, lymphadenitis, thrombosis, haemorrhagic diathesis and thrombocytopenia. A limit of 25,000 platelets/mm^3 generally applies.
– Tumourous regions must not be massaged because of the risk of transporting cancer cells in the blood vessels or lymph system and inducing metastasis. Massage treatments are no risk after surgical or radiological removal of the tumour, however. The same applies to heat or cold treatments. Lymphatic drainage should be avoided in subjects with involvement of the lymph system (e.g., in patients with cancerous lymph nodes).
– Particular caution should be exercised when applying heat treatment to breast cancer patients with latent lymphedema because the application of heat might increase the risk of swelling of the arm on the operated side. This occurs via rebound mechanisms even if the heat was applied to an entirely different area of the body.

Lymphatic drainage

Lymphatic drainage stimulates lymphatic flow. Manual lymphatic drainage significantly reduces excess limb volume and dermal thickness, is effective for edema-related pain and improves quality of life end points. Compression pain associated with lymphedema is effectively relieved by lymphatic drainage. A distinction is made between manual lymphatic drainage and drainage using compressive devices (Földi and Kubik, 1999). Physicians in the English-speaking world tend to prefer lymphatic drainage techniques using compression garments. Other countries tend to opt for manual lymphatic drainage, which is associated with considerably higher cost. Manual lymphatic drainage is performed by specially trained lymph therapists.

Lymphatic drainage needs to be repeated at regular intervals. Compression garments are worn between sessions. Compression garments should be worn from morning to night and removed at bedtime. There is no evidence to support the use of medical therapies, including diuretics (Kligman et al., 2004).

(See the section on breast cancer, for more information on the treatment of lymphedema.)

Thermal baths

Thermal baths may help to relieve pain through their relaxing effects. Thermal baths involve water temperatures of 36° to 38°C and are unsuitable for patients with cardiovascular problems. An effect on tumour growth and metastatic risk have not been proven but would be possible because of the associated enhancement of blood flow. Negative effects on the immune system are also conceivable.

Cold treatments and contrast hydrotherapy

Placing ice packs on inflammation and swelling has been successfully used for centuries as a means of relieving pain. Applying cold packs inhibits pain receptors, decelerates neurotransmission, and reduces the release of inflammatory and pain mediators.

Cold treatment may take the form of showers, wraps and packs, ice packs, ice wraps, ice sticks, cold air packs, brushing and friction, and Kneipp cold water treatments. Tense muscles and painful joints may become pain-free by applying ice treatments. Subsequent physiotherapy is easier and less painful. Local cold applications may provide relief of pain in subjects with painful bone metastases. These treatments should be applied approximately 3 to 4 times daily for 10 to 25 minutes. Short cold treatments have disadvantages. Their effect is based solely on a rebound phenomenon and produces rebound enhancement of blood flow with an at least theoretical risk of stimulating cancer cell dissemination.

Unlike heat treatment, cold treatment can be conducted in cancer patients with no risk involved. Cancer cell dissemination (i.e., the metastatic process) tends to be inhibited by cold therapy. Peripheral arterial occlusive disease is a contraindication.

Thermal treatment and fango mud packs

The word fango is from the Italian and means "healthful mud". Mud from volcanic ash is usually employed. Volcanic mud has a high thermal storage capacity and is an excellent conductor of heat.

Fango mud packs are mainly used to treat the pain associated with chronic degenerative joint disease, especially in accessible areas such as the knee and shoulder joints and in preparation for massage treatment.

Naturopathy uses hot water bottles, hayflower bags, peat bags and hot rolls to treat tense muscles and overstrained connective tissue.

Fango mud packs and other local thermal treatments should not be applied to cancerous areas of the body because of the risk of stimulating local tumour growth and metastatic processes.

Water treatments and Kneipp showers

Hydrotherapy and Kneipp water treatments use cold water applied at pressures of 1.5 to 2 bar. A mechanical effect and thermal stimulation come into play.

The water used for showering may be cold, lukewarm, warm, hot, or alternatively hot and cold. The steam shower is a special form involving the emanation of steam from the shower head under high pressure. Kneipp showers help to relax the muscles and the autonomic nervous system. They affect the circulation and may be hypnotic in agitated subjects and invigorating in fatigued subjects.

Kneipp showers have a stabilizing effect on the circulation and immune system. A prophylactic effect has therefore been imputed to them. Contra-indications for cancer patients are not documented.

Electrotherapy

Pain relief is one of the main therapeutic indications for electrotherapy. Electrotherapy involves exposing circumscribed areas of the body to electrical stimuli of a varying strength. It may relax the muscles and nerves and relieve various pain syndromes. Pain management techniques include low frequency, intermediate frequency, and high frequency diatherapy, magnetic therapy and ultrasound therapy.

No metal parts may be present in the treatment field because of the risk of overheating of the metal resulting in severe burns. This applies for example to women implanted with an intra-uterine device for contraception. Electrotherapy is contra-indicated in patients with cardiac pacemakers. Other contra-indications include skin lesions and acute febrile or inflammatory states.

Low frequency electrotherapies include Stanger bath treatment, diadynamic current therapy and transcutaneous electrical nerve stimulation (TENS).

Stanger bath treatment involves the application of direct current through metal electrodes attached to a special water bath. The pain relief provided is particularly promising in patients with polyneuropathy.

Diadynamic current treatment is a combination of low-frequency alternating current and underlying direct current, producing significant pain relieve and helping to relax tense muscles. This technique is mainly used in subjects with degenerative disease of the musculoskeletal system.

High frequency electrotherapies include short wave, ultra short wave and microwave therapy. They do not differ in principle from heat treatments. The various high frequency treatment methods available permit heat penetration of varying depths, ranging from shallow to very deep.

High frequency electrotherapy helps to relieve the pain associated with chronic joint disease, painful tendonitis and chronic inflammatory disease.

High frequency electrotherapy should not be applied to cancerous parts of the body because of a possible risk of stimulating tumour growth or exacerbating metastatic processes.

Electrical stimulation is based on the observation that pain is not perceived if peripheral electrical stimuli block pain receptor cells.

Electrical stimulation methods are primarily used for pain caused by destruction of nerve fibres. Electrodes implanted immediately beneath the skin block pain transmission by regular emission of electrical impulses.

Electrical stimulation is indicated for amputation-related pain and for other chronic poorly controlled pain states such as the pain of shingles.

There are three main types of electrical stimulation. These are transcutaneous electrical nerve stimulation (TENS), spinal cord or brachial plexus stimulation and stimulation of the brain, especially the diencephalon. Acupuncture is a particular form of electrical stimulation. Electrical nerve stimulation (TENS) involves the emission of short electrical impulses to the skin near the nerves involved in pain transmission.

TENS therapy is less suitable for cancer pain than for treatment-induced pain such as scar pain, shingles pain, phantom pain, pain induced by muscular tension, pain due to peripheral nerve injury, and sciatica. The effect differs from patient to patient. Some patients require only a few minutes of daily treatment for pain relief while others require continuous treatment. Efficacy is contingent not just upon the duration but also upon the form of stimulation applied.

Unless many pharmaceutical agents, TENS is impossible to overdose. Harmful side effects have not been documented. Patients with cardiac pacemakers may not receive TENS near the heart because of the associated risk of interference.

Acupuncture

The analgesic effects of **acupuncture** are based on the release of endorphins at three sites: the spinal cord, the mesencephalon and the hypothalamus.

The limited effect of acupuncture in cancer pain can be explained according to the guiding principle of classical acupuncture: "Acupuncture cures what is disturbed but not what is destroyed". It is effective however in managing the spasmodic states generated indirectly by the disease, and also shows efficacy in treatment-related neuropathic pain and the pain of shingles. This is especially important because neuropathic pain is often refractory to conventional treatment (Deng et al., 2004).

Acupuncture is contraindicated in the local area of an unstable spine, in persons with a severe clotting disorder, in neutropenic patients, and on limbs with lymphedema.

Magnetic field therapy

The value of **magnetic field therapy** among physical therapies is inconclusive. There is no scientific justification whatsoever for the therapeutic use of magnetic fields in cancer patients. Magnetic field therapy should not be applied to tumour tissue because of the possible risk of stimulating tumour growth and metastatic processes.

The effects of **ultrasound therapy** are mechanical and chemical. The basic principle is that ultrasound waves are converted to heat at the junctions between different tissues, in particular between muscle and bone. This suggests that pain where tendon meets bone (insertion tendonitis) and other musculoskeletal pain would respond well to ultrasound treatment. Ultrasound treatment has also demonstrated efficacy in managing scar pain. Ultrasound treatment should not under any circumstances be applied to the eye, the heart, or synthetic implants (such as silicon prostheses). Caution should be exercised after spinal surgery (laminectomy) and during or after radiotherapy. Ultrasound treatment should avoid the brain, spinal cord, abdominal and thoracic organs and the organs of reproduction. Caution should be exercised in patients with cardiac pacemakers. Ultrasound treatment should not be applied to tumour tissue because of the risk of stimulating metastatic processes.

Mental approach

Psychological pain management approaches capitalize on the interactions between mental symptoms and pain, and may help some cancer patients more than analgesics.

Chronic pain patients frequently suffer from insomnia, anxiety, hopelessness and despair. They are prone to depression. All these symptoms lower the pain threshold and result in more severe pain and a higher analgesic requirement (fig. 5.2). Psychosocial support should therefore always be considered as an adjunct to pharmacotherapy.

Cancer patients use a wide variety of nonpharmacological treatments regardless of effectiveness, which means clinicians should be aware of the common modalities for which there is available research. Several studies have demonstrated a lack of awareness of nonpharmacologic strategies in general among healthcare professionals, which suggests there is much to learn about which treatments are effective and which are not. The physician-patient relationship would benefit from the physician being able to discuss specific complementary treatments with patients, rather than avoid the topic or dismiss such treatments as elusive or not part of conventional cancer care.

Distraction and imaging strategies

Intensive occupation distraction and active interaction with other people help to lower the pain threshold. One way of achieving internal mental pain distraction is to pursue a hobby, arts and crafts for example (fig. 2.2, 2.3). Accordingly, art therapy is practised in most German cancer rehabilitation clinics.

Internal distraction techniques include various methods of focusing thought, for example on memories of happy holidays, taking inner thoughts for a walk, reciting a poem, concentrating on pictures, listening to a well-loved piece of music with the inner ear, or practising visual imaging techniques and thinking up fantasies. The deeper a person can become engaged with inner or external events, the more likely he or she will be able to forget the pain or keep it at bay.

Soothing and relaxation techniques, hypnosis

Some techniques aim for calm, even, aware breathing. Others aim to achieve muscular relaxation. Hypnosis and autosuggestion may be highly effective. All these techniques help to normalize the circulation, produce slower, more effective respiration, reduce oxygen consumption, lower the heart rate and the blood pressure, relax the musculoskeletal system and keep pain at a remove. Tension, depression and anxiety may disappear.

Numerous other methods promising a deep sense of relaxation exist in addition to autogenic training and progressive relaxation techniques. These include meditation, functional relaxation, focused motion exercises and yoga. There is no such thing as standard methods that produce relaxation in all situations and in all people.

One person achieves relaxation visually, while another achieves the same result through sounds, voices and auditory sensations. One person might experience a pleasant sense of relaxation and pain relief from hearing a poem, another might derive this effect from a physical experience perceived with a heightened awareness.

Hypnosis is one of the oldest relaxation techniques in pain management. If hypnosis is successful, the cause of pain is registered but only partly transmitted to the conscious self. Hypnosis modifies perception of pain so that the latter is no longer perceived as distressful. Third party hypnosis and self-hypnosis exist. Learning self-hypnosis is the better option for cancer patients, for several reasons. Third party hypnosis may be very effective and is also feasible in a group situation.

Hypnosis does not work for everyone. Few people are amenable to true hypnosis. Good concentration is a major requirement for hypnosis. Patients suffering from phantom pain may derive particular benefit from hypnosis.

Counteractivity

This term refers to measures and behaviours to override pain, similarly to distraction strategies. The basic principle is that you experience pain all the more intensely that you think about it. The same pain will be perceived less intensely in the presence of a distraction. There are numerous techniques for achieving this. One method is to increase your working capacity. Pain sufferers not uncommonly develop into workaholics by immersing themselves in work to distract themselves from their pain. Art therapy and occupational therapy are more positive examples of counteractivity.

Progressive relaxation is another counteractive measure. It is based on brief contraction of a muscle group. The basic principle is to achieve relaxation subsequent to muscular contraction.

Attitude therapy

This includes techniques aimed at keeping pain at a distance. The objective is to accept the pain and put the pain issue into perspective. Pain is easier to control if the patient knows why it is there and how it develops. This insight helps to show which measures might be effective in tackling the problem.

Monitoring-quality assurance

A pain diary kept by the patient has proved very valuable as a means of monitoring treatment. Pain diaries are an effective way of monitoring how pain responds over time and evaluating the patient's physical and psychological status. In addition, the patient is actively motivated to comply with treatment and becomes more involved. Patients rate the severity of their pain in this diary with the aid of a pain scale.

There are a variety of measures to determine severity of pain. Pain scales and assessment procedures to measure and to evaluate the effectiveness of pain management include numeric rating scales, visual analogue scales, verbal rating scales and emoticon (smiley faces) scales. (fig. 5.3, 5.4).

Pain questionnaires and quality of life questionnaires – e.g., SF 36, EORTC QLQ-C30, quality of life questionnaire (Coates *et al.*, 1997), BPI-C (Brief Pain Inventory) (Cleeland *et al.*, 1994), HADS (Hospital Anxiety and Depression Scale) (Bjelland *et al.*, 2002), PDI (Pain Disability Index) (Tait *et al.*, 1990), FESV (Geissner, 1996), ADS (Hautzinger, 1995; McGill Pain questionnaire) – are effective means of recording pain, monitoring outcome and evaluating the measures implemented (table 5.27).

Table 5.27 - Common questionnaires for assessment, monitoring and evaluation of pain and pain management.

– ADS = General Depression Scale
– BPI = Brief Pain Inventory
– PDI = Pain Disability Index
– RSCL = Rotterdam symptom checklist
– STAI = Spiegelberger Trait Anxiety Inventory
– FESV = Pain Coping Questionnaire
– FIM = Functional Independence Measure
– FIBECK = Freiburgs Inventory for Coping with Chronic Disease
– HDS = Hospital Anxiety and Depression Scale
– ADL = Activities of Daily Living
– VAS = Visual-Analogue-Scale

Pain has both physical – that is, medically quantifiable – and psychological causes. Sociocultural and family influences also play a large role. All these aspects must be taken into account during assessment, monitoring and evaluation of effectiveness. To address this problem, the Pain Research Group of the WHO Collaborating Centre for Symptom Evaluation in Cancer Care has developed the Brief Pain Inventory (BPI), a pain assessment tool for use with cancer patients. The BPI measures both the intensity of pain (sensory dimension) and interference of pain in the patient's life (reactive dimension). It also queries the patient about pain relief, pain quality, and his/her perception of the cause of pain (Cleeland, 1994).

Management of iatrogenic "cancer pain"

Many pain states are described as "cancer pain" although the cancer is not the specific cause. Not uncommonly, cancer treatment itself produces chronic pain.

Chronic pain syndromes caused by surgical interventions

Table 5.28 - Chronic pain as an after-effect of cancer surgery

– Post-mastectomy syndrome
– Post-gastrectomy syndrome
– Post-proctectomy syndrome
– Post-thoracotomy syndrome
– Post-amputation syndrome
– Phantom pain
– Lymphedema

Coccydynia (tailbone pain) may persist in rectally amputated colorectal cancer patients for months or indeed years after surgery (**post-proctectomy syndrome**). The pain is caused by the wound cavity gradually filling with connective tissue from the small intestine and neighbouring organs. The pain must not be mistaken for symptoms of progressive disease, which may be very similar. An MRI scan and/or PET is necessary for diagnostic purposes. Sitting baths may be helpful, or opioid patches if necessary (see section on rectal cancer).

Post-gastrectomy pain is common after potentially curative surgery for gastric cancer. It is due to the lower food reservoir and changes in motoricity and regulation. Individual dietary advice is the best pain management strategy in such cases (see section on gastric cancer).

Painful abdominal lesions may be an inevitable part of wound healing after surgery or radiotherapy. They are frequently mistaken for signs of disease progression. Good dietary advice may be very effective, but surgery may be necessary to detach the adhesions (see chapter on colorectal cancer).

Breast cancer patients often report headache, back pain und static pain after mastectomy (**post-mastectomy syndrome**). These symptoms are caused by unilateral weight loss. The best pain management strategy in such cases is good advice on an artificial breast to balance out the weight loss (see section on breast cancer).

Physiotherapy exercises and relaxation training are indicated in pneumectomised lung cancer patients complaining of chest pain (**post pneumectomy syndrome**).

Scars may cause pain for years, especially during a change of weather. This (usually) nagging pain may be referred to more remote regions. If ultrasound treatment, anaesthetic treatment and conventional analgesics have no effect, morphine-based painkillers may be necessary (see section on lung cancer).

Surgery or radiotherapy-related **lymphedema** in cancer patients may be extremely painful and is a major challenge for lymphatic therapists (see section on breast cancer).

Phantom pain after amputations responds only –if at all– to centrally acting analgesics. Pain in the remaining leg stump may be relieved by reworking the artificial limb or by infiltration of the scar with local anaesthetics. This type of pain must not be confused with the equally excruciating **neurinomas** caused by nerves sprouting from severed nerve ends in the amputation scar. These painful nerve networks are highly sensitive to mechanical, chemical and thermal stimuli. Pharmacotherapy options include antiseizure agents and major tranquilizers.

Long confinement to bed is enough to induce pain caused by **perfusion disorders** of the skin or spinal tension. Physiotherapy and massage are the best options for treating this kind of pain.

Chronic pain syndromes caused by chemotherapy

A number of highly effective antineoplastics such as taxanes, platinum and derivates cause treatment-limiting toxicity in the form of painful polyneuropathy (tables 5.29 and 5.30). Therapeutic intervention for acute pain is necessary if vinca alkaloids are administered paravenously.

Table 5.29 - Pain as a long-term side effect after chemotherapy/hormone therapy.

Site of pain	Symptoms	Drug culprit	Specific treatment
Head	Migraine-like pain	Vinblastine, gestagens, serotonin blockers	Migraine therapy
Mouth	Mucositis	Many antineoplastics	Local anaesthetics, mouth washes prophylaxis of infection
Eye	Conjunctivitis	5-FU, cytarabine	Local therapy with Cortisone ointments/ eyedrops
Nipples	Edema	Hormones	Prophylactic irradiation
Bladder	Cystitis	Alkylating agents, specially cyclophos-phamide	Mesna
Fingertips	Paraesthesia	Platinum, taxanes	Pyridoxine, B-vitamins,
Soles of feet	Neuropathic pain	Vinca alkaloids, thalidomide	Antidepressants, antiseizure agents, electrotherapy
Palms, soles	Palmar-plantar, erythrodysaesthesia	5- FU, capecitabine	Pyridoxine, B-vitamins
Bone	Flare, tenderness	Hormones	Cortisone
Muscles, joints	Myalgia, spasm	Taxanes, vindesine, interferon, oxaliplatin	Cortisone, no exposure to cold in case of oxaliplatin

Table 5.30 - Neurotoxic antineoplastics.

– Cisplatin
– Oxaliplatin
– Paclitaxel
– Thalidomide
– Vincristine
– Vinblastine

Chemotherapy-induced polyneuropathy is extremely intractable and resistant to many conventional pain management strategies. It may be worth attempting treatment with B-vitamins and glutamine infusions. Antidepressants and antispasmodics are used frequently with varying responses.

The positive impact of physical treatment approaches such as hydro-electric full blade or direct current is uncontested. Ice packs and contrast hydrotherapy may improve the patient's well-being. Temporary relief of pain symptoms in the hands and feet is achieved with particulate sand structures, but the relief provided by these physical measures unfortunately does not last.

Many patients say that autogenic training helps (see section on ovarian cancer.

Chronic pain syndromes caused by hormone therapy

Very severe pain (flare) in cancerous areas occasionally occurs during and shortly after hormone treatment. This pain may be interpreted as a good prognostic omen because it indicates a tumour response. Flare rarely lasts longer than a day. If it does, corticoids should be attempted.

Chronic pain syndromes caused by radiotherapy

Table 5.31 - Post-radiotherapy pain syndromes.

– Radiation fibrosis of the brachial and lumbar plexus
– Radiation myelopathy
– Radiation-induced peripheral tumours

Extremely painful cystitis may occur after radiotherapy of gynaecological tumours, colorectal or prostatic cancer. Symptomatic treatments such as phytotherapy should be attempted first. Heat treatments such as sitting baths provide pain relief but, like all water treatments, are prohibited in subjects with acute radiation inflammation.

Radiotherapy-induced proctitis may be very painful. It is frequently accompanied by spasmodic pain and painful bowel motions in the inflammatory phase. Antispasmodics and local application of xylocaine gel are indicated.

Post-radiation pain in the area served by the brachial plexus may occur for as long as 6 months to 20 years after treatment. It may be difficult to distinguish between radiation fibrosis and progressive disease. Pain occurs late and is often described as diffuse arm pain. Lymphedema in the arm is often present too.

Radiotherapy and chemotherapy both compromise the immune system, in turn promoting infections such as shingles. Shingles (herpes zoster) infection may be intractable, painful and refractory to treatment. Acupuncture, ultrasound therapy, cold packs, TENS and antiseizure agents/antidepressants may occasionally be effective.

Adverse effects of analgesics

Any effective drug may also cause unwanted side effects. Analgesics are no exception to this rule. Some of the potential side effects are described in the following.

Adverse effects of non-opioids

NSAIDs have many potential adverse effects (table 5.32). Non steroidal anti-inflammatory drugs must be combined with omeprazole in patients at risk of ulceration (table 5.33). Proton pump inhibitors (such as omeprazole) reduce the acidity of the gastric fluid. H2-receptor blockers inhibit histamine-mediated gastric acid and pepsin production.

A combination of two different NSAIDs is not allowed because of additive side effects.

Cox-2 inhibitors have many contraindications in cardiovascular risk patients. They are less ulcerogenic and do not inhibit platelet aggregation. They have less of a vasodilatory effect which may be one of the reasons for the higher risk of cardiovascular failure.

Table 5.32 - Side effects of NSAIDs.

– NSAIDs are contraindicated in patients with existing ulceration.
– Non steroidal anti-inflammatory drugs need to be combined with omeprazole in subjects with a history of ulcer, heavy smokers, older age, coumarin treatment. H2- blockers are not suitable for ulcer prevention. Though they reduce gastro-intestinal symptoms, they do not prevent ulcers and the associated risk of bleeding.
– NSAIDs are commonly associated with major side effects in gastrectomised subjects and Whipple surgery recipients because of the risk of mucositis.
– Renal function disorders may occur (interstitial nephritis, hyperkalaemia).
– Pseudo-allergic reactions are possible (asthma attacks).
– Platelet aggregation inhibition.
– Haematopoietic disorders.
– Hypersensitivity reactions.
– Watch out for antipyretic effects and masking of infection in immunosuppressed patients.
– Impairment of short-term memory in older patients.
– Cardiovascular risks (?)

Table 5.33 - Patients at high risk of ulcer.

– Heavy smokers
– Alcoholics
– History of ulcer
– Geriatric patients
– Coumarin therapy
– Corticoid therapy

All analgesics affect the blood count, especially those containing dipyrone.

Patients with existing liver damage should not take painkillers containing paracetamol. Renal function disorders may occur after long-term treatment with phenacetin analgesics. Non-steroidal anti-inflammatory drugs (NSAIDs) and morphine may also disrupt renal function.

Potential adverse effects of antiseizure drugs and antispasmodics include fatigue, gastro-intestinal intolerance, blood dyscrasia and skin rash. Regular hematologic tests are necessary during carbamazepine treatment because of the potential effects on the blood count.

Low-dose corticoids may have both positive and negative effects on mental status and appetite. Weight gain is not always welcome. Immunosuppressant and endocrine effects constitute treatment-limiting toxicities. Many side effects limit their use in severe (terminal) pain.

Dexamethasone has the lowest mineralocorticoid effect and is suitable for once-daily dosing because of its long half-life. Intravenous bolus doses should be administered over several minutes to reduce untoward reactions, such as burning sensations.

Adverse effects of antidepressants

Antidepressants may have many unwanted side effects (table 5.34). Side effects of tricyclic antidepressants at the start of treatment often prompt patients to discontinue this treatment. However, the side effects diminish as treatment progresses. Patients should be informed accordingly and started on very low doses. Antidepressants are best given in the evening because of their sedative effects. Clomipramine (starting dose of 25mg/day, escalating to a maintenance dose of 75 to 100mg/day) may be taken in the mornings because of its mildly drive-enhancing properties. Contrary to public opinion, antidepressants do not cause addiction or dependence; these are problems associated with benzodiazepines.

Table 5.34 - Possible side effects of antidepressants (tricyclic antidepressants).

– Sedation
– Dry mouth
– Sweating
– Headache
– Urinary retention
– Cerebral seizure
– Glaucoma
– Conduction defect
– Decrease of libido
– Immune reactions such as thrombocytopenia (very rare)

Table 5.35 - Precautions in subjects receiving analgesic antidepressants.

– Alcohol potentiates sedative effects.
– Patients with glaucoma, benign prostatic hyperplasia, or cardiac failure are more likely to develop complications.
– Warning for motorists. Drinking and driving are not allowed. The associated cognitive impairment is potentiated by the effects of alcohol.
– Tricyclic antidepressants must not be combined with MAO inhibitors because this may increase the risk and severity of seizures.
– Some antidepressants lower the seizure threshold. Therefore, particular caution is required in epileptics and patients with cerebral metastases.
– Some antidepressants (such as amitriptyline, doxepine, maprotiline and mirtazapine) cause weight gain while others (sibutramine, fluoxetine) are used for weight loss.

The significant side effects, especially in older patients, limit the use of these agents in palliative care, but their sleep-enhancing and mood-elevating effects may be beneficial enough to outweigh their disadvantages. The newer mixed SNRIs-selective serotonin reuptake inhibitors (SSRIs), such as venlafaxine and duloxetine, may offer some of the advantages of tricyclic antidepressants without the anticholinergic side effects.

Benzodiazepines have sedative, anxiolytic, muscle-relaxant and antispasmodic effects. However, they may be habit-forming. Consequently, and in view of their strong sedative effects and associated impairment of motor skills, they should be prescribed restrictively. Discontinuation of benzodiazepine treatment, especially if abrupt, may provoke a withdrawal syndrome (insomnia, anxiety, restlessness, cerebral seizure). The ability to drive motor vehicles and operate machinery is impaired.

Adverse effects of opioids

The only absolute contraindication to the use of an opioid is a history of a hypersensitivity reaction (e.g., rash, wheezing, and edema). Allergic reactions are almost exclusively limited to the morphine derivatives, and the prevalence of true allergic reactions to synthetic opioids is much lower. There is significant inter- and intra-individual variation in clinical responses to the various opioids, so dose titration is the best approach to initial management. Idiosyncratic responses may require trials of different agents in order to determine the most effective drug and route of delivery for any given patient.

Opioids cause mainly subjective symptoms. Unlike non-opioids, opioids rarely cause objective disorders or long-term target organ toxicity. The main reasons for "opiophobia" are a fear of habit-formation and abuse (table 5.36). The way of administration also influences the tolerability of opioids, i.e., a transdermal administration in general has a better tolerability profile compared to oral or parenteral administrations.

Table 5.36 - Reasons for reluctant use of strong opioids in pain patients.

– Fear of side effects (in particular respiratory depression)
– Fear of habit-formation and abuse
– Fear of withdrawal symptoms
– Complicated prescription modalities

All opioid drugs and their derivatives have central and peripheral effects of greater or lesser intensity (tables 5.37, 5.38 and 5.39). Tolerance differs from patient to patient. If side effects occur, it is better to try the patient on another opioid analgesic rather than dispense with opioid therapy altogether. Opioid rotation is indicated in cases of intolerance.

Table 5.37 - Central effects of opioids.

– Analgesia
– Respiratory depression
– Nausea and vomiting
– Euphoria
– Sedative/hypnotic side effects

Table 5.38 - Peripheral effects of opioids.

– Constipation
– Contraction of the Sphincter Oddi and sphincter of the bladder
– Histamine release
– Analgesia in inflamed tissue

Table 5.39 - Adverse effects of opioids

– Constipation
– Nausea and vomiting
– Sedative/hypnotic effects
– Dizziness
– Euphoria/depression
– Histamine release (itching) – sweating
– Dry mouth
– Contraction of sphincter of Oddi and sphincter of the bladder
– Respiratory depression
– Hypotensive crisis, cardiovascular failure
– Addiction
– Psychological dependence

Constipation is the most common side effect of opioid therapy. Constipation should be treated prophylactically. Gastro-intestinal tolerance does not develop. Opioid-induced constipation may be potentiated by the adjunctive use of co-analgesics. The rate of constipation can be decreased by choosing the transdermal administration of opioids.

Dietary measures such as high-fibre foods, plenty of liquids, and swelling agents (linseed, wheat bean) may be insufficient. Laxatives should be used for prophylaxis (e.g., lactulose syrup, sennoside, sodium picosulphate, bisacodyl). Lactulose works in the colon by volume enlargement which promotes bowel motion. Some patients report flatulence. Colicky pain is a significantly rarer side effect of lactose-containing laxatives. It is important to note that swelling agents work only if the patient takes plenty of fluids.

If constipation continues to be intractable, enemas and sometimes digital evacuation may be necessary.

Nausea and emesis tend to occur mainly during the first days of treatment and diminish spontaneously with time. Nausea is common and vomiting is an occasional adverse effect associated with opioids due to activation of the chemoreceptor trigger zone in the medulla, vestibular sensitivity, and delayed gastric emptying. In severe cases or when nausea and vomiting are not self-limited, pharmacotherapy is indicated. When treating opioid-induced nausea, it is important to administer the anti-emetic (5-HT3-antagonists and/or dexamethasone) at least twenty minutes before the opioid. If there is no relief within a few days, a different opioid is recommended. Opioid patches tend to be less emetogenic than tablets and capsules.

Excessive sedation may occur with the initial doses of opioids. If sedation persists after 24-48 hours and other correctable causes have been identified and treated, the use of psychostimulants may be beneficial. These include dextroamphetamine 2.5-5mg by mouth every morning and midday or methylphenidate 5-10mg by mouth every morning and 2.5-5mg midday (although higher doses are frequently used, and use later in the day may be required for wakefulness throughout the evening hours, if desired). Sedation is heavier and more frequent with some opioids than with others. It may be appropriate to switch the patient to another product (opioid rotation).

Insecurity and confusion may occur. These phenomena usually resolve within a few days. Hallucinations are rarer. Confused states are more common in anaemic subjects. Hallucinations are fairly rare in patients with buprenorphine.

Mental side effects differ in frequency depending on the product and duration of treatment. Mood swings are common. Euphoria and depressive mood swings are both possible. Slow influx and effective steady-state levels are maintained by the use of oral sustained release formulations and opioid patches. Use of these formulations minimises the euphoriant effect, which occurs only in association with intravenous injection. Euphoria and a risk of habit-formation are minimal in association with opioids with a slower onset of action, sustained-release formulations and transdermal patches that deliver the drug in a controlled fashion. The higher risk of addiction associated with rapid action opioids is one reason why subcutaneous or intravenous morphine treatment should be administered only in the final stages. Sustained- release formulations are otherwise preferable.

All centrally acting analgesics impair motor skills and concentration. The level of **cognitive impairment** is highest at the start of treatment. Patients should refrain from driving for the first ten days of treatment. After that period, it is important to be aware that opioid analgesics may impair judgment and motor skills. The physician must warn the patient that his or her **ability to drive** may be **impaired**. Most countries (Belgium is an exception) do not impose specific legislation regarding driving under the influence of opioids (Brandman, 2005), unlike their policy with regard to alcohol at the wheel.

Itching, hot flashes and sweating are very common side effects. An individual disposition applies depending on the particular opioid drug. Opioid rotation may be useful.

Pruritus can occur with most opioids, although it appears to be most common with morphine. Fentanyl and oxymorphone may be less likely to cause histamine release. Most antipruritus therapies cause sedation, so the patient must see this as an acceptable trade-off. Antihistamines (such as diphenhydramine) are the most common first-line approach to this opioid-induced symptom when treatment is indicated.

Dry mouth is common. Long-term sequelae include tooth decay and periodontitis with tooth loss. Recommended measures for dry mouth are synthetic saliva or at least lozenges, sage candy, and sugar-free chewing gum to stimulate endogenous salivation.

Approximately 5% of elderly men in most cases with benign prostatic hyperplasia develop urinary retention. This phenomenon is caused by **overstimulation of smooth muscle tissue**. This is also the reason for an increased incidence of biliary colic, pancreatic symptoms and bronchial symptoms. Supportive drugs such as benzodiazepines or tricyclic antidepressants may cause similar effects. Treatment with parasympathomimetics and/or antispasmodics may be necessary. Opioid rotation may be useful as the risk differs greatly from one opioid to the other.

Since most opioids have a mainly renal excretion, impaired renal function is likely to have an impact on the treatment management, i.e., the opioid dose needs to be adjusted to the degree of **renal function disorder** in order to avoid tolerability problems. Buprenorphine, which is mainly excreted via the faeces (Cowan *et al.*, 2005), can be administered to patients with renal impairment up to renal failure without the need for dose adaptation.

Changes involving the central and peripheral nervous system and drug pharmacokinetics are of special interest in the management of pain in **geriatric patients** (Balducci, 2003). Two of the most important pharmacokinetics changes are a declining glomerular filtration rate and reduced activity of the cytochrome P450 system, which is responsible for the activation and breakdown of a number of opioids. Hypoalbuminaemia is another factor that may contribute to enhanced opioid sensitivity. The effectiveness and toxicity of fentanyl may be increased as the drug is highly protein-bound.

Opioids reduce the sensitivity of the **respiratory centre**, possibly decreasing the respiratory rate to the point of apnoea. However, respiratory depression is rarely a clinically significant problem for opioid-tolerant patients who are in pain. When respiratory depression occurs in a patient with advanced disease, the cause is usually multifactorial. The antitussive effect is based on the suppression of the excitability of the cough centre and is not dependent on the respiratory depressant effect. Buprenorphine reaches a ceiling effect at fairly low doses and, as a result, virtually never causes clinically relevant respiratory depression (Dahan *et al.*, 2005). In the unlikely event that respiratory depression does occur, the effects of buprenorphine can be reversed relatively easily with naloxone.

Despite pulmonary function impairment, morphine derivatives have proved effective in lung cancer patients because of their concomitant antitussive effect. In pain patients the respiratory depressant effect of opioids is compensated by the stimulating effect of pain on respiration, with the result that the risk of respiratory depression is low in patients in pain.

Cardiovascular side effects may develop after intravenous or subcccutaneous administration but are extremely rare in association with sustained-release formulations. Postural hypotension and lowering of heart rate are mediated via inhibition of sympathetic centres in the brainstem.

Although side effects and complications have been few with neurolytic blocks, rare but serious complications can occur, even with imaging studies guiding needle placement. Common complications include **postural hypotension and diarrhoea** from decreased sympathetic nervous system outflow in the abdomen (Davies, 1993).

Whilst most opioids suppress the **immune system**, buprenorphine has no immunomodulatory effects (Budd, 2004). This lack of immunosuppressive effects may make buprenorphine an optimal agent in treating cancer-related pain patients, especially those having or needing imminosuppressive therapy.

Myoclonic jerking can occur with high-dose opioid therapy. If myoclonus develops, switch to an alternate opioid, especially if using morphine. Evidence suggests that this symptom is associated with metabolite accumulation, particularly in the face of renal dysfunction. A lower relative dose of the substituted drug may be possible, due to incomplete cross-tolerance. Clonazepam 0.5-1mg by mouth every 6-8 hours, to be increased as needed and tolerated, may be useful in treating myoclonus in patients who are still alert, able to communicate, and take oral preparations

Fear of **opioid tolerance, dependence, abuse and withdrawal symptoms is frequent. Tolerance** is defined as a necessity to raise the dose to achieve a desired effect and as a lowering of the analgesic effect upon repeated administration of the drug.

Physical **dependence** exists in patients who develop withdrawal symptoms on abrupt discontinuation. Psychological dependence is present in subjects with an irresistible desire for more after repeated administration of the substance (addiction). The habit formation and abuse risk correlates with the opioid's euphoriant effect. The risk of dependence is markedly greater in rapidly acting opioids than in sustained-release formulations. The risk of psychological dependence upon sustained-release opioids and fentanyl or buprenorphine patches in pain management is considered to be low. Regular timed dosing intervals for opioids minimize the risk of psychological dependence. Oral preparations and the new opioid patches reduce the risk of addiction. Slow influx and constant levels provided by oral sustained release formulations and opioid patches minimize the euphoriant effect.

Opioid patches can cause addiction only if misused. Misuse includes inhalation after steaming the patch, swallowing the patch, and intravenous injection. As up to 80% of the opioid may still be in the patch after three days on the skin, special caution is necessary for patch storage and disposal.

Opioids may cause **withdrawal symptoms** if administered daily (table 5.40). A stepwise reduction is therefore recommended.

Table 5.40 - Possible symptoms after abrupt withdrawal of opioids.

– Sneezing
– Tachypnea
– Yawning
– Hypotensive crisis, cardiovascular failure
– Sweating
– Goose-flesh, shivering
– Diarrhoea
– Bladder spasms
– Abdominal pain

Despite its rarity, **opioid-induced pain** should be considered as a possible diagnosis in subjects developing sudden exacerbation of their pain during opioid treatment if no other causes are apparent. Opioid-induced pain tends to be diffuse and of a less readily definable quality than the existing pain. Low pain threshold and pain in response to non-painful stimuli tend to be increased by enhancing the dose. Rapid reduction of the opioid dose and concomitant administration of an NMDA receptor antagonist (ketamine, for example) has been effective in these rare cases.

Opioid analgesics require a prescription. Prescriptions and possession are regulated by law. A patient requiring opioid treatment who travels between countries may experience problems with regard to the possession and supply of these analgesics. Cancer patients are therefore advised to carry a certification to carry narcotics that is applicable at least in Europe and also recognized in most non-European countries.

Table 5.41 - Frequent pitfalls in pain management of cancer patients.

- Tendency to always equate pain with cancer progression
- Assumption that pain in patients with infiltration of the spine is always due to tumour involvement and not to functional instability of the spine.
- Long-acting opioids are given "as needed" and not on a time-contingent dosing schedule
- Insufficient consideration of quality, quantity, aetiology, mechanisms and localisation of pain
- Insufficient consideration of co-analgesics and concomitant medication
- Insufficient consideration of emotional and psychosocial factors
- The belief that aspirin is a weak analgesic with few side effects
- The belief that severe pain automatically calls for opioids
- Useless combinations
- Administering two different NSAIDs
- Ignorance of the various ways of administering opioids to patients who cannot swallow (as first choice patches or rectal administration followed by parenteral application)
- Reducing the time interval instead of increasing the dose
- Unjustified fear of addiction with regard to morphine-based analgesics
- Administration of sustained-release drugs for acute pain attacks
- Chewing of sustained-release formulations
- Insufficient consideration of side effects
- No prophylaxis of constipation for patients on opioids
- Taking NSAIDs on an empty stomach
- Taking prostaglandin synthesis inhibitors without ulcer protection
- Insufficient consideration of non-medical pain management strategies
- Underestimation of physical therapies and overestimation of pharmacotherapy
- No consideration of metals in electrotherapy (hip joint replacement, cardiac pacemaker, coil/IUD)
- Reticent use of strong opioids and fear of addiction in patients who need morphine
- No pain diary for chronic pain patients
- Drug regimen not adapted to meet changing conditions

Bibliography

- Aronoff GM (1999) Evaluation and treatment of chronic pain. 3rd ed. Baltimore: Williams & Wilkins
- Balducci L (2003) Management of cancer pain in geriatric patients. J Support Oncol 1: 175-91
- Besson JM et al.(1999) The neurobiology of pain. Lancet 353: 1610-5
- Brandman J (2005) Cancer patients, opioids and driving. J Support Oncol 3: 317-20
- Budd K, Raffa RB (edit.) (2005) Buprenorphine - The unique opioid analgesic. Pharmacology and clinical application. Thieme Stuttgart, New York

- Budd K (2004) Pain, the immune system and opioimmunotoxicity. Reviews in Analgesia 8: 1-10
- Carter G, Gross AN (2003) Bisphosphonates and avascular necrosis of the jaws. Aust Dent J 48: 268
- Caraceni A, Portenoy RK (1999) An international survey of cancer pain characteristics and syndromes. IASP Task Force on Cancer Pain. International Association for the Study of Pain. 82: 263-74
- Cervero P, Laird (1999) JMA. Visceral pain 353: 2145-8
- Cleeland CS, Ryan KM (1994) Pain Assessment: Global Use of the Brief Pain Inventories Ann Acad Med Singapore 23, 2: 129-38
- Coates A, Porzsold F, Osaba D (1997) Quality of life on oncology practice: prognostic value of EORTC QLQ-C30 scores in patients with advanced malignancy. Eur J Cancer 33, 7: 1025-30
- Conradi E., Reißhauer A Physikalische und rehabilitative Medizin in der Betreuung von Tumorschmerzpatienten. In Zenz, Donner (Hrsg): Schmerz bei Tumorerkrankungen. Wissenschaftliche Verlagsgesellschaft. Stuttgart
- Cowan A, Fridericks E et al. (2005) Basic pharmacology of Buprenorphine. In Budd K, Raffe RB (edit) Buprenorphine-The unique opioid analgesic.Thieme Stuttgart, New York
- Dahan A, Yassan A et al. (2005) A comparison of the respiratory effects of intravenous buprenorphine and fentanyl in humans and rats. Br J Anesth 94: 825-34
- Davie D (1993) Incidence of major complications of neurolytic celiac plexus block. J R Soc Med. 86: 264-66
- Deng G, Cassileth B, Yeung K (2004) Complementary therapy for cancer-related symptoms. J Supportive Oncol 2: 419-29
- Edel H, Knauth K (1999) Grundzüge der Atemtherapie. Urban & Fischer, München
- Finlay IG, Mason MD, Shelley M et al.Radioisotopes for the palliation of metastatic bone cancer: a systematic review. Lancet Oncol 6, 6: 392-400
- Földi M, Kubik S (eds) (1999) Lehrbuch der Lymphologie für Physiotherapeuten und Mediziner. G. Fischer, Stuttgart
- Hall W, Christie M, Currow D (2005) Cannabinoids and cancer: causation,--remediation, and I palliation. Lancet Onco16 (1): 35-42
- Hamdy NA, Papapoulos SE(2001) The palliative management of skeletal metastases in prostate cancer: Use of bone-seeking radionuclides and bisphosphonates. Semin Nucl Med 1: 62-8
- Hans G (2005) Buprenorphine and neuropathic pain. In BuddK, Raffa RB (edit.) (2005) Buprenorphine - The unique opioid analgesic. Pharmacology and clinical application. Thieme Stuttgart, New York
- Hartsell WF, Scott CB, Brunner DW et al.(2005) Randomized trial of short- versus long-course radiotherapy for palliation of painful bone metastases. J Natl Cancer Inst 97, 11: 798-804
- Kligman L, Wong RK, Johnston M et al.(2004) The treatment of lymphedema related to breast cancer: A systematic review and evidence summary. Support Care Cancer 12, 6: 421-31
- Kressens JJ, Verhaak PF, Bartelds AJ et al.(2002) Unexplained severe pain in general practice. Eur J Pain 6 : 203-12

- McEwan AJ (2000) Use of radionuclides for the palliation of bone metastases. Semin Radiat Oncol 10, 2: 103-14
- McQuay H (1999) Opioids in pain management. Lancet 353: 2229-33 (9171)
- Meyers CA (2000) Neurocognitive dysfunction in cancer patients. Oncology 14: 75-9
- Paice J (2003) Mechanisms and management of neuropathic pain in cancer. J support Oncol 1, 2: 107-14
- Perkins FM, Kehlet H (2000) Chronic pain as an outcome of surgery. A review of predictive factors. Anesthesiology 93: 1123-33
- Plaghki L, Andriaensen H, Morlion B *et al.*(2004) Systematic overview of the pharmacological management of postherpetic neuralgia. Dermatology 208: 206-16
- Portenoy RK (1989) Painful polyneuropathy. Neuro Clin 2: 265-88
- Ripamonti C, Fulfaro F (2000) Malignant bone pain: Pathophysiology and treatments. Current science, 4: 187-96
- Sabino MA, Mantyh PW (2005) Pathophysiology of bone cancer pain. J Support Oncol 3: 15-24
- Sittle R (2005) Transdermal buprenorphine in clinical practice. In: Budd K, Raffa RB (edit.) (2005) Buprenorphine - The unique opioid analgesic. Pharmacology and clinical application. Thieme Stuttgart, New York
- Sloan P (2004) The evolving role of interventional pain management in oncology. J Support Oncol 2: 491-506
- Soden K, Vincent K, Craske S *et al.*(2004) A randomized controlled trial of aromatherapy massage in a hospice setting. Palliat Med 18: 87-92
- Tait RC, Chibnall JT, Krause S (1990) The pain disability index: psychometric properties. Pain 40, 2: 171-82
- Zech DF, Grond S, Lynch J *et al.*(1995) Validation of World Health Organization guidelines for cancer pain relief: A 10-year prospective study. Pain 63: 65-76
- Walsh D (2000) Palliative medicine. A supportive care of the cancer patient. Seminars in Oncology l: 1-108
- World Health Organization (1986) Cancer pain relief. WHO, Geneva

SECOND PART

Rehabilitation and palliation of breast cancer patients

Aims of rehabilitation and palliation: Significance and definition as distinct from curative tumour follow-up care

The chief goal of all medical, potentially **curative follow-up** care measures (recurrence prophylaxis, early detection and therapy of disease recurrence) is to lengthen survival time. The actual cancer disease therefore represents the focus of curative follow-up care (fig. 1.1, 1.3).

Rehabilitation and palliation, on the other hand, do not aim at influencing the illness, but rather reducing disabilities due to the tumour and therapy (fig. 1.2). Improvement of quality of life constitutes the aims of rehabilitative procedures (fig. 1.2). The negative effects of the disease and corresponding therapy in physical, psychic, social and vocational areas should be eliminated or at least mitigated by rehabilitation and palliation.

The requirements for the necessary therapeutic methods during rehabilitation are dependent primarily on the limitations of quality of life and not, as with curative therapy, on the extent, risk of recurrence and prognosis of the disease.

In theory, the goals of curative follow-up care can be differentiated simply and clearly from those of rehabilitation and palliation. In practice, however, there is a high degree of overlap in particular in tumour recurrence therapy and palliative measures. Potentially curative therapy does not only serve to prolong survival time, but also to alleviate symptoms (Giordano *et al.*, 2004).

The value of **curative tumour aftercare** in breast cancer patients is uncertain. It is doubtful whether potentially curative aftercare measures (early diagnosis of recurrence and treatment of recurrence) really prolong life.

The fact that therapy of disease recurrence may not actually cure the patient, even when routine diagnostics have detected growth at an asymptomatic stage, calls the value of routine follow-up diagnostics into question. Treatment of recurrence results brings only – if any at all – marginal gains in survival time. Whether treatment of advanced metastasized breast cancer has led to substantial improvements of survival in the last 20 years, is discussed controversially. (Schlesinger-Raab *et al.*, 2005). As long as the potentially curative measures (early detection and therapy of recurrence) have failed to show a significant survival benefit, rehabilitative and palliative measures in the follow-up care of breast cancer patients will remain the main focus.

The value of **palliative and rehabilitative follow-up care** is unambiguous, as opposed to the term of potentially curative follow-up care. The outcome of rehabilitative follow-up care involves primarily subjective and objective parameters such as improvement of pain, mobility, physical fitness, overcoming fears, coping with cancer disease, etc. (table 6.36). In general these parameters are not found in **outcome assessment and evaluation** of primary curative therapy such as response, remission and length of remission.

Rehabilitative measures

Rehabilitative measures can be considered for patients undergoing potentially curative as well as palliative treatment. A certain minimum amount of information (table 6.1) on disease status is required before initiating rehabilitative and palliative therapy. Without this information, valuable time is wasted in performing additional research, thus threatening the success of rehabilitation and palliation.

Table 6.1 - Minimum information required before initiating rehabilitative measures.

– Extent of tumour (e.g.,TNM before primary treatment and in the case of progression)
– Curative or palliative therapy approach? (e.g., R0, R1 or R2 resection of the tumour?)
– Localization of metastases (e.g., lymph nodes, bone, visceral involvement?)
– Hormone receptor status?
– Has hormone-, chemotherapy or radiation therapy taken place? (e.g., which cytostatic agents, which hormones and at what dosages were given. What were the results?
– Which radiotherapies have been performed? What dosages were prescribed and what were the results?
– Psychosocial information regarding the family structure, statements pertaining to degree of patient information, any problems with coping or compliance, support given by family members, social and occupational problems, etc.

Rehabilitative measures aimed at reducing physical problems ("rehabilitation before disability")

Physical rehabilitation aims at improving muscle strength and mobility of the shoulder, minimizing arm swelling, and facilitating resumption of all functional activities-ADL, recreation, and work. The spectrum of possible physical impairments and deficiencies is large. Physical impairments are often present against a background of co-morbidities and polypharmacy in older patients. Depending on extent of tumour ablation, hormone-radio- and/or chemotherapy, rehabilitative measures differ from patient to patient.

Therapy-induced polyneuropathies, pain of non tumour origin and recommendations for alleviation

Neuropathic pain is a common syndrome seen in women with breast cancer who have had special chemotherapy. Other aetiologies have to be considered as well (e.g., diabetes, alcohol, arsenic, shingles, paraneoplastic disease, vasculitis, vitamin B12 deficiency, folic acid deficiency, electrolyte misbalance, drugs like INH, amiodarone, phenytoin, metronidazole and others) (Paice, 2003).

Particularly neurotoxic are taxol and vinca-alkaloids which are often used to treat breast cancer.

Primary symptoms may include numbness/paraesthesia, tingling and burning in a symmetric stocking and glove distribution. Usually, the lower extremities are affected first, but a simultaneous onset in the upper and lower extremities has also been reported. Motor neuropathy is much less frequent than sensory symptoms and includes a mild distal weakness, especially in the toe extensor muscles. Diagnosis is usually made based on a clinical examination and electrophysiological measurements, while nerve biopsies provide a further diagnostic tool.

Mild sensory neuropathies appear often to be reversible within few months whereas more severe forms may persist significantly longer.

Tricyclic antidepressants and anticonvulsants are widely used in the treatment of neuropathic pain. Gabapentin, an anticonvulsant related to the neurotransmitter gamma aminobutyric acid with antihyperalgesic activity, offers promising efficacy in different neuropathic pain syndromes. It might relieve symptoms associated with paclitaxel-induced polyneuropathies.

Polyneuropathies induced by paclitaxel, docetaxel, platin, carboplatin and vinca-alkaloid are dose-related. Stopping taxol, symptoms often only improve slowly.

Gabapentin in a dose of 300-1,800mg per day and carbamazepine in a dose of 600-2,400mg per day are most often used for symptomatic treatment (Junker et al., 2004).

There is no irrefutable proof or efficacy regarding pyridoxine and vitamin B preparations, which are often prescribed. The use of alpha-liponic acid is contested and views on efficacy of the topical agent capsaicin are divided.

There are a few positive reports on prophylactic administration of vitamin E and glutamine but none when symptoms have already developed. Prophylactic treatment with nerve growth factor is being studied at present.

Improvement of symptoms with anti-epileptics (carbamazepine 600-2,400mg a day in slow release form and gabapentin 300-1,800mg a day) is proven. Additional treatments of anti-depressants can be useful (Amitriptyline), however this can lead to dry mouth, which can be disturbing.

Low frequency electrotherapy is one of the main treatments for pain relief. This includes Stanger bath treatment, diadynamic current therapy and transcutaneous electrical nerve stimulation (TENSE). Ice packs and contrast hydrotherapy may improve the patient's well-being. Temporary relief of pain symptoms in the hands and feet is achieved by manipulating structured sand but the relief provided by these physical measures unfortunately does not last. Many patients say that autogenic training helps.

Paraneoplastic neurologic syndromes due to breast cancer are rare (Altalia and Abraham, 2004). In the case of tumour-related neurologic disturbances, tumour therapies have to be applied (hormone-, chemo-, target- or radiotherapies).

Breast cancer patients often report headache, back pain and static pain after mastectomy (**post-mastectomy syndrome**). These symptoms are caused by unilateral weight loss. The best pain management strategy in such cases is good counselling on

breast protheses and post-mastectomy products or reconstruction to balance out the weight loss

Scars may cause pain for years, especially during a change of weather. This (usually) nagging pain may be referred to more remote regions. If ultrasound treatment, anaesthetic treatment and conventional analgesics have no effect, morphine-based painkillers may be necessary (see section on lung cancer). **Therapeutic ultrasound** is contraindicated over sites of possible metastasis in women with a history of breast cancer.

Surgery or radiotherapy-related **lymphedema** may be extremely painful. Pain and discomfort associated with lymphedema are common and should be managed primarily by controlling the lymphedema. Compression pain associated with lymphedema is effectively relieved by lymphatic drainage.

Aggravating conditions, such as infection and **recurrence of cancer** in the axillary lymph nodes or brachial plexus should be looked for and treated. In case of infection or recurrence lymphdrainage is contraindicated.

Breast resection is commonly followed by **unspecific back pain** that responds very well to physiotherapeutic exercises. Massage exerts mechanical tractive and compressive forces that can resolve painful tension, correct false posture that causes pain, and halt pathological processes.

Massage produces rebound vasodilation, thereby increasing the oxygen supply to the tissues and accelerating the removal and breakdown of pain mediators.

The mentally soothing and relaxing effects of massage act on the limbic system to lower the sensitivity to pain. The same applies to warm baths. Fatigue, distress, nausea and anxiety scores are significantly reduced (Deng *et al.*, 2004). Adding aromatic oil to massage oil enhances the effects of the massage. Underwater pressure massage combines the mechanical effects of massage with the lifting and warming effects of hydrotherapy.

Massage has no effect on pain caused by tumour growth. Massage should be applied judiciously. Contraindications must be observed (tables 6.2, 6.3, 6.4).

Table 6.2 - Contraindications for baths and massage.

– Baths are not suitable for subjects with severe heart failure, high blood pressure or acute inflammation.

– Opioid-containing transdermal patches should not come into direct contact with heat (thermal lamp, fango mud packs, etc.) because of the risk of releasing an elevated quantity of morphine into the skin.

– Massages should be avoided in subjects with dermatosis, phlebitis, lymphadenitis, thrombosis, haemorrhagic diathesis and thrombocytopenia. A limit of 25,000 platelets/mm^3 generally applies.

– Tumourous regions must not be massaged because of the risk of transporting cancer cells in the blood vessels or lymph system and inducing metastasis. However, massage treatments are no risk after surgical or radiological removal of the tumour. The same applies to heat or cold treatments. Lymphatic drainage should be avoided in subjects with involvement of the lymph system (e.g., in patients with cancerous lymph nodes).

– Particular caution should be exercised when applying heat treatment to breast cancer patients with latent lymphedema because the application of heat might increase the risk of swelling of the arm on the operated side. This occurs via rebound mechanisms even if the heat was applied to an entirely different area of the body.

Table 6.3 - Contraindications for electrotherapy.

– No metal parts in the treatment field because of the risk of overheating of the metal (e.g., intra-uterine device for contraception, endopthesis, pacemaker)
– Not in skin lesions, acute febrile or inflammatory states
– Pregnancy
– High frequency electrotherapy should not be applied to cancerous parts of the body because of a possible risk of stimulating tumour growth
– Cardiac pacemakers

Table 6.4 - Contraindications for ultrasound therapy.

– Not in skin lesions, acute febrile or inflammatory states
– Should not be applied in phlebitis
– Should avoid the brain, spinal cord, abdominal and thoracic organs and the organs of reproduction
– Should not be exercised in patients with cardiac pacemakers
– Should not be applied to the eye, the heart, or synthetic implants (such as silicon prostheses)
– Not after spinal surgery (laminectomy)
– Should not be applied to tumour tissue because of the risk of stimulating metastatic processes

Thermal baths may help to relieve pain through their relaxing effects. Thermal baths utilize water temperatures of 36° to 38° and are unsuitable for patients with cardiovascular problems. An effect on tumour growth and metastatic risk has not been proven but would be possible because of the associated enhancement of blood flow. Negative effects on the immune system are also conceivable.

Fango mud packs are mainly used to treat pain associated with chronic degenerative joint disease, especially in accessible areas such as the knee and shoulder joints and in preparation for massage treatment. Fango mud packs and other local thermal treatments should not be applied to cancerous areas of the body because of the risk of stimulating local tumour growth and metastatic processes.

Lymphedema and recommendations for treatment

Given the variation of therapeutic modalities used to define lymphedema and the variety of assessment techniques, it is not surprising to see wide variation in the reported incidence of lymphedema following breast cancer treatment. There is no consistent operational definition of "clinically significant lymphedema" in the literature. The lack of a consistent definition leads to confusion regarding the incidence of lymphedema after breast cancer treatment.

The reported incidence of lymphedema in the international literature ranges from 2% to 24% which depends upon the definition of lymphedema, the type of therapy, and the time elapsed since treatment.

The risk of lymphedema increases with irradiation of the axilla and by the extent of axillary dissection. Other factors that have been implicated in the development of lymphedema are obesity, extensive axillary disease and recurrent cancer in the axillary lymph nodes. Lymphedema is possible without axillary dissection as well.

Table 6.5 - Stages of lymphedema.

Stage I presents with pitting and is considered reversible; some women with this stage do not have increased arm girth or heaviness and no signs of pitting edema.
- As the edema progresses, it becomes brawny, fibrotic, nonpitting and irreversible (stage II).
- In advanced lymphedema (stage III), which rarely occurs following breast cancer treatments, cartilaginous hardening occurs, with papillomatous outgrowths and hyperkeratosis of the skin. In this guideline, we provide an evidence-based approach to the management of this difficult problem.

Early diagnosis and treatment is required in order to prevent progression of lymphedema. If left untreated, changes in tissues in the affected parts of the body take place which makes treatments more difficult. Chronic and severe lymphedema may very rarely give rise to lymphangiosarcoma. Clinicians should elicit symptoms of heaviness, tightness or swelling in the affected arm (table 6.6).
Pre-and postoperative measurements of both arms are useful in the assessment and diagnosis of lymphedema. Circumferential measurements should be taken at four points: The metacarpal-phalangeal joints, the wrists, 10cm distal to the lateral epicondyles and 15cm proximal to the lateral epicondyles. A difference of more than 2cm at any of the four measurement points may warrant treatment of the lymphedema, provided that tumour involvement of the axilla or brachial plexus, infection and axillary vein thrombosis have been ruled out. Other methods for assessing lymphedema, including lymphoscintigraphy, MRI, CT scanning and ultrasound, are being evaluated in research settings.

Table 6.6 - Early symptoms and warning signs of lymphedema.

- Swelling of the affected arm
- Symptoms of heaviness, tightness of the affected arm
- Feeling of tightness around the upper arm and/or the fingers
- Feeling or even pain of tension in the skin
- Weakness, pain, aching or heaviness in the arm
- Achy feeling in the arm
- A tight sensation arm
- Noticeable swelling in arms and hands in the case of physical effort
- Decreased flexibility of arms
- Sudden increase in weight, not associated with overeating
- Pitting is positive (occurs when a finger pressed against the skin indents and holds the indentation)
- Paresthesia in upper arm

Before any type of lymphedema treatment (table 6.7) is started, tumour involvement of the axilla or brachial plexus, infection and axillary vein thrombosis should be looked for and treated if present (table 6.8).

Table 6.7 - Therapies for lymphedema.

- Graded compression garments
- Pneumatic compression pumps
- Manual lymph drainage (complex decongestive physiotherapy or only complex physical therapy)
- Diuretics

Table 6.8 - Contraindications of manual lymph drainage and pump therapy in breast cancer patients with lymphedema.

- Should not be used over areas of active or potential breast cancer metastases, such as the ribs, chest wall or axillae. In the case of palliative care and generalized metastasis lymph drainage may be allowed.
- Contraindicated in the presence of active infection or deep vein thrombosis in the limb.
- Contraindicated during radiotherapy (however, lymph drainage is possible during chemotherapy).
- Lymph edema may be exacerbated in saunas, steam baths or hot tubs, in hot climates or travel.
- Many patients report worsening of their lymph edema during flight, which suggests that patients who use compression sleeves should probably use them during air travel.

Graded compression garments that deliver pressures of 20 to 60mm Hg are the mainstay of lymphedema therapy and can be used as primary therapy. Compression garments should be worn from morning to night and be removed at bedtime, (Klingman *et al.*, 2004). Compression garments may also protect the extremity from injuries such as burns, lacerations and insect bites. Good compression garments can be custom-made or prefabricated, and ideally they should be fitted by trained personnel. Some sleeves start at the wrist and end at the upper arm. Others incorporate the shoulder and fasten with a strap around the upper torso. A compression gauntlet, especially one incorporating the wrist, can be used if the hand is swollen. Compression garments should be replaced every four to six months, or when they begin to lose their elasticity.

Patients may be noncompliant with using compression garments because the garments are unsightly, uncomfortable, difficult to put on and expensive. Customized, lightweight and colourful garments may be an option for comfort and wear.

Pneumatic compression pumps provide additional benefit over compression garments alone. Multichambered pumps are more effective than monochambered pumps. The former produce a linear pressure wave from distal to proximal portions of the limb that reduces the tendency of fluid to collect in the hand. There are several commercially available pumps, ranging in complexity and cost.

The usual treatment is to initiate **manual lymph drainage** (also called complex decongestive physiotherapy or only complex physical therapy), bandaging, education plus fitting of special garments.

Manual lymph drainage must be repeated regularly. Meanwhile bandaging and compressing stockings are required in severe edema. Lymphatic drainage stimulates lymphatic flow. A distinction is made between manual lymphatic drainage and drainage using compressive devices (Földi and Kubik, 1999). Physicians in the English-speaking world tend to prefer lymphatic drainage techniques using compression garments. Other countries tend to opt for specially trained lymph therapists manually applying lymphatic drainage techniques. This method is considerably higher cost. Lymphatic drainage needs to be repeated at regular intervals. Compression garments are worn between sessions.

There is no evidence to support the use of medical therapies, including **diuretics** (Kligman *et al.*, 2004). Diuretics may help some in the short term as they remove excess fluid from the body via urination. They do not remove the excess protein deposits found in lymph edema and there is evidence that long-term use can be harmful by leading to connective tissue fibrosis. The diuretic effect in the rest of the body may cause adverse side effects, such as hypotension, dehydration and electrolyte imbalance.

Skin care is important. Scratches, sunburn, punctures or other injuries should be avoided. A skin moisturizer should be applied to prevent dryness and prevent the skin from cracking. Many studies have suggested that obesity or being overweight may predispose woman to develop lymphedema.

Surgery (e.g., microsurgical lymphovenous anastomoses, creation of a myocutaneous flap with latissimus dorsi muscle, omental transposition, grafting of lymphatic vessels with tubes or threads) has produced disappointing, inconsistent results and should be avoided.

Other physical therapy modalities, such as laser treatment, electrical stimulation, transcutaneous electrical nerve stimulation (TENS), cryotherapy, microwave therapy and thermal therapy, have been used for lymph edema in breast cancer patients (level V evidence). However, these modalities need further, rigorous evaluation before recommendations can be made.

Table 6.9 - Measures to prevent deterioration of lymph edema.

- Careful hand and arm care, e.g., proper hygiene and avoiding trauma to the arm can minimize risks for infection and lymph edema
- For recurrent infections, prophylaxis with oral antibiotics or monthly injections of penicillin should be considered.
- Scrupulous skin care should be encouraged. Women should avoid cuts, pin pricks, hangnails, insect bites, contact allergens or irritants, pet scratches and burns to the affected extremity.
- Wear protective gloves when doing household chores involving chemical cleansers or steel wool, gardening or yard work, and perhaps while washing dishes.
- Whenever possible patients should avoid medical procedures such as vaccination, blood drawing, intravenous access, blood pressure monitoring, acupuncture, venography and lymph angiography in the affected arm.
- Maintenance of ideal body weight should be encouraged. Obesity is a contributing factor for the development of lymph edema and may limit the effectiveness of compression pumps or sleeves.
- Constriction or squeezing of the arm may increase the pressure in nearby blood vessels, which may lead to increased fluid and swelling.
- Skin infection, which is often streptococcal, or on rare occasions staphylococcal, should be promptly treated with antibiotics such as a penicillin, a cephalosporin or a macrolide.
- Exercise involving the affected arm may be beneficial in controlling lymph edema. Although some clinicians have recommended avoiding of rowing, tennis, golf, skiing, squash, racquetball or any vigorous, repetitive movements against resistance, there is no published evidence to suggest that these activities promote or worsen lymph edema. Women with lymph edema are advised to wear a compression sleeve during arm exercises.
- It may be prudent to provide the patient who is subject to recurrent infections with an emergency home supply of an antistreptococcal antibiotic, to be taken at the first sign of infection. A patient traveling to a remote area should be encouraged to take along a supply of antibiotics

There are no arguments for performing preventive lymph drainage even in high risk patients. However lymphdrainage and other measures prevent deterioration of lymphedema.

In the case of advancing disease and axillary involvement, **chemotherapy and/or radiation therapy** may help the drainage by shrinking the tumours in the lymph nodes. Lymph drainage may not be used over areas of active or potential breast cancer metastases, such as the ribs, chest wall or axillae. (In the case of palliative care and generalized metastasis lymph drainage however may be allowed.)

Impairments of shoulder arm mobility and recommendations for treatment

The most common impairment after operation is breast and axilla scar tightness, axilla edema and neck shoulder pain. Limitation of shoulder mobility may occur in as little as two weeks following immobilization. Shoulder arm mobility is one of the most important sources of distress following breast cancer surgery, and it is one of the most troublesome long-term complications of breast cancer treatment, having a significant impact on the daily life of breast cancer survivors. Shoulder movement is impaired in the majority of patients in the immediate period after axillary lymph node dissection, but usually returns to near-normal values within twelve months of surgery.

Postoperative physiotherapy and upper extremity rehabilitation measures are very useful (table 6.10).

Table 6.10 - Upper extremity rehabilitation measures to mobilize upper extremity after surgery and axillary dissection in breast cancer patients.

– Postoperative physical therapy should begin the first day following surgery. Gentle ROM exercises should be encouraged in the first week after surgery.
– Active stretching exercises can begin one week after surgery, or when the drain is removed, and should be continued for six-eight weeks or until full ROM is achieved in the affected upper extremity. Women should be instructed in scar tissue massage.
– Postoperative assessments following surgery should include ROM, strength, sensation, limb circumference, and scar and chest wall tissue mobility.
– Progressive resistive exercises, i.e., strengthening, can begin with light weights (1-2lbs) within four-six weeks after surgery. A compression sleeve should be worn during any resistive exercises or strenuous upper body athletic activity.

Sport and advice

Women with breast cancer tend to exercise less after being diagnosed with the disease, even though physical activity is an important part of recovery. Overweight and obese women show greater decreases in physical activity after diagnosis when compared to lean women.

By getting less physical activity women are putting themselves at risk for weight gain, which may increase the risk of cancer recurrence. Studies have shown that exercise can help lessen the fatigue associated with cancer treatment, and help patients improve their physical functioning (Oldervoll, 2004).

Women who have had breast cancer should be encouraged to engage in an ongoing, regular program of moderate, aerobic exercise. There is growing evidence that regular physical activity may be beneficial not only for breast cancer prevention (table 6.11). Additional benefits of regular physical activity include prevention and management of heart disease and osteoporosis, as well as improved quality of life in women previously treated for localized breast cancer (Daley *et al.*, 2007). Regular physical activity is essential for weight management.

Table 6.11 - Interest of physical exercises in patients with breast cancer.

– Decreases physical and psychologic symptoms
– Enhances physical and mental well-being
– Helps to regain strength and mobility in affected shoulder and arm
– Decreases feelings of anxiety, depression, stress, and lead to improvements in self-esteem, self-efficacy, vigor, and satisfaction with life
– Induces positive mood changes
– Improves sleep and alleviates fatigue
– Improves self-confidence and control
– Enhances energy levels and helps to control weight
– Decreases stress and tension

Bicycle ergometer training, walking, weight training, aerobic exercises, and athletic activity are shown to have not only a positive effect on physical fitness and psychologic well-being, but also on fatigue symptoms (Oldevoll, 2004; Spruit *et al.*, 2006). A gradual increase in the training intensity is recommended, starting with 15 to 30 minutes three to five days a week. It is important to clarify to both the patient and to family that physical inactivity, which may be intended as rest, will be more likely to promote symptoms of fatigue than to alleviate them (Watson, 2004).

Particularly in Germany group activities such as "sport after cancer" are being supported by the health insurances. Apart from the positive effects on fatigue syndrome and general health, physical activities are expected to have positive repercussions on the social integration. Physical exercise has benefits both physically and psychosocially in cancer patients over time (Watson, 2004; Windsor *et al.*, 2004).

Breast protheses and post-mastectomy products

Many women do not wish to have surgical breast reconstruction after breast cancer surgery or decide to wait several months or years before having reconstructive surgery. For these women, breast prostheses and mastectomy bras are viable alternatives.

Any woman who has undergone breast cancer surgery that has removed a significant portion of tissue is a candidate for a breast prosthesis, which often needs to be worn with a post-mastectomy bra.

Usually, a patient's physician will recommend wearing a camisole (sleeveless undergarment made of soft material) with a non-weighted breast prosthesis after breast cancer surgery until the surgical site is completely healed. This typically takes between four and eight weeks but may be longer or shorter depending on the individual situation. After the chest area has healed, a woman may be fitted for weighted external breast prosthesis.

The main benefit of wearing a breast prosthesis (versus nothing) is that a weighted prosthesis can help balance the body and anchor the bra, preventing back or neck pain, shoulder sagging, or having a bra "ride up" in the back. Some women find that their prosthesis feels heavy at first since they are not used to wearing it. However, in time, most women feel comfortable with their prosthesis. Breast prostheses can also help protect the chest area and mastectomy scars.

There are several different types of prostheses. They may be made from silicone gel, foam, fiberfill or other materials that feel similar to natural tissue. Most are weighted so that they feel the same as the remaining breast (if only one breast has been removed). Some adhere directly to the chest area while others are made to fit into pockets of post-mastectomy bras. Different types of prostheses may also have different features, such as a mock nipple or special shape. In many cases, a woman will be fitted for prosthesis so that it can be custom-made for her body. Partial prostheses, called equalizers or enhancers, are also available for women who have had part of their breasts removed.

After a mastectomy, some women will be able to wear their regular bras with few or no adjustments. If the surgical area is especially sensitive after surgery, a bra extender can help increase the circumference around the body and make wearing a bra feel more comfortable. Bra shoulder pads can help prevent bra straps from digging into the shoulder.

If a woman chooses to wear a breast prosthesis that does not adhere directly to the skin, she will need to wear a special post-mastectomy bra with pockets for the breast form (special swimsuits also hold breast forms). Some women find that special sleep or leisure bras with or without pockets for prosthesis are comfortable to wear overnight.

While breast prostheses can provide physical and emotional benefits after breast cancer surgery, some women do not feel satisfied wearing breast forms. For them, surgical breast reconstruction is a more appropriate decision. Most women who undergo breast cancer surgery are candidates for reconstructive surgery, either during the same surgery as the breast is removed or at a later date. The two main types of reconstructive surgeries are implant insertion and muscle flap reconstruction (the latter involves using the patient's own tissue from another area of the body to reconstruct the breast).

Breast reconstruction

Women choose breast reconstruction for different reasons. Some want to make breasts look balanced when wearing a bra, others want to permanently regain breast contour or to give the convenience of not needing an external prosthesis (Kufe *et al.*, 2003; Resnick *et al.*, 2002)

Timing of reconstructive surgery is based on the woman's desires, other medical conditions, and cancer treatment. Whenever possible, plastic surgeons encourage women to begin breast reconstruction at the same time they are having their mastectomy. For many women, immediate reconstruction reduces the trauma of having a breast removed, as well as the expense and discomfort of undergoing two major operations.

It is also possible to do the reconstruction months or years after a mastectomy. For some women, this may be advised if radiation is to follow mastectomy.

Immediate reconstruction is done at the same time as the mastectomy when the entire breast is removed. A plus with immediate reconstruction is that the chest tissues are undamaged by radiation therapy or scarring. Also, immediate reconstruction means one less surgery.

Delayed reconstruction is done at a later time. For some women, this may be advised if radiation is to follow mastectomy. This is because radiation therapy that follows breast reconstruction can increase complications after surgery.

Decisions about reconstructive surgery will depend on many personal factors such as: Overall health, stage of breast cancer, size of natural breast, amount of tissue available (for example, very thin women may not have the excess body tissue to make flap grafts possible), desire to match the appearance of the opposite breast, desire for bilateral reconstructive surgery and the insurance coverage for the unaffected breast and related costs, type of procedure, size of implant or reconstructed breast

Several types of operations can be used to reconstruct the breast: Implant Procedures, Tissue Flap Reconstruction, TRAM (Transverse Rectus Abdominis Muscle), Flap (tummy tissue), Latissimus dorsi flap, DIEP (Deep Inferior Epigastric Artery Perforator) Flap, Gluteal Free Flap nipple and areola reconstruction.

Breast implants involve the least amount of surgery of all reconstruction options. Slim, small-breasted women tend to do best with breast implants, because they often don't have enough excess belly tissue to form a good tissue transplant.

Most implants that have been in place for 10-15 years have some leakage, but it's usually insignificant. Once a breast implant is in place, scar tissue forms all around it, forming what's called a tissue capsule. Most of the time, tissue capsules are soft-to-firm and unnoticeable. However, less than 15% of the time, a hard capsule forms that can be painful and distort the breast. In this case, a surgeon can break up the scar tissue and, if necessary, replace the implant.

There has been a lot of controversy about the use of silicone-filled implants. Silicone's advantage is that it is most like the normal breast in weight and consistency. An implant after mastectomy sits just under the surface of the skin and is what a person feels when he or she touches the breast area. A saline implant may feel like a water balloon, but a silicone-filled implant will feel more like natural breast tissue.

Some women believe they have been damaged by leaking silicone fluid – specifically, that they developed auto-immune diseases such as arthritis and lupus – and many lawsuits have been filed against the manufacturers of silicone implants. Based on a great deal of research it appears that – as a group – women with silicone implants are no more likely to get arthritis or lupus than women without the implants.

A leaking silicone implant should be removed. The body may react to leaking silicone by forming scar tissue. This may cause discomfort for the woman and an irregular shape to the breast. Though it rarely occurs, very small amounts of liquid silicone can travel to other parts of the body.

The most common problem with breast implants is **capsular contracture**. This can occur if the scar or capsule around the implant begins to tighten and squeezes down on the soft implant. There are four grades of capsular contracture known as Baker grades (Baker grade I-IV).

Capsular contracture can be treated in several ways. Grades III and IV require reoperation. It can result in having the implant removed or replaced.

Some breast implants may **rupture/deflate** in the first few months after surgery and some after several years. Others may take ten or more years to rupture/deflate. Magnetic resonance imaging (MRI) with equipment specifically designed for imaging the breast may be used for evaluating patients with suspected rupture or leakage of their silicone gel-filled implant. Plastic surgeons usually recommend removal of the implant if it has ruptured, even if the silicone is still enclosed within the scar tissue capsule, because the silicone gel may eventually leak into surrounding tissues.

When saline-filled breast implants deflate, the saline solution leaks either through an unsealed or damaged valve or through a break in the implant shell. Implant deflation can be immediate or progress over a period of days, months, or years and is noticed by loss of size or shape of the implant.

Table 6.12 - Potential local complications of breast implants.

– Asymmetry	– Inflammation/irritation
– Breast pain	– Malposition/displacement
– Breast tissue atrophy	– Necrosis
– Calcification/calcium deposits	– Nipple/breast changes
– Capsular contracture	– Palpability/visibility
– Chest wall deformity	– Ptosis
– Delayed wound healing	– Redness/bruising
– Extrusion	– Rupture/deflation
– Granuloma	– Scarring
– Hematoma	– Seroma
– Iatrogenic injury/damage	– Wrinkling/rippling

Trans-rectus abdominis muscle (TRAM) is the most popular of all reconstruction options, especially for a woman with excess belly fat or an abdomen that has been stretched out by pregnancy.

TRAM is not a good choice for thin women who don't have enough abdominal tissue, for women who smoke and therefore have blood vessels that are narrow and less flexible, for women who have multiple surgical scars on the abdomen (normal Cesarean-section scars are not usually a problem).

In general, **latissimus dorsi** is a good option for a woman with small- to medium-sized breasts, because there is so little body fat in this part of the back. An implant (inserted during the same operation) is almost always necessary to create a breast of moderate size.

Disadvantages of latissimus dorsi are that the skin on the back has a different colour and texture than breast skin and that Latissimus dorsi often results in some back asymmetry.

Nipple and areola reconstruction can use tissue taken from the labia just outside the vagina. Tissue can also be taken from the inside of the thigh.

Breast reconstruction restores the shape of the breast, but it cannot restore normal breast sensation. The nerve that supplies feeling to the nipple runs through the deep breast tissue, and is cut during surgery. In a reconstructed breast, the feeling of pleasure from touching the nipple is lost. A rebuilt nipple has much less feeling.

Sexual problems and recommendations for prevention and treatment

The negative impact of breast cancer treatment on the quality of life domain of sexuality for breast cancer survivors represents an important area for education, communication, support, and intervention, especially in younger women. Sexual counselling is an important task in rehabilitation (Krychman et al., 2007).

Breast surgery or radiation to the breasts does not physically decrease a woman's sexual desire. Nor does it decrease her ability to have vaginal lubrication, normal genital feelings, or reach orgasm. Within a year after their surgery, most women with early stage breast cancer have good emotional adjustment and sexual satisfaction unless they have therapy-induced hormonal changes. They report a quality of life similar to women who never had cancer.

Hormone and chemotherapy impair ovarian function. They have a major impact on female sexual function. Much of the loss of desire for sex in women with ovarian failure is linked to dyspareunia from vaginal atrophy. Hormonal changes influence libido and sexual behaviour (Ferell et al., 2003; Schover, 2005). Disturbances in sexual experience and behavior often emerge as an accompanying problem which may mean a significant loss in quality of life, self-esteem and satisfaction within their partnership. Breast cancer survivors who received systemic adjuvant therapy report less sexual satisfaction than healthy women, lower levels of sexual function, decreased libido, difficulty reaching orgasm, dyspareunia associated with vaginal dryness, and less sexual satisfaction, and they don't perceive themselves as feminine or sexually attractive as they did before treatment (Ganz et al., 2002).

If hormone replacement therapy is needed, it is safest to use low dose oestrogens in the form of vaginal ring or suppositories to treat pain that does not respond to appropriate use of water-based lubricants or vaginal moisturisers. Since little oestrogen escapes into the systemic circulation, these products can often dramatically improve dyspareunia with negligible risk of promoting cancer recurrence. Sexual rehabilitation cannot however be reduced to simple hormonal replacement or mechanical device.

Questions relating to sexual dysfunctions are complex in nature. In particularly problematic situations, psychotherapy can help women cope with difficult changes in sexual functioning (Anilo, 2000; Avis, 2004).

It can be assumed that only a small percentage of patients will bring up their sexual problems on their own. Most patients wait for questions from their physician or psychologist. The topic of sexuality, and in particular of "sexual incompetence", is accompanied by considerable inhibitions. Fears and feelings of guilt play a central role. These can be reduced through discussion. Under certain circumstances, it is advisable to include the partner in such a discussion, or to offer the partner individual counselling.

Hormonal problems and recommendations for prevention and treatment

Hormonal changes can have a significant impact on a woman's quality of life.

As a result of the therapy-induced castration particularly young women can develop typical symptoms of menopause (table 6.13a). Hot flashes are one of the main side effects of the commonly prescribed hormone therapies.

Ovarian toxicity is a predictable side effect of alkylating agent-based chemotherapy. It is influenced by the cumulative dose and the duration of therapy. Younger women who preserve their menses or who develop reversible amenorrhea will experience premature menopause but as a delayed effect rather than the immediate effect observed in older midlife women. In young women the incidence of amenorrhea ranges from 31% to 38% after treatment with CMF-chemotherapy; for women greater than 40 years of age, the incidence of amenorrhea is dramatically higher.

Hormonal substitution may avoid or at least alleviate acute and late side effects. Hormone replacement therapy is not recommended in receptor positive tumours. There are no arguments against hormonal substitution in receptor negative tumours. Sometimes gestagens (5-20mg) are given. However gestagens carry an increased risk of thrombosis.

Gabapentin (900mg/d) effectively reduces both the frequency and severity of hot flashes in breast cancer patients. Other non-hormonal treatments for hot flashes include selective serotonin reuptake inhibitors, e.g., venlafaxine (e.g., paroxetine 10mg/d) and clonidine (0,1mg/d).

Other non-medical interventions to alleviate hormonal symptoms include Kneipp baths, phyto-therapeutics, phytotherapy, sedative medication and beta blockers. Relaxation, meditation, and yoga may be useful in controlling mood swings. Exercise may help toward boosting mood and relieving anxiety.

Sometimes nervousness, depression, and anxiety need behavioural therapy or antidepressive therapy (Aapro and Cull, 1999; Hunter et al., 2004).

Table 6.13a - Complaints and complications of therapy-induced castration in breast cancer patients.

– Hot flashes
– Intense perspiration
– Vaginal dryness
– Urine incontinence
– Insomnia
– Reduction of physical fitness
– Irritability
– Loss of libido
– Fatigue
– Depression
– Troubles of dark-adaptation
– Osteoporosis with increased risk of bone fracture

Adjuvant therapy with tamoxifen has a symptom profile that includes vasomotor symptoms, vaginal complaints (dryness, itching, discharge), amenorrhea, hair and nail thinning, insomnia, and mood disturbances. Eye problems are a rare but possible side effect of tamoxifen.

Side effects of aromatase inhibitors include hot flashes, vaginal dryness, bleeding and discharge, decreased libido, breast tenderness, sleeping difficulties, fatigue, osteoporosis, increase in cholesterol levels, sore muscles, joint pain, and arthritis and stomach upset. (Fallowfield *et al.*, 2004). Removal of all the post-menopausal estrogen may be responsible for the increased risk of osteoporosis and fracture. Prescribing prophylactic of bisphosphonates is still under investigation in several studies (Morandi, 2004; Reidl, 2002).

Young and young midlife women with breast cancer are more vulnerable to psychosocial distress because of their developmental stage in life. The multiple demands of the cancer illness are layered on top of the multiple demands of a young woman's life cycle, and women become more vulnerable to psychological morbidity as they attempt to manage multiple stressors. Experiencing premature menopause can further increase a young woman's vulnerability, resulting in a greater risk for emotional distress and a poorer quality of life (Ganz *et al.*, 2003).

Fertility problems, pregnancy and recommendations for prevention and treatment

Pre-menopausal women treated with chemotherapy should be aware that treatment can cause infertility and/or premature menopause (table 6.13b) (Ganz *et al.*, 2003; Sonmezer *et al.*, 2004). This is especially true in older pre-menopausal women (typically in their forties) who are close to menopause (Gelber *et al.*, 2001; Lee *et al.*, 2006). Ovarian toxicity is a predictable side effect of alkylating agent-based chemotherapy and is influenced by the cumulative dose and duration of chemotherapy. The outcomes of women with chemotherapy-induced ovarian damage include menstrual changes, menopausal symptoms, changes in fertility potential, and infertility. In women below 40 years of age who receive a three-drug combination of cyclophosphamide and fluorouracil with either methotretxate (CMF) or an anthracycline (CAF, FAC) for six to nine cycles, the incidence of amenorrhoea ranges from 31 to 38%, and for women above 40 years of age, the incidence of amenorrhoea is dramatically higher (Goodwin *et al.*, 1999).

Table 6.13b - Gonadotoxic risks of cytostatics.

Drugs with high risk of ovarian toxicity
– cyclophosphamide
– chlorambucil
– melphalan
– busulfan
Drugs with medium risk of ovarian toxicity
– cisplatinum
– adriamycin
Drugs with low risk of ovarian toxicity
– methotrexate
– 5-Fluoruracil
– vincristin
– bleomycin
– actinomycin D

Contraceptive counselling is essential for women who experience menstrual changes associated with chemotherapy. Women on adjuvant endocrine therapy can become pregnant and should also be a targeted group for counselling. Pregnancy while on tamoxifen is not recommended because of possible teratogenic effects on the fetus, and women should be counselled to wait at least twelve weeks after discontinuation before attempting conception because of the half-life of the agent (Goldhirsch and Gelber, 2004).

The hormonal and metabolic changes that occur during pregnancy do not pose any increased risk of recurrent breast cancer. Pregnancy after successful treatment of breast cancer does not increase risk of recurrence (Saunders *et al.*, 2004; Blakely *et al.*, 2004).

Several details such as cancer type, degree of metastasis (spread), and amount of radiation and/or chemotherapy received should be considered before advising a woman whether it is safe to become pregnant. For women diagnosed with early-stage breast cancer, pregnancy is usually reasonable two or more years after diagnosis and treatment. Women with stage IV breast cancer or recurrent tumours may not be good candidates for future pregnancies. Apart from the high risk of recurrence, chemotherapy may have an adverse effect on the ovaries and lead to a higher rate of spontaneous miscarriages. Apart from these somatic problems the very difficult discussion of "what if the child is left motherless" is something to face.

Genetic particularities and counselling

The vast majority of cases of breast cancer does not show a strong familial tendency and appear to be sporadic. It is estimated that only 5 to 10% of cases of breast cancer are due to identifiable genetic factors. Most hereditary breast cancers arise from mutations in the genes BRCA1 and BRCA2. These are autosomal dominant genes that are thought to function as tumour suppressor genes (table 6.14).

In addition, the occurrence of rare malignancies or certain hallmark features may be suggestive of the presence of a specific syndrome associated with a breast cancer susceptibility gene other than BRCA1 or BRCA2. As an example, early onset sarcomas and breast cancers are suggestive of Li-Fraumeni syndrome, while the presence of hamartomas may indicate Cowden disease.

Table 6.14 - Features suggestive of a BRCA1 or BRCA2 mutation. Criteria for genetic counselling of relatives.

– Families with at least two patients suffering from breast and/or ovarian carcinoma, one of those below the age of 50 (this age limit does not apply to families with three or more patients)
– Women with more than one primary cancer, such as bilateral breast cancer or breast and ovarian cancer
– Families with one patient with one-sided breast carcinoma at the age of 30 or earlier
– Evidence of vertical transmission, including transmission in two or more generations as well as through male relatives (consistent with autosomal dominant inheritance)
– Families with one patient suffering from ovarian cancer at the age of 40 or earlier
– Families with one patient with bilateral breast carcinoma at the age of 40 or earlier
– Families with one patient with both breast and ovarian carcinoma
– Families with a male patient

Women concerned about the possibility of having inherited an increased risk of developing breast cancer should speak with a genetic counsellor. Based on the family history and, in some cases, genetic testing, an intensified programme of early detection, prophylactic surgery, and chemoprevention may be considered. They should be offered individualized psychologic support (Kuschel et al., 2000).

The decision to undergo genetic testing for breast cancer should not be made casually, but only after a woman has considered the implications of a positive or negative result. Pre-test and post-test genetic counselling is critical. The primary reason for its criticality is due to the complexities of test result interpretation and medical management options, as well as the potential psychosocial ramifications of testing. To help the patient decide about testing, the counsellor should explain there are three types of results and the patient must understand how each one would affect her. For example, would she change their surveillance behaviour? If a mutation were detected, would she share the result with the physician, partner, children, or other relatives? Would she consider prophylactic surgery?

Individuals who would not take any action regardless of the result should carefully consider whether the benefits of testing outweigh the burdens. Testing should be voluntary and not the result of coercion by a third party.

In general, individuals under 18 years of age should not be offered testing since there is no intervention to be offered prior to that age.

Detecting a mutation can provide various benefits. An important benefit may be the potential reduction in cancer morbidity and mortality. Such a reduction may be achievable by enhanced surveillance or by preventive measures in individuals with mutations. Surveillance strategies include breast self-examination, clinical examination by a health professional and sonography at six months intervals. Although the impact of mammography on the survival of women with BRCA1 or BRCA2 mutations is unknown, such women are generally advised to begin regular mammography between ages 25 and 35 (Burke *et al.*, 1997). For ovarian cancer, surveillance includes rectovaginal pelvic examination, serum CA-125 determination, and transvaginal ultrasonography at appropriate intervals. Ovarian cancer risk may be significantly reduced in BRCA1/2 mutation carriers with sustained use of oral contraceptives (Narod *et al.*, 1998).

Strategies aimed at prevention may be surgical (e.g., prophylactic skin sparing mastectomy and/or prophylactic oophorectomy) or chemical (e.g., tamoxifen prophylaxis). Tamoxifen prophylaxis and prophylactic oophorectomy do not completely prevent cancer. Potential benefits must be balanced against toxicity including menopausal symptoms in young women, and a risk, albeit small, of endometrial cancer and deep vein thrombosis in the case of tamoxifen prophylaxis. Participation in prospective registries and randomized clinical trials should be encouraged and facilitated regardless of whether or not individuals choose to undergo genetic testing.

Psychologic benefits may be important. Some may find the detection of a mutation valuable to resolve uncertainty about risk or to provide a needed explanation for one's personal or family history (Lerman *et al.*, 1997). An additional benefit is the opportunity to alert relatives to their possible risk. A frequently expressed reason to be tested is to determine whether children are at high risk although only adults are suitable candidates for testing. Finally, some members of affected families are motivated to advance research and believe knowing they have a mutation allows them to make a contribution and/or benefit directly by participating in outcome or intervention studies.

Osteopathy and advice for prevention

Ovarian insufficiency and premature menopause cause an increased risk of osteoporosis and bone fractures.

Physical activity, less alcohol and a diet rich in vitamin D and calcium should be recommended to prevent osteoporosis.

Whether or not prophylactic prescription of bisphosphonates is reasonable, is being investigated in several studies (Reidl, 2002). Bisphosphonates should not be given on a long term in patients with active periodontal disease, chronic corticosteroid treatment, uncontrolled diabetes, immune suppression, surgical manipulation of the oral cavity because of risk of avascular osteonecrosis of the jaws. (Carter, 2003).

Cardiovascular complications and recommendations for prevention and therapy

Premature menopause with its non-physiological premature hormonal withdrawal can cause late cardiac symptoms.

Cardiotoxicity is a major side effect of various anti-neoplastic agents, particularly anthracyclines and Trastuzumab (table 6.15). These patients require careful cardiac monitoring before, during, and after treatment (Chanan et al., 2004).

Cardiotoxicity induced by anthracyclines has been extensively studied. Recognized risk factors for cardiac toxicity include advanced age, prior chest-wall radiation therapy, prior anthracycline exposure, hypertension, diabetes, and known underlying heart disease; (Chanan et al., 2004).

Anthracyclines induce an acute/subacute toxicity and a chronic progressive cardiotoxicity (tables 6.16, 6.17). **Chronic progressive cardiomyopathy** can have an early onset within a year of the treatment or progress slowly to become manifest only years to decades after chemotherapy completion. It is characterized by a decrease of left ventricular function, changes in exercise-stress capacity and overt signs of congestive heart failure.

The most important prognostic factor is a cumulative dose of anthracyclines. The probability of doxorubicin-induced cardiotoxicity is estimated 3% or less with a cumulative dose of $400mg/m^2$, 7% with $550mg/m^2$ and 18% with $700mg/m^2$. Liposomal doxorubicin (myocet) or pegylated liposomal doxorubicin (caelyx) are less cardiotoxic than doxorubicin (Chanan-Khan et al., 2004; Zielinski, 2003). The coprescription of the iron chelator dexrazoxane has been shown to decrease the risk of doxorubicin-induced cardiac toxicity (van Dalen et al., 2005). The risks of cardiac toxicity may also be reduced by administering doxorubicin as a continuous intravenous infusion.

Table 6.15 - Cardiotoxic effects of cytostatics.

– Anthracyclines (cumulative effect, induces cardiomyopathy)
– Trastuzumab (no cumulative effect, induces cardiomyopathy, optimum duration of trastuzumab therapy remains to be determined)
– 5-Fluouracil, capacitabine (no cumulative effect, induced spasme of coronary arteries)
– Cyclophosphamide (high doses (superior to 100mg/kg) induce hemorrhagic necrosis of myocard)
– Paclitaxel (no cumulative effect, induces arythmias)

The optimum duration of trastuzumab therapy remains to be determined. It is uncertain whether the long-term incidence of cardiotoxicity will increase in breast cancer survivors who have received trastuzumab.

Concerns have been raised that aromatase inhibitors used in postmenopausal patients with estrogen-receptor-positive or progesterone-receptor-positive tumours may increase the risk of coronary artery disease.

Table 6.16 - Risk factors for anthracyclin-induced cardiotoxixity.

– High cumulative anthracycline doses (superior to 450mg/m^2 adriamycin)
– High single doses
– Pre-existing cardiac disease
– Short infusion time/bolus administration (threshold adriamycin dose with continuous infusion 700mg/m^2)
– Concurrent or previous mediastinal radiation treatment
– Advanced or very young age

Table 6.17 - Measures to reduce anthracycline cardiotoxicity

– Respect the cumulative dose-epirubicin. Cardiotoxicity occurs at a higher cumulative dose (superior to 900mg/m^2) compared with 550mg/m^2 with conventional doxorubicin).
– Prolong the time of administration (a prolonged continuous intravenous infusion over more than 48-96 hours is less cardiotoxic).
– Patients submitted to anthracyclines should be monitored.
– High risk patients (e.g., high blood pressure, pre-existing cardiac disease, advanced age) should get liposomal anthracyclines such as liposomal doxorubicin (Myocet®) or pegylated liposomal doxorubicin (Caelyx®).

Radiation of remaining left breast tissue after breast-conserving surgery with inclusion of the left or right internal mammary chain and left axillary or chest wall radiation may raise heart disease risk (Hoonig *et al.*, 2007). With the possible exception of older women with small hormone-receptor-positive breast cancers who will be receiving adjuvant hormonal therapy, whole breast irradiation is still the standard of care for all women undergoing breast conservation surgery for early stage breast cancer. Modern techniques (i.e., three-dimensional conformal tangential irradiation) have significantly reduced the incidence of radiation-induced cardiotoxic sequelae such as pericarditis and pericardial effusion. Radiotherapy techniques that reduce cardiac dosage, such as respiratory gating and intensity-modulated radiation therapy with multileaf collimators, may further reduce long-term cardiotoxicity.

Nevertheless irradiated breast cancer patients should be advised to retain from smoking to reduce their risk for cardiovascular disease.

Pulmonary toxicity and advice for prevention and treatment

For more details see chapter: "bronchial carcinoma".

Chemotherapy and radiation therapy may both cause lung toxicity.

Classically, radiation pneumonitis manifests from two weeks to six months after completion of radiation therapy. Radiological changes are often discovered in asymptomatic patients. Today, modern techniques (i.e., three-dimensional conformal tangential irradiation) have significantly reduced the incidence of radiation-induced pneumonitis and heart disease.

In **asymptomatic pneumonitis** treatment is not necessary. In **symptomatic pneumonitis** (grade II) bronchodilators and corticoids therapy may provide symptomatic relief. In **severe pneumonitis** (grade III-IV) bed rest, oxygentherapy and even respirator assistance may be necessary.

About 10% of patients receiving well-established antineoplastic chemotherapy develop pulmonary toxicity. The diagnosis depends upon a history of drug exposure, and most importantly, the exclusion of other causes leading to lung damage, including infections, fluid overload, pulmonary edema, pulmonary embolism radiotherapy and lung involvement from the underlying neoplasm. Infiltrative lung disease is the most common form of antineoplastic agent-induced respiratory disease.

Nutrition and recommendations

Magazine articles, books, Internet, family, and friends present cancer survivors with a wide range of options and choices about what to eat and what types of supplements or herbal remedies might improve the outcome of standard cancer therapy. The value of this information is at best minimal.

Very few controlled clinical trials have been done to test the impact of diet, nutritional supplements, or nutritional complementary methods on cancer outcomes among cancer survivors. The scientific evidence from many recommendations comes only from *in vitro* and laboratory animal data or anecdotal reports from poorly designed clinical studies.

Breast cancer patients do not need special dietary recommendations. Neither dietary modifications nor nutritional supplements such as vitamins, anti-oxidants, retinol, and garlic alter the disease course of patients with breast cancer. On the other hand, "encouraging a healthy diet" is certainly important because many patients with breast cancer will live a long time and may die of other diseases related to diet (table 6.18).

Table 6.18 - Nutritional advices to prevent breast cancer.

– The nutrition should be low-calorie.
– The nutrition should be low-fat and high-fiber.
– Excess weight should be avoided.
– Less meat and more fruits and vegetables.
– Alcohol only in small quantities (inferior to 10gr/d).
– Daily physical activity.

Older women with early-stage breast cancer are actually at higher risk of death from heart disease than from breast cancer, so it is especially wise for breast cancer survivors to follow a heart-healthy diet that is low in saturated fat, high in fruits and vegetables, and accompanied by regular physical activity. Less red meat intake, particularly processed meat, and physical activity may have beneficial effects on the course of the disease, protect against diabetes and cardiovascular diseases.

The majority of women treated with adjuvant chemotherapy gain weight during treatment. Since obesity has been associated with poorer outcomes in women with breast cancer, diet and exercise programmes are important components of adjuvant therapy (table 6.19).

Table 6.19 - Arguments against overweight in breast cancer patients.

– An unhealthy weight may elevate the risk for progression (only for postmenopausal women).
– Obesity is a contributing factor for the development of lymph edema and may limit the effectiveness of compression pumps or sleeves.
– Excess weight increases lethargy.
– Physical activity may reduce the risk of disease recurrence.
– Excess weight makes radiotherapy planning and metabolism of cytostatics more difficult and complications therefore occur more frequently.
– Overweight aggravates breast reconstruction and renders providing for breast prosthesis more difficult.
– Overweight enhances the risk of osteoporosis.

Although many studies have examined the relationship between the incidence of breast cancer and dietary fat intake, a strong relationship between dietary fat consumption and the primary occurrence of breast cancer has not been demonstrated. Even less is known about the impact of dietary fats on breast cancer growth after diagnosis and treatment. The few studies on the relationship between dietary fat and recurrence of breast cancer suggest that low levels of fat in the diet might be associated with lower recurrence rates and better survival (American cancer society, 1999).

Research has shown that consumption of alcohol is associated with an increased risk of breast cancer. The adverse effects of alcohol on breast cancer risk may be due to the effects of alcohol on estrogen levels in women. As the effects of alcohol on breast cancer survival are unknown at this time, it would be prudent to avoid high levels of alcohol (more than one to two drinks per day). For women with estrogen-responsive breast cancers, total avoidance of alcohol may be the best choice (American association of cancer, 1999).

Fatigue, anxiety, depression as well as problems resulting from therapy can all contribute (in addition to tumour progression) to loss of appetite and weight loss.

Appetite can be influenced by psychopharmacological drugs, especially tricyclic anti-depressants. If all dietary measures are unsuccessful, one may attempt hormonal treatment with gestagens or cortisone. These can improve the appetite and lead to weight gain.

While corticoids (e.g., prednisolone 10 to 30mg/d or dexamethasone 2 to 4mg/d) have a short-term appetite-stimulating effect of two to four weeks as well as a reconstituting effect. After the two to four week period side effects become predominant and the weight-increasing effects of megestrol acetate (160 to 480mg/d) lasts significantly longer.

Complementary therapies and advice

Many patients with breast cancer are exploring complementary therapies. Complementary medicine is often used together with conventional medicine (table 6.20). Patients often believe that complementary methods will cure disease. This is not true. Complementary therapies may help control symptoms and improve well-being.

They can reduce stress, lessen side effects from cancer and cancer treatments, and enhance well-being.

Survivors may believe that such therapies are "natural" and therefore harmless; this assumption may not be correct. It is important for health care providers and survivors to discuss the use of complementary or alternative therapies so survivors are fully informed regarding both possible benefits and risks. Some complementary and alternative therapies may interfere with standard treatment or may be harmful when used with conventional treatment.

There is much support for the use of hypnosis in managing pain associated with medical procedures and some support for its use in managing chronic cancer pain. There is less evidence to support the use of modalities such as acupuncture, meditation and massage for management of chronic pain. However, there is some compelling data to support the use of acupuncture for nausea and vomiting associated with cancer treatments, and there are some data suggesting that qigong, neuro-emotional techniques, meditation techniques, and massage can decrease pain levels and improve the sense of well-being.

Table 6.20 - Complementary Therapies.

– Biofeedback
– Distraction
– Hypnosis
– Imagery
– Massage therapy
– Meditation and prayer
– Muscle tension and release
– Physical exercise
– Rhythmic breathing
– Visualization
– Yoga
– Art therapy
– Journaling
– Qigong
– Reiki
– Music therapy
– Pet therapy
– natural products (vitamins, herbal medicines, teas)
  - deep breathing exercises
  - chiropractic
  - diet-based therapies
  - acupuncture

Alternative therapies and advice

Patients with breast cancer tend to use more alternative therapies than do other cancer patients. Most of them use complementary and therapies as well as conventional medical treatment. Doctors should always ask the patients for all complementary and alternative therapies to manage cancer related symptoms. Some complementary and alternative therapies may interfere with standard treatment or may be harmful when used with conventional treatment (American association of cancer 2000, Wells *et al.*, 2007).

"Alternative" refers to treatments that are promoted as cancer cures. They are unproven because they have not been scientifically tested, or were tested and found to be ineffective (table 6.21). Personal testimonials are often offered as evidence of the efficacy and safety of these methods and the treatment is often claimed to be effective in other diseases as well as cancer.

So far there has not been a scientific study which has proven any tumour-inhibiting effects of mistletoe preparations. The assertion that the patient's quality of life can be improved through its use is very difficult to confirm. Yet these mistletoe preparations are not only used by those practicing alternative and nature-oriented forms of medicine, but also by some oncologists. The primary reason for resorting to these treatments is basically not related to their effectiveness, but more to the opportunity to offer the patient an additional therapy option. Experience has shown not only that "faith can move mountains", but that it can also improve the quality of life. One should not shatter these patients' faith in a particular therapy form with evidence-based arguments. (Deng, 2004).

Table 6.21 - Characteristics of alternative charlatan therapies.

– Pretends to be unique. Therapy is mysterious, often esoteric and spiritual.
– Pretends to be effective in all sorts of malignancies.
– Pretends to be always successful.
– Brings classic therapies into bad repute.
– Therapy never has been objectively demonstrated in a peer-reviewed scientific literature to be effective. No scientific background. Shows no inclination for evaluation.
– Pretends to have no side effects.
– Is not reimbursed by medical aid.

Lack of information and patient education (discussion groups and health training)

Education and information are important aids in overcoming illness. This involves the patient's understanding of what is happening to her body and why a certain form of therapy has been chosen. Many women want information pertaining to the disease, treatment, and self-care issues. Many patients express they would like to participate in a counselling programme to discuss psychologic issues caused by suffering from breast cancer (Liang *et al.*, 2002).

The majority of women do not wish to make decisions about tumour therapy by themselves. They also want and need to know why a particular form of therapy has been chosen among others.

Health education takes place in discussion groups in which psychologists, physicians and social workers all take turns moderating the groups (Bourbonniere et al., 2004; Jeziorowski, 1995).

Education counselling programmes include general information on breast cancer, different therapeutic approaches including alternative and complementary therapies, psychosocial and vocational consequences of the disease, cancer therapies, and recommendations about what to do in the case of problems.

Consequences of therapy on sexuality (Black, 2004), prevention of recurrent disease, aftercare, coping with anxiety, how to cope with pain and treatment of relapsing disease will be discussed and information on entitlement to social care, legal aspects and career consequences will be given (table 6.22).

Questions relating to nutrition, side effects of therapy and hormonal symptoms, social provisions and psychological strategies for relaxation to combat fear are all important topics which must be discussed and material prepared to help the patient learn more about the disease, and related curative and palliative quality of life measures.

It is useful for patients and their families to have access to printed versions of information and advice which they have received in health education sessions (e.g., in the form of differentiated self-help literature which should not be industry-affiliated). This printed material should of course never take the place of consultations with a physician but should rather provide the basis for productive discussions with the attending physician.

The Internet, seen as a platform for communication and collaboration, will inevitably contribute to the building of communities and partnerships for improved patient care (Rowett, 2000). Never underestimate the patients' thirst for knowledge. Patients will conduct their own literature searches. They will find books and of course use the Internet. It is often difficult for the lay patient to recognize whether the information available is factual or not. Physicians must take an active role and recommend fact-based Internet sites that he/she considers to be serious, informative and helpful. Further, explanations regarding this information will most likely be required. Further explanations may be facilitated in health education discussions within the context of a one-on-one meeting or in a group discussion.

In some countries specialist breast cancer nurses fulfill rehabilitative and educative duties as well. They are both vital in providing information about the disease and its treatment, as well as advice and support for patients and their families (Yates et al., 2007; Lauver et al., 2007).

Carriers of BRCA1 and 2 mutation and their families need special attention because they have an increased risk of developing cancer. They have to be informed about the increased risk of breast and ovary cancer and about the necessity of frequent aftercare visits (Vadaparampil et al., 2004; Watson et al., 2004). The availability of genetic counselling by human geneticists needs to be mentioned.

Table 6.22 - Subjects of education counselling programmes for patients with breast cancer.

– Information about the disease, about the various possibilities of treatments.
– Information on necessity of aftercare, content and time table of follow-up examinations.
– Information about physical therapies to limit shoulder-arm immobility.
– Information about lymph edema. (how to avoid it?).
– Information about breast prothesis.
– Information about symptoms of recurrences (are there possibilities to avoid them?
– Information about therapies in the case of recurrences (possibilities to join clinical trials.
– Information about alternative therapy forms and complementary therapies.
– Information about adverse effects of radio-, hormone-, chemotherapy (prevention and therapy of side effects).
– Information about pain (how to treat and how to cope pain).
– Information about immune defence.
– Information about dietary recommendations. Are nutritional supplements necessary? What is a healthy nutrition? Information about overweight.
– Measures designed to improve general physical and mental performance.
– Significance of physical activity. Which sport activities should be avoided?
– Complementary therapies to combat tension, anxiety, depression, fears.
– Information about the fatigue syndrome and possibilities to combat fatigue. How to cope with fears, anxiety, depression and fatigue symptoms?
– Information about sexual problems, partner problems.
– Information about interpersonal and social consequences of the disease.
– Information about questions concerning medical care, nursing care, social-legal issues, life insurance and practical issues.
– Information about rehabilitation clinics, further care at home, hospice, palliative care, nursing home, etc.
– Information about self-help groups.
– Effects of cancer therapies and restrictions of working incapacity. Workloads to be avoided.
– Aids and measures for vocational reintegration; vocational protective measures.
– Providing contact addresses (self-help groups, counselling centres, etc.).

Rehabilitative measures aimed at reducing psychic problems ("rehabilitation to combat resignation and depression")

See also chapter: "Psychologic support and self–help groups in cancer rehabilitation and palliation".

Table 6.23 - The most important psychosocial factors during aftercare.

– Emotional problems (anger, depression, anxiety, aggression, suicidal thoughts, hopelessness, pessimism, loss of purpose, fatigue, problems with self-esteem and identity)
– Problems with partner and family (communication and relational problems, change of role sexuality, dyspareunia associated with vaginal dryness and decreased libido as a consequence of hormonal alterations)
– Professional problems (strains and changes of the professional situation, restrictions on working capacity, unemployment, early retirement and others)
– Social problems (isolation, incertitude in dealing with friends and acquaintances, changing behaviour during leisure time and other, financial problems, securing adequate care at home)
– Compliance problems (avoidance of diagnostic and therapeutic measures, coping with cancer, with social and occupational problems)

Need for psychologic support

In many women the assessment of psychic symptoms, interpersonal or social consequences of the disease and of the treatment is as important, if not more important, as the assessment of physical complaints. It is the task of all members of the rehabilitation team to alleviate these problems as well (Avis *et al.*, 2004). Coping with cancer poses enormous mental strain. Fear of progress, reduced physical activities, pain, immobility and social and vocational uncertainty are some of the reasons for psychologic help (fig. 5.2) (Lauver *et al.*, 2007; Manuel *et al.*, 2007). Younger women often face very different issues and problems than older women, including concerns about children, concerns about having children when faced with a life- threatening illness, premature menopause leading to loss of fertility, sudden unset of vasomotor symptoms, and long term consequences of early ovarian decline, greater concerns about body image and sexuality, concerns related to career and work (Manuel *et al.*, 2007).

Although vasomotor symptoms and vaginal dryness are often reported as the only true physiologic effects of estrogen withdrawal, there are data suggesting a neuroendocrine link to other symptoms, such as cognitive changes, mood swings, and related symptomatology, such as insomnia due to hot flashes. Women's emotional, physical, and functional well-being are negatively impacted by the persistence and severity of menopausal symptoms after treatment. Young and young midlife women with breast cancer are more vulnerable to psychosocial distress because of their developmental stage in life. Experiencing premature menopause can further increase a young woman's vulnerability, resulting in a greater risk for emotional distress and a poorer quality of life (Knobf, 1999; Fallowfield *et al.*, 2004).

Although more recent studies do not confirm earlier claims that psychosocially treated patients have a longer survival time, they do show that psycho-oncologically treated patients experience an improvement in mood (depression/melancholy, tension/fear, anger/hostility, and confusion/dismay) and a reduction of perceived pain; in short, an improvement in their quality of life (Goodwin *et al.*, 2001).

Perceptions that mental factors alone, such as stress, depression, the loss of a loved one, or a patient's personality, may play an etiological role in the development of cancer are popular myths that lack any scientific foundation. Measures for psychologic assistance are always of a supportive nature and never curative. They must never be performed independently of other measures of somatic, social, and professional support. Insufficiently treated somatic symptoms are an obstacle for successful psycho-oncological care.

Depressions

Depression occurs very frequently. It is important for the ensuing therapy to first perform a differential diagnostic assessment in order to discriminate between feelings of sadness, despondence, listlessness, and fatigue and a full, clinical depression (Love, 2002; Norton *et al.*, 2004; Hahn *et al.*, 2004). Mental impairments such as depressions can also be caused by somatic, social, or professional factors (fig. 5.2). Should sudden changes in mood occur, the possibility of cerebral metastasization or hypercalcemic syndrome should be considered. Hormone therapies and hormone withdrawal may also accompany mental alterations. Somatic causes must therefore be ruled out before psychologic care is implemented. Interdisciplinarity is necessary in both assessment and therapy.

The focus of therapy is personal and psychosocial care. Fears and depression should not be automatically treated with antidepressants, but rather combated with supportive and clarifying conversations. The specific implementation of psycho-oncological measures can make the use of psychotropic drugs unnecessary for many cancer patients.

The choice of antidepressant in cancer patients with depression requires consideration of psychic and behavioral symptoms, adverse effect profile, route of metabolism, drug half-life, and drug-drug interactions.

If a medicinal therapy is necessary, the first choices are often tricyclic antidepressants. Their doses should be increased step by step from 75mg to 150mg to achieve an antidepressive effect. It is important to heed that in contrast to the sedative effect the entry of the antidepressive effect may last up to two weeks. Their usefulness is limited in the late stage of a tumour illness. The side effects, such as sedation and dry mouth, may then be potentially dominant and limit the benefit of the drugs.

Anxiety, restlessness

Causes of anxiety disorders can be very complex (Love, 2002; Norton et al., 2004). Anxiety and fear of follow-up diagnostic tests, fear of progression or recurrence, fear of the uncertain future, and also family, economic and social problems, are frequent. Survivors experience chronic fear of recurrence, sexual dysfunction and identity disturbances (Black, 2004). Hormonal changes cause vegetative disturbances with depressive cases, insomnia, distress and nervousness (Ganz et al., 2002; Fallowfield et al., 2004).

In cases of disease progression anxiety, depression and fears are often linked to pain. Increased attention, conversations, "taps on the shoulder", and social activities on their own are often not sufficient to solve psychic problems. It may be necessary to involve a psycho-oncologist (see chapter about psychologic support and self-help groups).

Fears and depression, as well as restlessness and pain, can be reduced through the use of complementary therapies such as relaxation techniques progressive muscle relaxation, autogenic training, imagination methods (Luebbert et al., 2001), non-verbal expression of emotions, ergotherapy, art therapy (Devlin, 2006), music therapy (Haun, 2001; Rose et al., 2004), dance and movement therapy (Dibbel-Hope, 2000), bibliotherapy (Stanton et al., 2002), painting therapy (Deane et al., 2000), (table 6.24) (fig. 2.2, 2.3). They may contribute to relaxation and, at least temporarily, improve the patient's quality of life.

Table 6.24 - Complementary therapies to combat tension, anxiety, depression, fears.

– Attitude therapy (includes techniques aimed at keeping problems such as pain at a distance; the objective is to accept the pain and put the pain issue into perspective).
– Biofeedback (controls body functions such as heart rate, blood pressure, and muscle tension).
– Distraction (takes off worries or discomforts). Talking with friends or relatives, watching TV, listening to the radio, reading, going to the movies, doing needlework or puzzles, building models, or painting are all ways to distract. Music or creative art therapies, dance therapies can be very helpful. Include various methods of focusing thought.
– Hypnotherapeutic procedures (modifies perception of pain so that the latter is no longer perceived as distressful; helps to reduce discomfort and anxiety; helps to lower the pain threshold).
– Imaginative procedures (takes away tension).
– Counter activity (overrides pain, similar to distraction strategies; art therapy, music therapy and occupational therapy are typical examples of counter-activity).
– Massage therapy (achieves muscular relaxation).
– Meditation and prayer (is especially helpful when mind and body are stressed from cancer treatment).
– Muscle tension and release (normalizes the circulation, produces slower, more effective respiration, reduces oxygen consumption, lowers the heart rate, lowers the blood pressure, relaxes the musculoskeletal system and keeps pain away).
– Progressive muscle relaxation (achieves relaxation subsequent to muscular contraction).
– Physical exercise (reduces pain, strengthens weak muscles, restores balance, and decreases depression and fatigue).
– Rhythmic breathing (relaxes).
– Visualization (similar to imagery).
– Yoga.
– Humour, journaling, reiki, pet therapy.

Medications for anxiety include the benzodiazepines and the antidepressants. Lorazepam is often the first choice in managing anxiety. As with depression, physical causes for the anxiety must be explored at the same time that anxiolytes are provided. Adequate sleep medication can also reduce daytime anxiety.

Fears

Fears are frequent (table 6.25). The mere diagnosis of cancer leads to fear, completely independent of the severity of the illness and any therapeutic intervention. Fears and stressors are most after treatment which suggest that women need more support immediately after their treatment, to cope effectively with the stressors in this phase of survivorship (Lauver et al,. 2007). Many patients suffer from fear and depression long after the conclusion of a successful primary therapy (Bottomley, 1998; Montazeri et al., 2001; Bukovic et al., 2004). It is the task of the physician and the psycho- oncologist to deal with these fears.

Table 6.25 - Fears in cancer patients.

- Fear of a progression of the illness
- Fear of helplessness, of death
- Fear of the side effects of the therapy
- Fear of pain
- Fear of an agonizing death
- Fear of a deterioration of the partner relationship
- Fear of becoming unemployable
- Fear of not being able to provide for the family
- Fear of social isolation
- Fear of being unalluring
- Fear of being a burden to others
- Fear of being dependent on nursing care

Important fundamentals of therapeutic intervention measures for fear include conversations in a stress-free, calm environment, taking one's time, listening, and conveying a sense of trust. This must be required of the entire rehabilitation team, not only of the psychologists. If the fear is connected with medical, social, or professional problems, then explanations, information, and counselling can aid in achieving a lessening of the fear. If the fear is accompanied by pain, adequate measures to alleviate the pain must first be undertaken before psychotherapy is possible.

An adequate therapy of the fears and depression is a prerequisite for other rehabilitation measures (e.g., vocational).

Medicinal support may be considered, but it cannot replace cognitive therapy. Benzodiazepines should be preferred to other substances due to their tolerability. Neuroleptic drugs also have strong anxiolytic qualities. Tricyclic antidepressants are primarily considered when fear emerges in conjunction with depression. However, these drugs may not become effective for up to two weeks. Anxiolytic drugs (such as lorazepam 1-2mg/per day) may be indicated in insomnia. (Aapro and Cull, 1999).

Diminished self-esteem

The course of cancer is often accompanied by the patient's loss of self-esteem. There are many potential reasons for this. One may be the patient's isolation from her environment and friends. Not only do the people in the patient's environment pull back, but the patient herself may also withdraw. The experience with the intimidating, overwhelming medical system can also create a feeling of helplessness and of being at the mercy of the medical specialists, with a reduction in the patient's feeling of self-worth. Other factors that may lead to a reduction of self-esteem are the uncertain outcome of the illness, the fear of test results, and the fear of therapies that the patient may not understand and last not least hormonal and sexual alteations.

One of the tasks of psychology can be to prevent diminished self-esteem. In addition to classical psychologic rehabilitation, the geographical location of a rehabilitation clinic can contribute to mental relaxation.

Coping strategies

Many women want information about coping strategies (Stewart *et al.*, 2000). There is not a standardised approach to coping with the disease; every patient reacts in a different way. Their needs must be addressed individually (table 2.6) (Manuel *et al.*, 2007; Lauver *et al.*, 2007). Some, often those with a firm religious belief, may do very well without any professional psychologic help.

Self-help groups (support groups) are also a possible source of emotional support and therefore can contribute to quality of life of patients with breast cancer. Knowing that others had similar symptoms and reactions, and that those experiences are normal, is very important for self-help group participants.

Fatigue syndrome

Cancer-related fatigue is defined as sustained, agonizing, physical and mental exhaustion that can emerge even years after the conclusion of treatment. In contrast to normal exhaustion, cancer-related fatigue does not improve with rest, adequate nutrition, and sleep (Watson, 2004; Evans, 2007). The triad of tiredness, inefficiency, and depression that is typical for fatigue syndrome has somatic, functional, and mental aspects. The genesis is multifactorial (Flechtner and Bottomley, 2003) (table 6.26). Patients with a combined chemo-, radio-, and hormonal therapy display the highest degree of fatigue (Weis and Bartsch, 2000). However, there seems to be no significant correlation between disease burden and fatigue.

Table 6.26 - Possible etiologic factors of fatigue.

– Anemia.
– Chemotherapy and radiotherapy.
– Immune therapies, targeted therapies. Fatigue is a common side effect of target therapies.
– Loss of nutrients as a result of anorexia, nausea, vomiting or hyper-metabolism.
– Emaciation
– Ccytokines. During tumour activity, a disrupted balance of endogenous cytokine levels and their natural antagonists can occasionally influence cancer-related fatigue, which is why a reduction of fatigue symptoms can be expected to accompany successful tumour therapy.

When assessing cancer-related fatigue, the health-care provider needs to include both subjective and objective data. As in all aspects of subjective experience, an objective measurement of fatigue symptoms is difficult (table 2.9). Underlying factors that contribute to fatigue should be evaluated and treated when possible. Contributing factors include anemia, depression, anxiety, pain, dehydration, nutritional deficiencies, sedating medications, and therapies that may have poorly tolerated side effects. If anemia is the cause, transfusions of erythrocyte concentrates or a physiological increase of hemoglobin with erythropoietin can lead to improvement. However, the effects are marginal if hemoglobin values are greater than 12g/dl. A balanced and vitamin-rich diet is important, since fatigue symptoms are occasionally caused by improper and unbalanced nourishment. Some centres successfully use megestrol acetate for the treatment of both emaciation and fatigue symptoms. Many studies indicate the positive effects of physical activity. Bicycle ergometer training, walking, weight training, aerobic exercises, and athletic activity are shown to have not only a positive effect on physical fitness and psychic well-being, but also on fatigue symptoms (Delay *et al.*, 2007; Oldevoll, 2004). It is important to clarify to both the patient and to family that physical inactivity, which may be intended as rest, will be more likely to promote symptoms of fatigue than to alleviate them (Watson, 2004).

Many patients experience a feeling of relief when informed about the somatic causes of fatigue syndrome. They are often distraught because they believe they are suffering from depression with mental causes. When it is explained to them that the symptoms can emerge in conjunction with, for example, chemotherapy, they are very relieved and motivated to begin with physical training.

Psychotropic drugs have been used successfully to treat fatigue. Sometimes, however, fatigue symptoms are linked to the antidepressant medications themselves.

Table 6.27 - Non- pharmacological interventions in fatigue.

- Education and support groups. With appropriate educational grounding, patients can prepare for side-effects and adopt management strategies.
- Exercise. The theory supporting exercise as a treatment for fatigue proposes that the combined toxic effects of cancer treatment and the decreased degree of physical activity during treatment cause a reduction in the capacity for physical performance.
- Rest and sleep. Patients with cancer report significant disruptions in sleep. The essential issue may be sleep quality rather than quantity.
- Energy conservation and activity management. Decreasing activity to save energy could contribute to deconditioning and decreased activity tolerance.
- Stress reduction and stress management. Cancer-related fatigue could be a response to stress, or the emotional state of a patient could affect the way he or she perceives and reports fatigue. Although a strong correlation exists between emotional distress and fatigue, the precise relation is not clearly understood.
- Ergotherapy for cancer patients has more creative aspects than merely occupying the patient or providing physical-rehabilitative tasks, or even employment-oriented rehabilitative goals. The focus is placed on group work (therapeutic painting, therapeutic sculpting with clay, walks on therapy trails, cosmetics classes, etc.).
- Tailored behavioural interventions.

Self-help groups

Participation in support groups can be an important source of emotional and informational support for patients. Providing contact addresses of self-help groups is helpful. There are various motives for becoming and remaining member of a patient association. Motives for membership reflect both benefits for the individuals and the welfare of others. Many patients say they want to use the association's information and activities. These comments are very common in members of a breast cancer association (Carlsson *et al.*, 2005).

A support group may help to cope with the practical and emotional aspects of the disease. Talking with other women with breast cancer may also help ease feelings of isolation. Moreover, they have the effect of motivating the patient and contribute to a reduction of fear and depression (Montazeri, 2001; Keller, 2000).

In addition to providing psychologic support, self-help groups often provide their members with specific knowledge about medications and resources as well as social laws. Self-help groups play an important role with regard to the aims of follow-up.

The concept behind self-help groups is based on the idea that sharing of mutual experience and situations offers a person strength. The participants discover they are not alone in their experiences and emotions, and other patients experience the same problems. These common experiences and feelings are intended to strengthen the patient's feeling of self-worth. The patients are to adopt an active attitude towards themselves, their illness, and their environment. The members of self-help groups have first-hand knowledge of the illness and its resulting medical, mental, social, and professional problems ("experts in their field"). Thus they are often more successful than professional healthcare providers at winning the trust of the other patients and offering them support with their physical, emotional, and social problems. Self-help groups help to absorb some of the patient's mental distress. Even close family members, relatives, or friends – and of course even physicians and psychologists – have limits to how much they can offer in this regard. Through activities of many different kinds, self-help groups show the patient that a meaningful and fulfilling life is possible even after cancer. Members who have overcome their illness in a positive way serve as a positive role model for newly ill patients. Cancer patients can better overcome the isolation caused by the illness in this way. Enormous reassurance and support is received by the interaction of individuals with the same conditions, when they have the chance to discuss their feelings and how they deal with family, friends, fellow-workers, and society at large. Membership in a self-help group is not suitable for all cancer patients.

Self-help groups can particularly address the specific rational and emotional needs of people with cancer using support options that are oriented towards specific target groups developed from their own experience with the illness. They organize talks with others affected by the same illness and provide information on certain difficulties that are specific to a given impairment or illness. They also offer knowledge on the chances for success of various treatment and rehabilitation options as well as on the adequate use of cancer resources. Internet chat groups and telephone support groups fulfill similar needs. They connect patients who are homebound, isolated, or otherwise unable or unwilling to travel to meet together (Colon, 1996).

Not every self-help group can be recommended, especially since some groups have a very particular, individual focus. Participation in self-help groups is to be discouraged when the group interferes with the patients' trust in their physician or in the medical system, or when they advise participation in alternative or supplementary therapy forms that have been scientifically shown to be ineffective or even potentially harmful. As a basic principle, however, physicians should consider self-help groups to be partners and not rivals in the medical and psychosocial rehabilitation of their patients. Experience shows that patients from these groups turn to non-traditional medical disciplines when they are not taken seriously enough or sufficiently advised by traditionally oriented physicians.

Self-help groups for breast cancer patients exist in most countries. Regional self-help groups are frequently short-lived, especially since their activities are often dependent on the initiative and capacities of individual cancer patients. In this respect, the address lists must be continually updated. The national cancer societies generally have address lists that are regularly updated.

Support for family members

Cancer not only places strain on the patient but also has direct effects on the partner and entire family (Keller, 1995). Research surveys show that depression and anxiety are almost as common among patients' partners as among patients themselves. It is helpful if care givers can be seen alone from time to time, perhaps by the family doctor, asked how they are coping and invited to talk over any emotional distress.

Cancer can cause considerable distress for the healthy partners of cancer patients. They lose the security provided by continuity in their relationship prior to the cancer. Plans for a "peaceful retirement" are shattered, prospects for their life in old age must be reconsidered and redeveloped. The physical exertion involved in caring for the patient as well as the financial costs of old and new burdens may pose substantial problems for some families. The transition in role allocation from "being provided for" to "being the provider" places high demands on the family's ability to adapt to the new situation. In addition to conflicts between the family members' own needs, the desire for autonomy and obligations to the ill parent, conflicts also often arise between caring for the patient and fulfilling responsibilities in the adult child's own family or professional career. The partners of older cancer patients particularly experience emotional distress, while the adult children of cancer patients more frequently describe their stress as the result of confusion in roles. This particularly applies to middle-aged daughters, who fulfill the responsibilities of several roles simultaneously, who more commonly experience stress and fear, and who are less able to fall back on support from their social environment.

Psychologic care of BRCA gene carriers

Patients and their family who carry BRCA1/2 gene need special psychologic attention because they have an increased risk of developing cancer (Vadaparampil et al., 2004; Watson et al., 2004; Dooren et al., 2005; Buddeberg, 1991). They experience significant challenges. These include decision making regarding surgical options and notification to offspring and family along with a sense of isolation which may lead to psychic and emotional distress.

Rehabilitative measures aimed at reducing social problems ("rehabilitation to combat the need for care")

See also chapter entitled "Social support in rehabilitation and palliation"

One of the aims of rehabilitative measures is to strengthen the patient's own resources and to prevent the risk of the need for care, or at least reduce such a need (table 3.2).

Securing adequate care at home

If the patient is no longer able to care for himself/herself, support must be organized. Early organization of assistance and support is crucial in patients with poor prognosis and rapidly progressing disease. The planning of further care must be arranged with both the patient's and the family's consent. Patients themselves are often not aware of social deficits or do not declare them. Forms of assistance such as "meals on wheels", household assistance, home nursing care, care assistance and sometimes nursing home care or hospice placement have to be arranged. Providing contact addresses (self-help groups, counselling centres, etc.) is helpful.

Self-help groups play an important role with regard to the aims of follow-up on the social level; their impact is often limited, however, by the complexity of problems patients are facing.

Specialist nursing support at home can have a significant impact on a patient's experience of living with breast cancer (Stanley *et al.*, 2004). In Great Britain mainly specialised nurses (specialist breast cancer nurses and community nurses) fulfill rehabilitative duties. They are both vital in providing information about the disease and its treatment, as well as advice and support for patients and their families. Their role is crucial in guiding the patient through the complexities of the multidiciplinary team and in accessing help from other services, such as social work, community follow-up and physiotherapy. Patients and carers feel reassured that the nurse is an approachable point of contact at any stage in their illness.

Experienced physicians, psychologists and representatives of self-help groups share their experiences, information and helpful advice. Some of the maisons de repos in France, and the bridge clinics in Italy have similar functions.

Rehabilitation institutions

If home care cannot or cannot yet be arranged, the time spent in hospital can be followed up by a temporary stay in an institution for follow-up care. In Germany there are rehabilitation hospitals ("AHB hospitals") which are designed especially to meet the needs of patients with gynaecological tumours and in which plans are made for the patients' social assistance, in addition to medical and psychologic guidance. A subsequent stay in a rehabilitation hospital, directly following the standard hospital stay is recommended for all patients with breast cancer in Germany where every cancer patient has a legal claim to a three-five week stay in such an institution. About 40% of all German cancer patients who have had a treatment for breast cancer prefer staying at such a rehabilitation hospital. It cannot be denied that inpatient rehabilitation in a beautiful environment can have a positive influence on the mood of some patients. The distance from household problems can be a sensible aid for coping with the illness.

Adjuvant and additive cancer therapies, supportive therapies, psychologic support, counselling of the patients and their families are some of the tasks of these AHB clinics. Experienced physicians, psychologists and representatives of self-help groups share their experiences, information and helpful advice.

Most German cancer rehabilitation clinics offer the spouse/partner the option of residing in the clinic with the patient for the cost of room and board. A number of German cancer rehabilitation clinics that have a basis on therapy close to the patient's residence explicitly integrate psychosocial care into both their inpatient and their outpatient/semi-outpatient treatment concepts. Self-help groups for family members have also been established. In some regions of Germany there are special centres and organizations (Alpha) that promote the support of family members of the terminally ill.

Rehabilitative measures aimed at reducing vocational problems ("rehabilitation before retirement")

See also chapter entitled "Vocational integration in cancer rehabilitation"

Harmful occupational substances

According to our current state of knowledge, work does not affect tumour growth, does not influence the risk of recurrence or prognosis. Association between certain harmful occupational substances and breast cancer have not been conclusively demonstrated, although breast cancer appears to occur more frequently in certain occupations (Teitelbaum, 2003).

Restrictions on working capacity

Incapacity to work is generally encountered during tumour therapy and in the subsequent recovery phase. Recovery phase includes physical weakness, problems with wound healing, anaemia from bleeding, reversible problems caused by chemotherapy and reversible side effects of radiation. Work is impossible during these early side effects. In this phase, rehabilitation therapies predominantly consist of toughening measures and measures designed to strengthen functions so that those affected are fit to resume their original jobs as early as possible. A full restoration of working capacity can usually be expected after the acute side effects have receded.

Dependent on the type of treatment and on individual disposition (WHO, ECOG and/or Karnofsky index), the recovery phase can differ in duration. The average duration of working incapacity following potentially curative treatment and uncomplicated progress without adjuvant chemo- or radiotherapy is about one-two months after a tumourectomy (lumpectomy) and three months after breast amputation with axillary lymph node resection. In the USA the median days missed are 22, the median days missed by women treated with surgery and chemotherapy is 40 (Bradley *et al.*, 2006). However, these are average values that may be subject to considerable deviations in individual cases, in different societies and in different countries.

For breast cancer patients who have been treated potentially curatively, professional limitations are mainly due to chemotherapy and hormonal changes and negative coping as well (Maunsell *et al.*, 1999; Johnsson *et al.*, 2007). The patient's long-term restriction performance is highly dependent on the patient's individual recovery.

Extended cancer for which there is no treatment generally involves an incapacity to work. These patients should ask for early retirement on grounds of ill health as soon as possible. However, there are numerous exceptions.

For many women, their profession and work mean more than just a way to meet their existential requirements. To many women, work is the only possibility for social contact and is a confirmation of their self-esteem. It represents a form of diversion, distance and suppression of the feeling of a constantly threatening Damocles' sword. It can therefore be perfectly legitimate to support cancer patients – even those with extended cancer disease or greatly reduced working capacity – in resuming their previous jobs. For psychologic considerations alone, an incurable tumour should basically not be equated with vocational inactivity. Patients afflicted with chronic cancer can work to a limited degree if the vocational activity pursued is not accompanied by discomfort and a drop in performance. In the case of these patients, however, vocational rehabilitation aids are restricted to aids designed to maintain workplaces (Manuel *et al,*. 2007).

Table 6.28 - Negative predictors for return to work in breast cancer.

– Previous time-limited pensioning
– Unemployment prior to falling ill
– Limited labour market
– Patient's desire to be given a pension
– Progression of cancer disease
– Adjuvant chemo- and radiotherapy
– Lymph edema
– Limitation of shoulder mobility
– Advanced age

Type of work to be avoided in the case of lymph edema

There are certain limitations for cured patients with lymph edema. These are mainly works demanding physical exertion (table 6.29). White collar workers can more easily return to their work, although hormonal changes may hamper sometimes occupational activities.

Table 6.29 - Occupational activities that cured breast carcinoma patients with manifest lymph edema (R0) should avoid.

– Work done by clerks, workmen and cleaners
– Activities carried out under unfavourable heat radiation or lengthy exposure to the rays of the sun
– Activities accompanied by an excessive load on the affected arm
– Activities involving a possible risk of injuring the affected arm
– Easy, monotonous activities with the affected arm lasting several hours
– Activities in which restrictive clothing is required or shoulder straps have to be placed on the shoulder on the affected side
– Activities in a water bath or thermal bath higher than 33° C

How to return to work

Whether and to what extent the intended goals of vocational integration are reached or not depends not only on the quality of the vocational rehabilitation measures but also on many predictors (table 6.30). Humanitarian and political labour-market reasons must also be added to these.

Table 6.30 - Factors that can influence the introduction, implementation and the result probability of vocational rehabilitation measures in the case of cancer patients, independent of their vocational performance and the quality of the rehabilitation measures conducted as well as the type and scope of the tumour disease.

– Risk of relapse
– Lifetime forecast
– Age and gender of the patients
– Social status
– Unemployment prior to falling ill
– Level of education, earning status
– Patient's motivation and willingness to participate
– Patient's desire to be given a pension
– Time elapsed since primary therapy
– Sponsors' expectations
– Employer's motivation and willingness to participate
– Attitude of the workforce and close colleagues
– Pressure on workforce in the company
– Previous time-limited pensioning
– General and special labour market

There are numerous forms of assistance both for employees as well as for employers that are intended to facilitate vocational reintegration. Primarily, these are measures designed to keep jobs. Retraining is rarely considered and – if it is – it is only for younger patients with good lifetime forecasts. Many cured cancer patients of advanced age no longer have the mental flexibility, the stamina and the ability to adapt that are required for successful retraining. In Germany, the only retraining measures that are financed by sponsors – if at all – are for patients with a good prognosis being under the age of 40.

Gradual reintegration into the work process is one vocational rehabilitation measure that is frequently practiced. Resumption of work can, for example, be done with the person concerned initially only working two to three hours every day; after a certain time, this is increased to four to six hours and then to six to eight hours until work returns to full working hours. In Germany and France, cancer patients receive their full wages from the medical insurance for the full period of this increasing workload although they are not working full shifts. Unfortunately, this sensible vocational rehabilitation approach is only possible in a few countries and even there often only in large companies and in the civil service.

Palliative measures

Informing the patient in the event of disease progression; breaking bad news

The attending physician must inform the patient about disease progression in a personal conversation (table 2.11). Even when prognosis is desperate, positive aspects have to be mentioned (e.g., improved palliative therapies, improved pain management, etc.).

One must always inform about relative risk and consequences of necessary treatments. Even palliative tumour and symptomatic therapies can have subjective and objective side effects of varying severity, which must be taken into consideration, especially in elderly patients. More than 30% of breast cancer cases occur in women aver age 70 (Balducci, 2001). Toxicity associated with some palliative treatments can be important (Dunton, 2002; Earle et al., 2001; Ershler, 2003), and resource implications may be considerable (Doyle, 2001).

Choice of treatment modalities

Answering the question: "How much therapy and which one?" not only requires oncological expertise (tables 6.31, 6.32). Ethical competence and communication skills are just as important. Under no circumstances should therapeutic decisions be made exclusively depending on response in terms of likelihood of remission. Goals such as reduction of physical symptoms, emotional stabilisation, and maintenance of daily activities are very important (table 3.10). Treatment must be tailored to the individual patient.

Table 6.31 - Factors that need to be considered before initiating potentially curative tumour therapy.

– Treatment will depend on whether the recurrence is local, regional or distant.
– Altered pharmacodynamics mainly in old patients and in patients with over- or under weight.
– Comorbidity.
– Toxicity.
– Response rates.

Table 6.32 - Factors that need to be considered (besides potential tumour regression) before initiating palliative tumour therapy.

- Quality of life scores.
- Coping.
- To which extent can the patient tolerate cancer therapy?
- To which extent will the patient suffer from side effects of this therapy for the rest of her life?
- To which extent home care can be influenced by therapy?
- Can therapy be administered on an outpatient basis, or will admission be necessary for example due to insufficient support at home?
- What influence will concomitant conditions (such as diabetes, renal failure, cardiovascular disease, poor nutritional status) and functional disability have influence on outcome?
- Will insight, will to survive, coping strategies, and social provision influence the preferred therapeutic option?

Localization of recurrences

Breast cancer carcinoma can spread by cutaneous infiltration, by lymphatic invasion, and by hematogenous dissemination.

Following primary surgical treatment of breast cancer with mastectomy or breast-conserving surgery (lumpectomy plus radiation), patients may experience a local recurrence which is defined as cancer recurring within the previously affected breast, chest wall, or skin over the breast. A regional recurrence involving the supraclavicular, internal mammary, or axillary lymph nodes is more serious than local recurrence because it usually indicates that the cancer has spread past the breast and the axillary lymph nodes.

Regional breast cancer recurrences can occur in the pectoral (chest) muscles, in the internal mammary lymph nodes under the breastbone and between the ribs, in the supraclavicular nodes (above the collarbone), and in the nodes surrounding the neck.

Distant metastases may recur in almost all common locations including the liver, bones, lungs, brain, and skin. A systemic recurrence is typically treated with chemotherapy, hormonal therapy, or combinations of therapy. Local-regional recurrences may require surgery, radiation, and/or systemic therapy.

Local, regional and distant recurrences and recommendations for treatment

Type of treatment in loco-regional recurrences

The type of treatment for local breast cancer recurrences depends on the initial treatment. In the case of previous lumpectomy, local recurrence is usually treated with mastectomy. If the initial treatment was mastectomy, recurrence near the mastectomy site is treated by removing the tumour whenever possible, usually followed by radiation therapy.

Local recurrence of breast cancer following initial treatment with mastectomy may be effectively controlled with additional radiation treatment. Surgical treatment of locally recurrent cancer prior to radiation therapy may also be beneficial in selected circumstances.

The size of the cancer, the amount of radiation delivered and the size of the radiation field all influence the ability to prevent additional local recurrences. Because the majority of patients with local recurrence ultimately develop a systemic recurrence of their cancer, many doctors believe additional treatment with chemotherapy or hormonal therapy can be useful.

Locally recurrent cancer following initial treatment with breast-conserving surgery (lumpectomy and radiation) is best controlled with mastectomy. Surgery with or without radiation therapy can also effectively provide local control of patients with regional recurrence of breast cancer. Even more so than locally recurrent breast cancer, the majority of patients with regionally recurrent cancer will ultimately relapse systemically.

Distant metastases and recommendations for treatment

Metastases of breast cancer are often responsive to therapy, though treatment is rarely curative at this stage of disease. The hormone receptors (ER and PR levels), HER2/neu positivity at the time of recurrence, and previous treatment should be considered when selecting therapy. ER status may change at the time of recurrence. If ER and PR status is unknown, then the site(s) of recurrence, disease-free interval, response to previous treatment, and menopausal status are useful in selecting chemotherapy or hormonal therapy.

Supraclavicular recurrences and recommendations for treatment

Although complete remission can be obtained in most patients with isolated supraclavicular recurrence, the prognosis for these patients is poor.

There still is debate as to whether breast carcinoma patients with isolated supraclavicular recurrence should be considered to be patients with disseminated disease or patients for whom aggressive treatment with curative intent is justified. Nevertheless, all patients presenting recurrence in supraclavicular nodes should be treated with definitive loco-regional treatments (involving field radiotherapy) and systemic therapy because the outcomes are better.

Osseous metastases and advice for prevention and treatment

More than 50% of patients with breast cancer will eventually develop bone metastases.

Lung cancer patients with bone metastasis have median survivals of less than six months; however, patients with breast cancer can have prolonged survival with bone metastases.

The goal of treatment for bone metastases is palliative, to relieve pain and reduce the risk of complications such as fracture (table 6.33).

Table 6.33 - Possible complications of osseous metastasis.

– Pain
– Fractures
– Immobilisation
– Cord compression, nerve root compression
– Hypercalcemia
– Myelosuppression, pancytopenia

The management of bone metastases depends on a number of factors: The hormone receptors, the location and extent of bony destruction, the severity of morbidity, the availability of effective systemic therapies (hormonal or chemotherapy), and the overall status of the patient. Breast cancer patients may have a high response rate when treated with hormonal agents or combination chemotherapy.

Prophylactic **orthopedic/surgical stabilization** is required if there is an increased risk in fracture. Metal rods, plates, screws, wires, nails, or pins may be surgically inserted to strengthen or provide structure to the bone damaged by metastasis. An increased risk in fracture of the long bones can be anticipated with 50% destruction of the cortex and a defect size superior to 2.5cm. There is a risk of vertebral fracture if there is destruction of the middle/central or anterior and posterior pillar of over 60% in the axial plane.

Radiation therapy has a major role in the palliation of painful bony metastases. For metastatic lesions that do not represent an immediate risk of fracture, radiation is effective for reducing bone pain and progression of the cancer. Radiation is especially useful when metastatic lesions are limited to a single area. Radiation therapy should also be given following fixation of pathologic fractures.

Hormonal therapy should generally be considered as initial treatment for a postmenopausal patient with newly diagnosed bone metastasis if the patient's tumour is receptor-positive or receptor-unknown. Hormonal therapy is especially indicated if the patient's disease involves only bone and soft tissue and if the patient has either not received adjuvant antiestrogen therapy or has been off such therapy for more than one year. **Chemotherapy, bone-seeking radiopharmaceuticals and/or bisphosphonates** are indicated in the case of diffuse osseous involvement and receptor negativity.

Very severe pain (flare) in cancerous areas occasionally occurs during and shortly after hormone treatment. This pain may be interpreted as a good prognostic omen because it indicates a tumour response. Flare rarely lasts longer than a day. If it does, corticoids should be attempted.

Parenteral administration of **bisphosphonates** is indicated in symptomatic and oral administration in asymptomatic bone metastases. They should be given in an asymptomatic stage because of reducing the risk of pathologic fractures. Bisphosphonates do not influence tumour cell growth but decrease the proliferation and functional activity of osteoclasts and may also be beneficial in subjects with predominantly osteoblastic metastatic processes (Hamdy, 2001). Side effects are minimal. **Radio-isotopes** such as strontium-89 and samarium-153 have been shown to decrease pain in patients with osteoblastic metastases in contrast to osteolytic metastases which respond better to bisphosphonates.

If X-ray shows a metastatic lesion in a long bone with cortical destruction, particularly the femur or humerus, pathologic fracture must be prevented if possible. Generally this will require local irradiation and **internal fixation** with or without systemic therapy. If the patient develops a pathologic fracture, internal fixation followed by radiotherapy is a most effective approach, assuming the patient can undergo the operative procedure. If bone metastases are not complicated by pathologic fracture or do not involve the spinal cord or nerve roots, treatment is dictated by symptoms, by the risk of pathologic fracture, and by the potential for effective systemic therapy.

In symptomatic bone metastasis **percutaneous cement injection** and **thermal ablation** are alternative or additive treatment options to standard therapy. Thermal ablation could achieve spontaneous pain relief due to the destruction of sensitive nerves surrounding the tumour. Thermal ablation and percutaneous cement injection seem to be a reasonable combination as thermal ablation destroys sensible nerve ends, whereas cement injection increases stability.

Kyphoplasty is a treatment option for chronically painful, osteoporotic, vertebral compression fractures (concavity, biconcavity or wedge-shaped fracture). Several authors have reported pain relief after kyphoplasty in uncontrolled and retrospective observational cohort studies (Grafe *et al.*, 2005).

Patients with bone metastasis can and should avail of **physiotherapy**. Some physiotherapy exercises are possible even in subjects with extensive skeletal involvement. Painful positions adopted for protective reasons can be resolved by suitable physiotherapy.

Cutaneous metastases and advice for treatment

Cutaneous involvement is usually associated with advanced stages of the disease. Nodular carcinoma, inflammatory or erysipeloides carcinoma, telangiectatic and *"en cuirasse"* carcinoma are the typical clinical manifestations of the lymphatic dissemination to the skin. Unusual and nonspecific clinical appearances of cutaneous metastatic breast carcinoma have been described (Mordenti *et al.*, 2000).

The prognosis of patients with cutaneous metastasis depends on the type and biological behavior of the underlying primary tumour and on its response to treatment.

Systemic chemotherapy is the most commonly used treatment whereas the specific protocol depends on the histopathologic type of the primary tumour and staging of the patient. Surgical excision, radiotherapy, intralesional chemotherapy or immunotherapy can be used when solitary lesions develop or in the late stages of the disease in order to improve the quality of life of the patient. Topically applied 6% miltefosine solution, either used alone or in conjunction with other therapies for distant metastases, is an effective and tolerable local treatment.

Liver and lung metastases and recommendations for treatment

Solitary liver and lung metastases are rare. Therefore, neither surgical removal of metastases nor isolated regional chemotherapy or embolisation can be expected to bring about any significant benefit in survival time. In the case of asymptomatic multiple liver metastases, hormonal therapy should be considered. Chemotherapy should be applied in symptomatic liver metastasis.

The response rates to regional chemotherapy are significantly higher than systemic therapy; however this is not identical to prolongation of life and certainly not with an improvement in quality of life.

Liver metastases which do not respond to systemic chemotherapy can be an indication for placement of a hepatic artery port. Partial tumour remission can be achieved in a few patients with local alcohol injections or cryoablation. A less costly non surgical treatment alternative that requires only very short hospitalization, if any, is high frequency-induced thermotherapy (HiTT®). It is given in combination with classical imaging techniques (ultrasound, CT or MRI).

A resection of **solitary lung metastases** followed by chemotherapy is indicated if the metastasis occurred more than a year after the diagnosis of the primary tumour and if there is no other organ involvement. In the case of multiple or diffuse metastasis or if lung metastases appeared before, chemotherapy has priority.

Brain metastases and advice for treatment

Based on autopsy reports, the incidence of central nervous system (CNS) metastases among patients with breast cancer is as high as 23% but only 10-15% of these patients will develop clinically overt (CNS) manifestations (Di Stefano *et al.*, 1979). Brain metastases occur more frequently in young women with large and/or aggressive tumours and in the late stages of the disease. There are also data indicating an increased risk in breast cancer patients receiving trastuzumab and patients who received a taxane-containing chemotherapy regimen (Slimane *et al.*, 2004).

Headaches characteristic of increased intracranial pressure, such as early morning headaches, or headaches exacerbated by coughing, bending, and straining, are present in less than half of patients with brain metastases. They are often indistinguishable from tension headaches and may be associated with nausea, vomiting, and transient visual obscurations. Focal neurologic dysfunction is the presenting symptom in 20% to 40% of patients. Hemiparesis is the most common complaint, but the precise symptom varies depending on the location of the metastases. Cognitive dysfunction, including memory problems and mood or personality changes, are the presenting symptoms in one-third of patients, while seizures are the presenting symptom in another 10% to 20%.

Neurosurgical resection and the ablation by gamma knife or total brain radiation can be considered in the case of **single brain metastasis**. The role of surgery in patients with **multiple brain metastases** is usually limited to resection of large lesions or symptomatic lesions or life-threatening lesions. Whole-brain radiotherapy and symptomatic therapy are indicated in **multiple brain metastases**. The main goal of radiation therapy is to improve neurological deficits caused by the tumour deposit. Symptoms such as headache, focal neurological dysfunction, cognitive dysfunction, and seizures will improve.

Symptomatic therapy includes the use of corticosteroids for the treatment of peritumoural edema, anticonvulsants for control of seizures, and anticoagulants or inferior vena cava filters for the management of venous thromboembolic disease (Nguyen and De Angelis, 2004). The overall response rate to chemotherapy is more than 50% (Rosner, 1993). The kinase inhibitor Lapitinib penetrates the CNS and may be effective in brain metastasis.

Venous thromboembolic disease is common in patients with brain metastases, occurring in approximately 20% of patients. Anticoagulation may be more effective than inferior vena cava filter placement, and is acceptably safe when the prothrombin time is maintained within the normal range, especially in patients with brain metastases that generally do not hemorrhage, such as breast cancer.

There is increasing evidence that brain tumour patients who receive corticosteroids are at increased risk of developing Pneumocystis carinii pneumonia. This complication can be prevented by treating patients who are on prolonged courses of a corticosteroid, especially those over the age of 50 years, with trimethoprim/sulfamethoxazole prophylaxis.

Spinal cord compression syndrome and recommendations for treatment

Spinal metastases represent a difficult problem. Cord compression, nerve root compression, and leptomeningeal metastases can develop. About 95% of cases with spinal cord compression are caused by the epidural infiltration of vertebral metastasis. Most patients having paralysis experience pain coming from the spinal cord or spinal roots several weeks or several months before onset of paralysis.

Depending on the results of myelography, CT myelography, or MRI and the patient's status and short-term prognosis, decompressive laminectomy followed by radiotherapy or radiotherapy alone may be selected. Patients who present with spinal instability often require internal fixation.

Acute spinal cord compression syndrome requires prompt treatment within a few hours. Paralysis is inevitable unless radiotherapy is initiated within two or three days. Radiation therapy should also be given following surgery for decompression of intracranial or spinal cord metastases.

Patients with corresponding symptoms (progressive back pain, spinal cord compression syndrome) should be promptly referred to a centre which can offer complete diagnostic tests and has the appropriate departments (neurosurgery, radio-oncology, orthopedics, and hematology). Meanwhile the patient should get corticosteroids.

Pleuritis carcinomatosa, malignant effusion and recommendations for treatment

Pleuritis carcinomatosa with pleural effusion is the most frequent cause of dypnea, cough and chest pain in the advanced stage.

Intervention only makes sense in symptomatic pleuritis and effusion. Small collections that do not cause symptoms should be observed.

Options include thoracentesis, chest-tube placement, video-assisted thoracoscpy (VATS) and pleurodesis. Intermittent needle drainage at about 500-1000mL is preferred in many cases.

The pleural cavity needs to be thoroughly drained during pleurodesis, before instilling fibrosing substances. If there is a large residual effusion at the time a sclerosing agent is administered, the likelihood of success is low, and the possibility of turning a simple effusion into a multi-loculated collection requiring further interventions is high.

Chemical pleurodesis is achieved by instilling a sclerosing agent into the pleural space to incite an inflammatory reaction, which ultimately causes the visceral pleura to adhere to the parietal pleura, thereby eliminating the potential pleura and thus the pleural space in which fluid can accumulate. Any cytotoxic effect will only affect the uppermost cellular layers. Disadvantages of local instillation therapy are possible pain on inspiration, and reformation of encapsulated collections, that are more difficult to access.

Most commonly used substances with success rates between 54% and 98% are bleomycine, tetracycline, mitoxantrone, fibrin and talkum. When tetracycline is used (10-20mg/kg body weight in 50ml solution), local and possibly systemic preventative pain medication is necessary. (e.g., 10-20mL xylocain 1% intrapleurally)

Surgical pleurodesis with adhesion of both pleurae is sometimes the only option to treat particularly persistent breathlessness.

Peritoneal carcinosis and malignant ascites and recommendations for treatment

See also chapter entitled: "Rehabilitation and palliation of patients with ovary cancer".

Malignant ascites causes significant patient morbidity, discomfort and distress to many patients in advanced stages.

It is important to know whether ascites is ex-sudative or trans-sudative in nature. Ex-sudative ascites is most often due to tumour spread and needs targeted therapy aimed at the underlying reason. Cholesterol levels above 60mg/dL, and CEA levels above 12ng/mL in the ascites are a strong indicator of malignancy as well as raised serum levels of the tumour-marker Ca15-3.

Systemic hormonal therapy and/or chemotherapy should be attempted first, although experience has shown that this is less effective in cases of peritoneal carcinosis than in other metastatic locations

Intraperitoneal chemotherapy can limit ascites production for a short period of time, but tends to have only a local – if indeed any – effect due to cavity formation. If local chemotherapy is done, substances with good response rate in systemic application should be chosen (Sood *et al.*, 2004). Hyperthermic peritoneal chemotherapy may have an added effect on chemotherapy but this is not without risks (Hildebrandt *et al.*, 2004).

Larger instillation volumes are used than for pleurodesis in order to prevent adhesions. If cytostatic are left in the peritoneal cavity instead of eliminating them after several hours application time, there is increased systemic absorption with toxicity.

Therapy-induced symptoms have to be taken into account. Chemically induced peritonitis often limits cytostatic treatment. Intraperitoneal application of vinblastin can cause severe paralytic ileus; adriamycin may lead to painful peritonitis.

Intraperitoneal radio-isotopes with 32Phosphorus, 90Yttrium, 198Au37 or 32CrP38 have been used with some success, with the same limitations as local chemotherapy caused by unequal distribution due to intra-abdominal adhesions. They have little effect when retro-peritoneal lymph nodes are affected.

Diuretic therapy and dietary modifications have a limited role as most patients continue to accumulate ascites. **Paracentesis** show good temporary relief of symptoms. Rapid re-accumulation can necessitate frequent procedures. Repeated large volume paracentesis without plasma volume expansion may be associated with significantly higher incidence of hypotension and renal impairment

Alternatively, permanently implanted drainage catheters and shunting procedures represent another group of treatment options. Shunts offer advantages such as conservation of electrolytes and proteins. Palliative drainage catheters have a lower associated risk of electrolyte imbalance than serial large volume paracenteses, minimize procedural risk associated with either repetitive paracentesis or shunt procedures.

It is agreed by most authors that a shunt should only be used when other treatment options like diuretics have failed and when the life expectancy of the patient is long enough to derive benefit.

Systemic palliative therapies

Hypercalcemia and advice for treatment.

One important cause of hypercalcemia is metastatic bone disease. Care must be taken not to confuse clinical symptoms of hypercalcemia (table 6.34) with the terminal stage symptoms of cancer. Unless treated promptly, hypercalcemia is life threatening.

Table 6.34 - Major clinical symptoms of hypercalcemia.

– Extreme muscle weakness
– Fatigue
– Loss of appetite
– Nausea, vomiting
– Polydipsia and polyuria
– Constipation
– Anorexia
– Weakness
– Changes in heart rate
– Sleepiness
– Confusion
– Coma

The standard treatment for moderate and severe cases is the intravenous infusion of bisphosphonates. Newer bisphosphonates, such as zolendronate and ibandronate, give a longer duration of maintenance of normocalcemia action than clodronate (Pavalakis and Stockler, 2002).

In addition, breast cancer patients may develop hypercalcemia while being successfully treated with hormonal agents, particularly estrogens and tamoxifen. Response is associated with elevated serum calcium. Patients who develop hypercalcemia in this setting should be treated with intravenous fluids and, in some cases, plicamycin. The hormonal agent may be withheld during the acute hypercalcemia but reinstituted once the calcium normalizes.

Saline rehydration will usually effect a median reduction of 0.25mmol/L but its effect is transient. Rehydration is useful for treating mild degrees of hypercalcemia, but should be accompanied by bisphosphonate therapy.

Role of hormone therapies

Hormonal therapy is especially indicated if the patient's disease involves only bone and soft tissue and if the patient has either not received adjuvant antiestrogen therapy or has been off such therapy for more than one year. Chemotherapy is the treatment of second choice. About 30% of recurrences in premenopausal and 80% of recurrences in postmenopausal recurrences will respond to hormonal therapy.

Women whose tumours are receptor-positive or unknown who have received an antiestrogen within the past year should be given second-line hormonal therapy. Examples of second-line hormonal therapy in postmenopausal women include selective aromatase inhibitors, megestrol acetate estrogens; androgens or fulvestrant. In comparison to megestrol acetate, aromatase inhibitors have demonstrated at least equal efficacy and better tolerability.

Premenopausal women should undergo oophorectomy (surgically, with external-beam radiation therapy or with LHRH agonists). Patients with pulmonary lymphangiosis, major liver involvement, and/or central nervous system involvement should not receive hormonal therapy as a single modality.

Patients with structural compromise of weight-bearing bones should be considered for surgical intervention and/or radiation in addition to systemic therapy. Patients with vertebral body involvement should be evaluated for impending cord compression even in the absence of neurologic symptoms. Increasing bone pain and increasing alkaline phosphatase within the first several weeks of hormonal therapy do not necessarily imply disease progression. Patients with extensive bony disease are at risk for the development of symptomatic hypercalcemia early in the course of hormonal therapy. Early failure (e.g., before six months) on hormonal therapy suggests that cytotoxic chemotherapy should be the next modality employed

Very severe pain (flare) in cancerous areas occasionally occurs during and shortly after hormone treatment. This pain may be interpreted as a good prognostic omen because it may indicate a tumour response. Such flare rarely lasts longer than a day. If it does, corticoids should be attempted.

Corticosteroids are successful in joint pain and in subjects with headache and vomiting caused by brain metastases. Patients rapidly become pain-free on the first day of treatment. In subjects with rapidly growing liver metastases, corticosteroids reduce painful peritumoural inflammation and swelling. Corticoids are indicated in painful peritumoural edema but are effective for a limited period only.

Role of chemotherapies

The efficacy of chemotherapy for the relief of symptoms and improvement in quality of life makes these drugs a fundamental part of palliative care. Patients whose tumours have progressed on hormonal therapy, with hormone receptor-negative tumours and those with visceral metastases or diffuse bone involvement are candidates for cytotoxic chemotherapy (table 6.35).

Table 6.35 - Indications for chemotherapy in breast cancer recurrences.

– Tumours which have progressed on hormonal therapy
– Recurrences which are very active and progressive
– Visceral metastasis which are symptomatic (e.g., pain, dyspnea, cough)
– Lymphangiosis
– Receptor-negative tumours

There are more than 100 chemotherapy drugs and combinations to treat breast cancer recurrences (Caponigro *et al.*, 2004). The toxic potential should be considered in the selection of chemotherapeutic regimens.

The presence or absence of comorbid medical conditions, and physician/patient preference will influence the choice of therapy in individual patients. Whether single-agent chemotherapy or combination chemotherapy is preferable is unclear. Response rate and time-to-progression might be better for the combination; survival, however, doesn't differ significantly (Fossati *et al.*, 1998; Overmoyer, 2003). At this time, no data support the superiority of any particular regimen. Sequential use of single agents or combinations can be used for patients who relapse. Combinations of chemotherapy and hormonal therapy have not shown an advantage over the sequential use of these agents.

Role of targeted therapies

Targeted therapies are treatments such as herceptin (Trastuzumab) which are aimed at a target within the cancer cell that has been identified. Herceptin has as its target the HER-2/neu receptor. Herceptin can work only if the woman carries the HER-2 gene in those tumour cells. In patients previously treated with cytotoxic chemotherapy whose tumours overexpress **HER2/neu**, administration of herceptin as a single agent resulted in a response rate of 21%. About 25% of breast cancer patients are considered HER-2 positive.

When combined with doxorubicin, herceptin is associated with significant cardiac toxicity. Consequently, patients with metastatic breast cancer with substantial over expression of HER2/neu are candidates for treatment with the combination of herceptin and taxanes or other chemotherapeutic agents. Lapatinib is another promising tyrosine kinase inhibitor with activities against HER-2.

The anti-angiogenic agent Bevacizumab has been associated with a significant survival advantage when added to Paclitaxel.

Special features of pain therapy

See also chapter entitled: "Pain management in cancer rehabilitation and palliation".

Pain can lead to depression, loss of appetite, irritability, withdrawal from social interaction, insomnia, anger, loss of sleep, inability to cope, etc., which will influence sensibility of pain receptors as well. Uncontrolled pain can destroy relationships with loved ones and the will to live.

Fortunately, pain can almost always be controlled. The first step in reducing pain is to evaluate the cause and source of pain. It is important to differentiate malignant from non-malignant aetiology. It is important to differentiate causal and symptomatic pain therapy.

There are many different types of treatments used in the control of pain, including causal therapies (hormone-, chemo-, radio-, radionuclide therapy), symptomatic analgesics (peripherally and centrally acting pain medications, non-opioids, opioids, antidepressants, coanalgesics), specialized techniques to relieve pain (acupuncture, biofeedback, TENS devices, nerve blocks, and epidural injections), physical therapies (physiotherapy, manual methods, massage and warm baths, lymphatic drainage, thermal baths, hydrotherapy, fango mud packs), mental and relaxation techniques (table 5.25).

Compression pain associated with lymph edema is effectively relieved by lymphatic drainage. Compression garments should be worn between sessions.

The analgesic (causal) effect of **sexual hormonal therapy** depends mainly on the hormone sensitivity of the tumour and its metastases. Pain relief occurs just a few days after initiation of hormonal therapy in subjects with these hormone sensitive cancers.

Very severe pain (flare) in cancerous areas occasionally occurs during and shortly after hormone treatment. This pain may be interpreted as a good prognostic omen because it indicates a tumour response. Flare rarely lasts longer than a day. If it does, corticoids should be attempted.

Corticoids are indicated in painful peritumoural edema but are effective for a limited period only.

Percutaneous (external) radiotherapy is effective in palliating pain from solitary bone metastases. Two different mechanisms apply. The first mechanism is that of reducing tumour volume (curative radiotherapy or causal pain therapy), involving elevated cumulative therapeutic doses and fractionation (e.g., 5 x 4Gy or 10 x 3Gy). The analgesic effect of fractionated radiotherapy correlates with cancer cell kill and occurs after several days or weeks of treatment.

The second mechanism is that of symptomatic radiotherapy, requiring lower doses and only one shot (e.g., 1 x 8Gy). Pain relief is rapid. The "only" effect is reduction of peritumoural inflammatory acidosis, i.e., reduction of tumour swelling but not of actual tumour size.

Both regimens are equivalent in terms of pain and narcotic relief at three months and are tolerated with few adverse effects (Hartsell *et al.*, 2005).

Treatments aimed at the tumour itself such as **chemotherapy** may decrease pain by causing the tumour to shrink.

Pharmaceutical symptomatic therapy of bone pain includes **non-steroidal analgesics and opiates** (tables 5.18, 5.21). Non-steroidal anti-inflammatory drugs are often more effective for bone pain than opioids. However, they are associated with side effects, and tolerance to these agents necessitates treatment with other modalities (table 5.32). Morphine preparations have fewer side effects in the long run (tables 5.37, 5.38, 5.39). In several studies it has been shown that the physical and mental fitness of patients with tumour-related pain tends to increase with opioids. Periphery-acting pain medications frequently have only short-term effects, if any at all; for this reason they should be administered very early together with long-term morphine preparations.

Long-acting morphines should be preferred in palliative situations. A requirement for successful therapy with morphine preparations is using a controlled-release formula (table 5.21). The advantages of using transdermal application are less problems and potential fewer side effects (table 5.23). Pain peaks can be covered with short-acting morphine preparations (e.g., Sevredol®, Temgesic sublingual® or Actiq®). The patches only have to be changed every 48 to 72 hours.

Bisphosphonates are excellent painkillers in osteolytic metastases. Clinical experiences show however beneficial effects in osteoblastic metastasis as well. Parenteral administration of bisphosphonates is indicated in symptomatic bone metastases (Saad, 2004; Smith, 2003; Rosen *et al.*, 2004).

Systemic **beta-emitting, bone-seeking radiopharmaceuticals** represent a good alternative or adjuvant to external beam radiotherapy for palliation of painful diffuse osteoblastic bone metastases. Pain relief starts within one-four weeks after the initiation of treatment, continues for up to eighteen months, and is associated with a reduction in analgesic use in many patients (Finlay *et al.*, 2005; McEwan, 2000; Hamdy, 2001).

Relative contraindications for treatment include osteolytic lesions, pending spinal cord compression or pathologic fracture, pre-existing severe myelosuppression, urinary incontinence, inability to follow radiation safety precautions, and severe renal insufficiency.

Some **antidepressants** can be used for their analgesic effect alone or in combination with other analgesics (mainly opioids). Side effects have to be respected (tables 5.34, 5.35).

The doses used for pain management are considerably lower than those used for psychiatric treatment. In addition to their antidepressant and analgesic effect, some antidepressants (amitriptyline and doxepine, for instance) also have sedative effects and may be indicated for patients with sleep disorders. Some antidepressants are associated with weight gain (e.g., amitriptyline, doxepine, maprotiline, mirtazapine) while others are used for weight loss (e.g., sibutramine, fluoxetine).

Antidepressants are best given in the evening because of their sedative effects.

Anorexia and cachexia

There is no satisfactory drug therapy for cachexia. Corticosteroids may reduce anorexia but have no effect on the metabolic abnormalities of cancer cachexia. Megestrol acetate may exert an anabolic effect and reduce or prevent weight loss (Mateen and Jatoi, 2006).

Quality assurance and rehabilitative measures

To guarantee quality of rehabilitation and palliation you have to ensure quality of structures, quality of rehabilitative and palliative measures and to evaluate outcome.

As with acute therapy, certain guidelines and quality assurance procedures should also apply to rehabilitation and palliation (Delbrück, 1997; Barat and Franchignoni, 2004). Unfortunately there are only few guidelines on this subject for breast cancer patients. There are hundreds of national and international guidelines for general breast cancer but only few of them include rehabilitational problems (NHMRC, 2001; Kwaliteitsinstituut voor de Gezondheidszorg, 2001; Scottish Intercollegiate Guidelines, 2001; Deutsche Krebsgesellschaft, 2004).

Quality of structural features

Rehabilitation in breast cancer patients can only be achieved through the work of a qualified rehabilitation team (fig. 1.4). Special experience and a specialised infrastructure are essential. Due to the experience necessary, the rehabilitative institution should care for at least 100 breast cancer patients per year.

The rehabilitation team should be coordinated by a physician experienced in rehabilitation and palliation with demonstrable oncological knowledge. Physiotherapists and lymph edema therapists play an important role in this team. The collaboration of psycho-oncologists is very useful. Social workers are essential because of the social aids that are often needed. Cooperating and exchanging information with the previously and subsequently treating physicians are important.

Breast cancer rehabilitation services include critical components of assessment, physical reconditioning, skill training, and psychosocial support. They may include vocational evaluation and counselling.

Rehabilitative care can be offered either on inpatient or outpatient basis. Breast cancer patients who have undergone surgery, radiotherapy and/or chemotherapy are often weakened. For this reason, patients in Germany – as opposed to most other countries – are usually offered inpatient rehabilitation in specialised hospitals following primary therapy.

Quality of medical and therapeutic processes

Verifiability of the quality of rehabilitation and palliative therapies must be guaranteed.

All members of the breast cancer rehabilitation team should participate in the patient's assessment. The initial evaluation should include the medical history, diagnostic tests, current symptoms and complaints, physical assessment, psychologic, social, or vocational needs, nutritional status, exercise tolerance, determination of educational needs, ability to carry out activities of daily living and interests and compliance.

In rehabilitation and palliation it is not the rehabilitation team alone, but also the patient who takes on the task of assessing many treatment measures (Wan *et al.*, 1997) although expectations of a successful treatment are often very different in patients (Doyle *et al.*, 2001). Many patients accept rehabilitative and palliative therapies for reasons that are possibly quite different from those of the physicians.

The rehabilitation program must be tailored to meet the needs of the individual patient, addressing age-specific and cultural variables, and should contain patient-determined goals, as well as goals established by the individual team.

Outcome assessment and evaluation

The evaluation of rehabilitative measures in breast cancer patients is directed not at survival time, but rather at quality of life criteria. This involves primarily subjective and objective parameters such as improvement of pain, mobility, physical fitness, overcoming fear's, etc. (table 6.36). In general these parameters are not found in outcome assessment and evaluation of primary therapy (response, remission and length of remission).

The evaluation of rehabilitative and supportive measures is much more difficult than checking the outcome of intervention procedures generally used in potentially curative follow-up care (length of recurrence-free period, detection of early recurrence).

Outcome assessment in most clinical trials is affected by a purely medical understanding of the disease. This is reflected in the predominant use of oncological symptoms as the content of outcome measures. The assessment of other health aspects, like psychic symptoms, interpersonal or social consequences of the disease, seems to be similarly, if not more, important and should be considered in quality control of rehabilitation (table 6.36).

Quality of life questionnaires of the European Organization for Research and Treatment of Cancer (such as EORTC-BR23, EORTC QLQ C-30) and the functional assessment of cancer therapy breast cancer (Fact-B) can be used. Both are internationally validated questionnaires and have been used in multiple studies. They are composed of multi-item scales and yes/no questions assessing physical, role functioning, cognitive, emotional, and social effects.

Table 6.36 - Possible therapeutic aims and their effectiveness parameters in the rehabilitation of breast cancer patients.

Therapy goal	Parameter of effectiveness
Reduction and avoidance of lymph edema	Volume measurements, reduction of symptoms, improvement of ADL
Relief of physical and psychic symptoms in the palliative situation	Questionnaires: POS
Pain relief	Pain diary, reduction of analgesic drugs, pain sensitivity scales, questionnaires: PDI, BPI, EORTC QLQ-C-30, SE 36, SDS, RSCL
Improvement of shoulder-arm mobility	Measurements of abduction/adduction
Reduction of disorders resulting from surgery, chemotherapy, radiotherapy	WHO- toxicity scale, CTC-classification, FACT, CIRS-G, assessment of organ functions
Improvement of physical fitness	Ergometry, Karnofsky Status, WHO- and ECOG-Performance Status, EORTC-Performance-Status, walking distance, shuttle walking test, muscle force (hand-held dynamometry), exercise capacity (symptom limited, bicycle ergometry), muscle force (hand-held dynamometry). Questionnaires: ADL, IADL, FACT, FACT-An, Nottingham health profile, ESAS, (EORTC) LC-13, LC-13, LCSS, QLQ-C- 30, FLIC
Reduction of complaints resulting from hormonal therapy	Reduction of symptoms (e.g., hot flashes, insomnia)
Informations on curative follow-up and rehabilitation/palliative measures, counselling for family members	Questionnaires, tests
Reduction of anxiety, depression, fatigue	Rating scales, questionnaires: POMS, STAI, BDI, BFI, BSI, HADS-D, GDS
Coping with illness	Questionnaires: FKV, FKV-LIS, BEFO, TSK, FIBECK
Clarification and improvement of vocational fitness	Resumption of work, length of period of inability to work, FLI-C
Reduction of necessity of nursing care	Reduction of required level of nursing. Questionnaires: Barthel index, FIM, ADL, IADL, CIRS-G, FLIC-C

Abbreviations of questionnaires:
ADL = Activities of Daily Life; BFI = Brief Fatigue Inventory; BPI = Brief Pain Inventory; CCM = Cancer Care Monitor; CIRS-G = Cumulative Illness Rating Scale Geriatric; DDC = Daily Diary Card; EORTC-QLQ = European Organization for Research and Treatment of Cancer Quality of Life; ECOG = European Cooperative Oncology Group-Scale; ESAS = Edmonton Assessment Scale; FIM = Functional Independence Measure; FLI-C = Functional Living Index-Cancer; GDS = Geriatric Depression Scale; HADS-D = Hospital Anxiety and Depression Scale; IADL = Instrumental Activity Daily Living; KPS = Karnofsky Performance Scale; MFI = Multidimensional Fatigue Inventory; PDI = Pain Disability Index; POMS = Profile of Mood Status; POS = Palliative Care Outcome Scale; FACT-An = Functional Assessment of Cancer Therapy Anaemia (Cella, 1997); FLIC = Functional Living Index; PDI = Pain Disability Index; RSCL = Rotterdam-Symptom Check List; SDS = Symptom Distress Scale; SF-36 = Medical outcome study short form-36

Measurements of quality of life

Studies of quality of life in breast cancer patients have been performed mainly in therapeutic trials in order to assess the disease and treatment of specific symptoms. The studies mainly used performance status as a proxy regarding quality of life, even though there is only a weak association between the performance status such as the Karnofsky performance scale and the quality of life as measured by the EOTC QLQ-C30 (Montazeri *et al.*, 1998). Palliation of symptoms, psychosocial interventions, and understanding patient's feelings and concerns all contribute to improve quality of life in lung cancer patients.

Activities of daily life play an important role in rehabilitation. Widely used measures to assess activities of daily life are the functional independence measure or the Barthel Index (Mahoney and Barthel, 1965).

Basically, improvement in quality of life aimed at in rehabilitation is achieved when less nursing care is necessary ("rehabilitation to combat the need of care"), when the patient can be vocationally reintegrated ("rehabilitation to combat early retirement"), when he/she feels secure ("rehabilitation to combat resignation and depression") and when the patient's physical handicaps and functional limitations are at a minimum ("rehabilitation to combat disability").

Comparisons with patient-reported symptoms from the quality of life questionnaire have shown that physicians fail to report approximately one half of the symptoms identified by the quality of life questionnaire as adverse events, and the quality of life questionnaires did not detect approximately one half of the symptoms (Fromm *et al.*, 2004).

Different outcome scales in palliative care of cancer patients have been developed (Aspinal *et al.*, 2002; Bausewein *et al.*, 2005). The scales cover physical and psychic symptoms, spiritual considerations, practical concerns, emotional concerns of the patient and family, and psychosocial needs of the patient and family. The Palliative Care Outcome Scale (POS) is a multidimensional instrument covering these physical, psychosocial, spiritual, organizational, and practical concerns.

Bibliographie

- Aapro M, Cull A (1999) Depression in breast cancer patients: The need for Treatment. Ann Oncol 10: 627-36
- Ahles TA, Saykin AJ, Furstenberg CT *et al.* (2002) Neuropsychologic impact of standard-dose systemic chemotherapy in long-term survivors of breast cancer and lymphoma. J Clin Oncol 20: 485-93
- Anilo LM (2000) Sexual life after breast cancer. Journal of Sex & Marital Therapy 26,3: 241-8
- Altaha R, Abraham J (2004) Paraneoplastic neurologic syndrome associated with occult breast cancer. Breast J 9, 5: 417-9
- Aspinal F, Hughes R, Higginson I *et al.* (2002) A user's guide to the palliative care outcome scale. Palliative care & policy publications. Kings College, London

- Avis N, Crawford S, Manuel J (2004) Psychosocial problems among younger women with breast cancer. Psycho-oncology 13, 5: 295-308
- Bausewein C, Fegg M, Radbruch L *et al.* (2005) Validation and clinical application of the German version of the palliative care outcome. J Pain Symptom Manage 30: 51-62
- Balducci L, Extermann M, Carrera I (2001) Management of breast cancer in the older women. Cancer control 8, 5: 431-41
- Barat M, Franchignoni F (2004) Assesssment in physical medecine and rehabilitation. Maugeri Foundation books. PI-ME Press Pavia
- Bartsch HH, Delbrück H, Kruck P *et al.* (2000) Zur Prozessqualität in der onkologischen Rehabilitation. Rehabilitation 39: 355-8
- Blakely J, Bulder A, Loleda JS *et al.* (2004) Effect of pregnancy after treatment for breast cancer. Cancer 100, 3: 465-9
- Bottomley A (2000) Quality of life data interpretation: Key issues in advanced breast cancer. In: Nabholtz JM, Tonkin K, Aaapro M S *et al.* (edit) Breast cancer Management. Application of evidence to patient care. M Dunitz London 363-72
- Buddeberg C, Wolf C, Sieber M *et al.* (1991) Coping strategies and course of disease of breast cancer patients. Psychother: Psychosom 55: 151-7
- Bourbonniere M, Kagan SH (2004) Nursing intervention and older adults who have cancer: Specific science and evidence based practice. Nurs Clin North Am 39: 529-43
- Bradley C, Oberst K, Schenk M (2006) Absenteeism from work: The experience of employed breast and prostate cancer patients in the months following diagnosis. Psycho-oncology 15, 8: 739-47
- Bukovic D, Fajdic J, Hrgovic Z *et al.* (2004) Sexual dysfunction in breast cancer survivors. Onkologie 28, 1: 29-34
- Bundesarbeitsgemeinschaft für Rehabilitation (BAR) (2003) Rahmenempfehlungen zur ambulanten onkologischen Rehabilitation
- Burke W, Daly M, Garber J *et al.* (1997) Recommendations for follow-up care of individuals with an inherited predisposition to cancer II BRCA1 and BRCA2. Cancer Studies Consortium; Ethical, Legal, and Social Implications Branch; National Centre for Human Genome Research. JAMA 277: 997-1003
- Calabrese C, Distante V, Orzalesi L *et al.* (2001) Immediate reconstruction with mammaplasty in conservative breast cancer treatment: Long-term results. Focus Rec Breast Cancer Surg, Osp Ital Chir 7: 38-46
- Carlsson C, Baigi A, Killander D *et al.* (2005) Motives for becoming and remaining member of patient associations: A study of 1,810 Swedish individuals with cancer associations. Support Care Cancer 20
- Caponigro F, Basile M, Rosa VD *et al.* (2004) New drugs in cancer therapy. Anticancer Drugs 16, 2: 211-21
- Carter G, Gross A (2003) Bisphosphonates and avascular necrosis of the jaws. Aust Dent J 48: 268
- Cella D (1997) The functional assessment of cancer therapy anaemia (FACT-An) scale: A new tool for the assessment of outcomes in cancer anemia and fatigue. Semin Hematol 34 (suppl 2): 13-9
- Chanan-Khan A, Srinivasan S, Czuczman MS (2004) Prevention and management of cardiotoxicity from antineoplastic therapy. J Support Oncol 2, 3: 251-6

– Cuzick J, Stewart H, Peto R et al. (1987) Overview of randomized trials of postoperative adjuvant radiotherapy in breast cancer. Cancer Treat Rep 71: 15-29
– Daley, A (2007) Exercise progress improves well being in survivors of breast cancer. J Clin Oncol 25, 1713-21
– Delbrück H, Witte M (2006) Onkologische Nachsorge und Rehabilitation in Ländern der europäischen Gemeinschaft. (in press)
– Deng G, Cassileth B, Yeung K (2004) Complementary therapy for cancer-related symptoms. J Supportive Oncol 2: 419-29
– Deutsche Krebsgesellschaft (2004) Interdisziplinäre S3-Leitlinie für die Diagnostik und Therapie des mammakarzinoms der Frau. W Zuckschwerdt Stuttgart
– Di Stefano, Yap H, Blumenschein G (1979) The natural history of breast cancer patients with brain metastases. Cancer 44: 1913-8
– Dooren SV, Seynaeve C, Rijnburger AJ et al. (2005) The impact of having relatives affected with breast cancer on psychologic distress in women at increased risk for hereditary breast cancer. Breast Cancer Res Treat 89 (1): 75-80
– Ernst E (edit) (2001) The desktop guide to complementary and alternative medicine. An evidence based approach. Mosby
– Evans H, Lambert C (2007) Physiological basis of fatigue. An J Phys Med Rehabil 86, 1: 29-6
– Extermann M, Overcash J, Lyman GH et al. (1998) Comorbidty and functional status are independen in older cancer patients. J Clin Oncol 16: 1582-7
– Fallowfield L, Cella D, Cuzick J et al. (2004) Quality of life of postmenopausal women in the Arimedex, Tamoxifen, Alone or in Combination (ATAC) adjuvant breast cancer trial. J Clin Oncol 22: 4261-71
– Fossati R, Confalonieri C, Torri V et al. (1998) Cytotoxic and hormonal treatment for metastatic breast cancer. A systematic review of published randomized trials involving 31,510 women. J Clin Oncol 16, 10: 3439-60
– Fromme E, Eilers KM, Mori M et al. (2004) How accurate is clinician reporting of chemotherapy adverse effects? J Clin Oncol 22, 17: 3485-90
– Ganz P, Desmond K, Leedham B et al. (2002) Quality of life in long-term disease – free survivors of breast cancer: A follow-up study. J Natl Cancer Inst 94: 39-49
– Ganz P, Greendale G, Petersen L et al. (2003) Breast cancer in younger women: Reproductive and late health effects of treatment. J Clin Oncol 21: 4184-93
– Geels P, Eisenauer E (2000) Palliative effect of chemotherapy. J Clin Oncol 18: 2395
– Gelber S, Coates S, Goldhirsch A et al. (2001) Effect of pregnancy on overall survival after the diagnosis of early-stage breast cancer. J Clin Oncol 19(6): 1671-5
– Giordano SH, Buldak AU, Smith TS (2004) Is Breast cancer survival improving? Cancer 100, 1: 44-52
– Goldhirsch A, Gelber R(2004) Life with consequences of breast cancer: Pregnancy during and after endocrine therapies. Breast 13: 443-5
– Goodwin P, Blau R, Gazder P et al. (1999) The risk of premature menopause induced by chemotherapy. J Womens Health Gend Based Med 8: 949-54
– Grafe I, Fonseca KD, Hillmeier J (1999) Reduction of pain and fracture inicidence after kyphoplasty. Osteoporosis Int 16: 2005-12
– Højris I, Overgaard M, Christensen JJ et al. (1999) Morbidity and mortality of ischaemic heart disease in high-risk breast-cancer patients after adjuvant postmastectomy systemic

treatment with or without radiotherapy: analysis of DBCG 82b and 82c randomised trials. Lancet 354: 1425-30
- Hillner BE *et al.* (2004) American society of clinical oncology 2003 update on the role of bispohosphonates and bone health issues in women with breast cancer. J Clin Oncol 21: 4042-57
- Hokin PJ, Yarnold JR, Roos DR *et al.* (2001) Second workshop on Palliative Radiotherapy and Symptom Control: Radiotherapy for bone metastases. Clin Oncol (R Coll Radiol) 13: 88-90
- Hunter MS, Grunfield E, Mittal S *et al.* (2004) Menopausal symptoms in women with breast cancer: Prevalence and treatment preferences. Psycho-oncology 13, 11: 769-78
- Jeziorowski M, Leuschner G, Schwerdtfeger R (1995) Gesundheitstraining in der onkolo-gischen Rehabilitation. In Günther H, Ehninger G (edit) Individuelle Therapieentscheidungen bei unbegrenzten Möglichkeiten. Pechstein Verlag
- Johnsson A, Fornander T, Olsson M *et al.* (2007) Factors associated with return to work after breast cancer. Acta Oncol 46, 1: 90-6
- Kienle G, Kiene H, Albonico H (2006) Anthroposophic medicine. Effectiveness, utility, costs, safety. Schattauer, Stuttgart
- Kligman L, Wong PK, Johnston M *et al.* (2004) The treatment of lymph edema related to breast cancer: Asystematic review and evidence summary. Support Care Cancer 12, 6: 421-31
- Knobf M (1999) The influence of symptom distress and preparation on responses of women with early stage breast cancer to induced menopause. Psycho oncology 8: 88a
- Koski S, Venner P (2000) Chemotherapy-induced nausea and vomiting. In: Nabholtz JM, Tonkin K, Aapro MS, Buzdar AU (edit) Breast cancer management. Application of eviden-ce to patient care. M Dunitz London 317-29
- Krychman M, Pereira L, Carter J (2007) Sexual health issues in women with cancer. Oncology 71,1-2, 18-25
- Kufe DW, Pollack RE, Weichselbaum RR *et al.* (2003) in Cancer Medicine, 6th ed. Hamilton, Ontario
- Kuroi K, Shimozuma K (2004) Neurotoxicity of taxanes: Symptoms and quality of life assessment. Breast cancer 11, 1: 92-9
- Kwaliteitsinstituut voor de Gezondheidszorg (2001) Behandeling van het Mammacarcinoom. CBO, http://www.cbo.nl
- Laurer D, Connolly-Nelson K, Vang B (2007) Stressors and coping strategies among fema-le cancer survivors after the treatment. Cancer nurs. 30, 2: 101-11
- Lee S, Schover LR, Partridge A *et al.* (2006) American Society of Clinical Oncology Recommendations on Fertility Preservation in Cancer Patients. J Clin Oncol 20, 24(18): 2917-31
- Liang W, Burnett CB, Rowland JH *et al.* (2002) Communication between physicians and older women with localized breast cancer: Implications for treatment and patient satisfac-tion. J Clin Oncol 20: 1008-16
- Lerman C, Biesecker B, Benkendorf JL *et al.* (1997) Controlled trial of pretest education approaches to enhance informed decision-making for BRCA1 gene testing. J Natl Cancer Inst 89: 148
- Levine ERG, Eckhardt J, Targ E (2005) Change in post-traumatic stress symptoms follo-wing psychosocial treatment for breast cancer. Psycho-oncology 13

– Limper AH (2004) Chemotherapy-induced lung disease. Clin Chest Med 25: 53-64
– Love W, Kissane D, Bloch S et al. (2002) Diagnostic efficiency of the hospital anxiety and depression scale in women with early stage breast cancer. Australian New Zealand J Psych 36: 246-50
– Manuel J, Burwell S, Cranford S et al. (2007) Younger women's perceptions of coping with breast cancer. Cancer nurs 30, 2: 85-94
– Maunsell E, Brisson C, Dubois L et al. (1999) Work problems after breast cancer: An exploratory qualitative study. Psycho-oncology 8, 6: 467-73
– MacDonald N (edit) (1998) Palliative Medicine, a Case-Based Manual. Oxford, NY: Oxford University Press
– Morandi P, Rouvier R, Altundag K (2004) The role of Aromatase inhibitors in the adjacent treatment of breast cancer. Cancer 101, 7: 1482-9
– Mordenti C, Peris K, Couletta Fargnoli M et al. (2000) Cutaneous metastatic breast carcinoma. Acta dermatovenerologica 9, 4
– Moser MT, Weis J, Bartsch HH (2001) Effects of oncological inpatient rehabilitation programs on quality of life. Psycho-oncology 10: 21
– Nguyen T, DeAngelis L (2004) Treatment of brain metastases. J Support Oncol 2: 405-16
– Nitz U (2004) Disease-management-Programm Mammakarzinom. Der Onkologe 10: 404-8
– Overmoyer B (2003) Combination chemotherapy for metastatic breast cancer: Reaching for the cure. J Clin Oncol 21 (4): 580-2
– Paterson A, Lindasy MA (2000) Erythropoetin in the management of cancer patients. In: Nabholtz JM, Tonkin K, Aaapro MS, Buzdar AU (edit) Breast cancer Management. Application of evidence to patient care. M Dunitz London 311-6 In: Nabholtz, JM. K Tonkin, M S Aaapro, A U Buzdar (edit): Breast cancer Managment. Application of evidence to patient care. M Dunitz London 363-72
– Pavlakis N, Stockler M (2002) Bisphosphonates in breast cancer (Cochrane Review). In: The Cochrane Library, issue 1, Oxford: Update software
– Rabaglio M, Egli G, Castaglione M (2004) Edema after cancer treatment. Ther Umschau 61, 11: 649-54
– Reidl IR (2002) Intavenous zoledronic acid in postmenopausal women with low bone mineral density. N Engl J Med 346: 653-61
– Resnick B, Belcher AE (2002) Breast Reconstruction. Am J Nurse. 102: 26-33
– Rosner D, Flowers A, Lane WW (1993) Chemotherapy induces regression of brain metastases in breast carcinoma patients: Update study (abstract). Proc Am Soc Clin Oncol 12: A508
– Rowett L (2000) The Internet, health professionals and the health consumer. In Nabholtz JM, Tonkin K, Aaapro MS, Buzdar A (edit) Breast cancer management. Application of evidence to patient care. Dunitz, London 539-47
– Saunders C, Hickey M, Ives A (2004) Breast cancer during pregnancy. Int J Fertil Womens Med 49, 5: 203-7
– Schlesinger-Raab A, Eckel R, Engel J (2005) Metastasiertes Mammakarzinom: Keine Lebensverlängerung seit 20 Jahren. Dtsch. Ärztebl. 102, 40: 2706
– SIGN (1998) Breast cancer in women. http:www.sign.ac.uk/guidelines/published/index.html

– Slimane K, Andre F, Delaloge S (2004) Risk factors for brain relapse in patients with metastastic breast cancer. Ann Oncol 15: 1640-4
– Sonmezer M, Oktay K (2004) Fertility preservation in female patients. Human Reproduction Update 10: 251-66
– Stevinson C (2001) Why patients use complemetary and alternative medecine. In: Ernst E (edit.) The desktop guide to complementary and alternative medecine. An evidence-based approach. Mosby
– Stoeckli R, Keller U (2004) Nutritional fats and the risk of type 2 diabetes and cancer. Physiol Behav 83, 4: 611-5
– Storey P (1998) Symptom control in dying. In: Berger A, Portenoy RK, Weissman D, eds. Principles and Practice of Supportive Oncology Updates. Philadelphia, Pa: Lippincott-Raven Publishers, 741-8
– Teitelbaum SL, Britton JA, Gammon MD (2003) Occupation and breast cancer in women 20-44 years of age. Cancer Causes Control 14, 7: 627-37
– Tennant A (2004) Principles and practice of measuring outcome in Barat M, Franchignoni F (edit) (2004) Assessment in physical medicine and rehabilitation. Maugeri Foundation books, PI-ME Press Pavia
– The American Cancer Society Advisory Committee on Diet, Nutrition, and Cancer Prevention (1999) Guidelines on diet, nutrition, and cancer prevention: Reducing the risk of cancer with healthy food choices and physical activity. CA Cancer J Clin 46: 325-41
– Thorsen L, Skovlund E, Stromme SB et al. (2005) Effectiveness of physical activity on cardiorespiratory fitness and health-related quality of life in young and middle-aged cancer patients shortly after chemotherapy. J Clin Oncol 23, 10: 2378-88
– Twycross R, Lichter I (1998) The terminal phase. In: Doyle D, Hanks GWC, MacDonald N, eds. Oxford Textbook of Palliative Medicine. 2nd ed. Oxford, England: Oxford University Press, 985-6
– Van Dalen E, Caron H, Dickinson H et al. (2005) Cardioprotective interventions for cancer patients receiving anthracyclines. Cochrane Database Syst Rev: CD 003917
– Van Gils, Peeters PH, Bueno-de-Mesquita HB et al. (2005) Consumption of vegetables and fruits and risk of breast cancer
– Watson M, Forster C, Eccles D et al. (2004) Psychosocial impact of breast/ovarian (BRCA1/2) cancer-predictive genetic testing in a genetic testing in a U.K. multi-centre clinical cohort.
– Watson M, Haviland JS, Greer S et al. (1999) Influence of psychologic response on survival in breast cancer: A population-based cohort study. Lancet 354: 1331-6
– Watson T, Mock V (2004) Exercise as an intervention for cancer related fatigue. Phys Ther 84: 736-43
– Wells M, Sarna L, Cooley M et al. (2007) Use of complementary and alternative medecins to control symptoms in women living with lung cancer. Cancer Nurs 30, 1: 45-55
– WHO (2001) International classification of functioning, disabilities and health. www.WHO.int/classification/ICF
– Yates P, Evans A, Moore A et al. (2007) Competency standards and educational requirements for specialist breast nurses in Australia. Collegium 14, 1: 11-5
– Zielinski CC (2004) Gemcitabine, anthracycline, and taxane combinations for advanced breast cancer. Oncology 17, 12: 36-40

Rehabilitation and palliation of ovarian cancer patients

Goals of rehabilitation and palliation: Significance and definition as distinct from curative tumour follow-up care

The chief aim of all medical, potentially **curative follow-up** care measures (recurrence prevention, early detection and therapy of disease recurrence) is to lengthen survival time (fig. 1.1). The cancer disease thus represents the focus of curative follow-up care.

Rehabilitation and palliation, on the other hand, do not aim at influencing the illness, but rather reducing disabilities due to the tumour and therapy (fig. 1.2). Improvement of quality of life constitutes the goals of rehabilitative procedures. It is the intention to alleviate the negative effects of the cancer disease and therapy, not only physically, but also psychologically, socially and vocationally. The ICF (International Classification of Functionality, Disability and Health) is the basis for assessment, therapy and quality assurance of rehabilitation (Barat and Franchignoni 2004). It is considerably more comprehensive than the ICD – the standard classification system used in curative cancer care –, as it includes psychological aspects in addition to biological ailments.

In theory, the aims of curative follow-up care can be differentiated simply and clearly from those of rehabilitation and palliation. In practice, however, there is much overlapping. This involves in particular tumour recurrence therapy and palliative measures. Potentially curative therapy for recurrences does not only serve to prolong survival time, but also to alleviate symptoms.

Experiences show that in most patients the disease recurrence is no longer potentially curatively treatable even when it has, by means of routine diagnostics, been detected at an asymptomatic stage, thus very "early". This questions the value of routine follow-up diagnostics. The value of prophylactic forms of therapy (adjuvant therapy) is controversial, and therapy of disease recurrence brings about only – if any at all – marginal gains in survival time. As long as the potentially curative measures (recurrence prevention, early detection and therapy of recurrence) have failed to show a significant survival benefit, rehabilitative and palliative measures in the follow-up care of ovary carcinoma patients will remain the main focus.

Rehabilitative measures in follow-up care

Rehabilitative measures are necessary for patients undergoing potentially curative as well as palliative treatment.

A certain minimum amount of information on disease status is required before administering rehabilitative and palliative forms of therapy (table 7.1). Without this knowledge, valuable time is wasted searching for information and performing additional research, thus jeopardising the success of rehabilitation. Before carrying out rehabilitative measures, a rehabilitative assessment has to take place, with rehabilitation planning and documentation of the goals to be achieved (Barat and Franchignoni, 2004).

Table 7.1 - Minimum informations required before initiating rehabilitative measures.

– Extent of tumour (for example TNM).
– Curative or palliative therapy approach (for example, R0, R1 or R2 resection of the tumour)?
– Has chemotherapy or radiation therapy taken place (for example, which cytostatic agents at what dosages and with which results)?
– Have other organs been removed during the operation (e.g., spleen)?
– Psychosocial information (for example, about statements given pertaining to degree of patient information about any problems with coping or compliance, amount of support given by family members, about social and occupational problems, etc.).

Rehabilitative measures aimed at reducing physical problems ("rehabilitation to combat disability")

Polyneuropathies, pain of non tumour origin and recommendations for alleviation

Neuropathic pain is a common syndrome seen in women who have been treated for ovarian cancer. Chemotherapy is a possible cause (mainly with vinca alkaloids, platinum derivates or taxans) but other aetiologies have to be considered (e.g., diabetes, alcohol, arsenic, shingles, paraneoplastic disease, vasculitis, vitamin B12 deficiency, folic acid deficiency, electrolyte misbalance, drugs like INH, amiodarone, phenytoin, metronidazole and others) (Paice, 2003). Most often, however, chemotherapy has to be blamed for these sometimes disabling sensory and motor disturbances (Dunton, 2002).

Taxol and platinum preparations are particularly neurotoxic as well as vinca-alkaloids. These substances are often used to treat ovarian cancer. Vinca-alkaloids and taxol preparations cause axonal degeneration; cisplatin induces demyelination. These disturbances may predominately be proximal or peripheral (paclitaxel), sensory (cisplatin) or sensory motor (vinca-alkaloids).

Neurotoxicity, mainly seen as cumulative sensory peripheral neuropathy represents the most important non hematological toxicity associated with paclitaxel administration. Factors affecting the development of neuropathy could include application of paclitaxel as a single agent or in combination with other chemotherapeutics, single and cumulative dose levels, schedules and individual features of the subjects studied (e.g., age, pretreatment, comorbidities).

Primary symptoms may include numbness/paraesthesia, tingling and burning in a symmetric stocking and glove distribution. Usually, the lower extremities are affected first, but a simultaneous onset in the upper and lower extremities has also been reported. Motor neuropathy is much less frequent than sensory symptoms and includes a mild distal weakness, especially of the toe extensor muscles (Dubois, 1999; Mielke et al., 2006). Diagnosis is usually made based on a clinical examination and electrophysiological measurements, whilst nerve biopsies provide a further diagnostic tool.

Mild sensory neuropathies often appear to be reversible within a few months whilst more severe forms may persist significantly longer. Tricyclic antidepressants and anticonvulsants are widely used in the treatment of neuropathic pain. Gabapentin, an anticonvulsant related to the neurotransmitter gamma aminobutyric acid with antihyperalgesic activity, with promising efficacy in different neuropathic pain syndromes, might relieve symptoms associated with paclitaxel-induced polyneuropathies.

Polyneuropathies induced by paclitaxel, docetaxel, platin, carboplatin and vinca-alkaloids are dose-related. Sometimes symptoms can further deteriorate after discontinuing Cisplatin. Also, after stopping taxol symptoms often only improve slowly.

Cisplatin leads to a mainly sensory polyneuropathy when cumulative doses of 200mg per square metre are reached. In typical cases this progresses for a further three months after discontinuing therapy ("coasting").

Regarding oxaliplatin, acute and chronic neurotoxicity need to be distinguished. Directly after administration of oxaliplatin (after 30-60min) neurological symptoms (such as paraesthesias, dysaesthesias, hyper-sensitivity to low temperature, muscle pain e.g., in the jaw) can be avoided by not exposing the patient to low temperatures on the day of administration. Acute neurotoxicity is not dose-dependent.

More problematic and more difficult to avoid is the late onset sensory neuropathy which often manifests itself after a cumulative dose of 510mg per square metre. Virtually all patients treated with oxaliplatin develop sensory motor neuropathy at this dose. It is reassuring however that these neurological disturbances improve very soon after discontinuing chemotherapy as opposed to platin-induced neuropathies.

Gabapentin in a dose of 300-1,800mg per day and carbamazepine in a dose of 600-2,400mg per day are most often used for symptomatic treatment (Junker et al., 2004).

There is no equivocal proof or efficacy for pyridoxine and vitamin B preparations, which are often prescribed. The use of alpha-liponic acid is contested and views on efficacy of the topical agent capsaicin are divided.

There are a few positive reports on prophylactic administration of vitamin E and glutamine but none when symptoms have already developed. Prophylactic treatment with nerve growth factor is being studied at present.

Improvement of symptoms with anti-epileptics (carbamazepine 600-2,400mg a day in slow release form and gabapentin 300 1,800mg a day) has been substantiated. Additional administration of anti-depressants (amitriptyline) can be useful, however, causes a dry mouth, which can be disturbing.

Amifostin and glutamine infusions can be given to prevent and treat cisplatin-induced neurotoxicity. There is no doubt that the combination of carboplatin and docetaxal is less neurotoxic than that of cisplatin and paclitaxel.

Pain relief is one of the main therapeutic indications for low frequency electrotherapy. This includes Stanger bath treatment, diadynamic current therapy and transcutaneous electrical nerve stimulation (TENSE). Ice packs and contrast hydrotherapy may improve the patient's well-being. Temporary relief of pain symptoms in the hands and feet is achieved by manipulating structured sand but the relief provided by these physical measures unfortunately does not last. Many patients state that autogenic training has helped.

Painful abdominal lesions may be an inevitable part of wound healing after surgery. They are frequently mistaken for signs of disease progression. Good dietary advice may be very effective but surgery may be necessary to detach adhesions.

Cardiovascular problems and advice for prevention and treatment

For more details see chapter: Rehabilitation and palliation of patients with breast cancer.

Premature menopause with its non physiological premature hormonal withdrawal can cause late cardiac symptoms. Hormonal substitution is, for this reason, indicated, especially for young patients with good prognosis.

Cardiotoxicity is a major side effect of various anti-neoplastic agents, particularly anthracyclines and trastuzumab treatment. The spectrum of cardiac side effects varies with the anti-neoplastic agent dose and schedule. Important risk factors associated with cardiac toxicity are cumulative dose, infusion schedule and pre-existing cardiac disease (Chanan-Khan *et al.*, 2004).

Renal problems and recommendations for prevention and treatment

Sometimes extended tumour operations are necessary, causing loss of one kidney; hydronephrosis caused by adhesions or tumour compression of the urinary tract is not rare. Platinum preparations are nephrotoxic. Cisplatin induces renal toxicity by damaging the tubuli. It is acute and cumulative as opposed to carboplatin-induced toxicity.

An important protective measure with cisplatin therapy is sufficient hydration and forced diuresis. Nephrotoxic antibiotics should not be administered at the same time. As opposed to cisplatin, sufficient hydration and forced diuresis are not necessary with carboplatin therapy.

Toxic cyclophosphamide metabolites causing haemorrhagic cystitis and cyclophosphamide may induce secondary malignancies of the bladder.

Toxic metabolites are bound and inactivated by prophylactic administration of mesna.

In the case of renal failure and pain, buprenorphine should be preferred to other morphine-containing analgesics.

Hormonal problems and recommendations for prevention and treatment

As a result of the therapy-induced castration, particularly young women can develop typical symptoms of menopause (hot flushes, insomnia, fatigue, depression, vaginal dryness, loss of libido and urinary incontinence). This can have a significant impact on a woman's quality of life.

For this reason, and also to prevent possible late complications such as osteoporosis and cardiovascular disease, estrogen should be substituted locally or even systemic. There are no good arguments against hormonal substitution for these patients.

Hormone substitution does not increase risk of tumour relapse (apart from endometrioid carcinomas). Selective serotonin reuptake inhibitors, e.g., venlafaxine, are a non hormonal treatment that is often effective in patients complaining about hot flashes.

Other non hormonal interventions to alleviate these symptoms include Kneipp baths, phyto-therapeutics, phytotherapy, sedative medication and beta blockers. Sometimes gestagens are given. Megestrol acetate and MPA carry an increased risk of thrombosis.

Osteopathy and advice for prevention

Shutting down ovarian function and premature menopause cause an increased risk of osteoporosis and bone fractures. In addition to hormonal substitution, a sensible diet rich in vitamin D and calcium should be recommended. Whether or not prophylactic prescription of bisphosphonates is reasonable is being investigated in several studies.

Diarrhoea and advice

After extended bowel resections and particularly resections of the small intestine, diarrhoea is frequent. Individual dietary advice is important (Lim and Ho, 2001). For more details see chapter: Rehabilitation and palliation of patients with colon carcinoma.

Peritoneal carcinosis should always be considered as a possible cause as well. This condition manifests itself through paradoxical diarrhoea.

Constipation and advice for prevention

Constipation is the most common side effect of opioid therapy. Opioid-induced constipation should be treated prophylactically (see chapter: Pain management in cancer rehabilitation and palliation). Sudden onset constipation could also be a side effect of pain relief or anti-cancer medication. Tumour progression, e.g., intestinal obstruction, should be considered as well.

Non malignant bowel obstruction and recommendations for treatment

Extensive surgical debulking, pelvic or abdominal irradiation and intraperitoneal chemotherapy are some of the factors that predispose patients to non-cancerous causes of bowel obstruction (Jatoi *et al.*, 2004). Adhesions can cause chronic abdominal symptoms to the point of acute ileus.

The therapeutic decision is whether conservative management should eventually, after an unspecified period, culminate in surgery or not in patients who do not recover. Surgical resection may be necessary.

In cases of partial obstruction, nutrition has to be modified to prevent ileus. Diet rich in fibres, mushrooms and nuts should be avoided. Gas-producing food can cause substantial symptoms, both for this reason cabbage, roasted onions, lentils and sugar substitutes should be avoided. Sugar substitutes can cause symptoms because they are only incompletely absorbed and reach lower segments of the gut in digestion where bacteria decompose them thereby liberating gases.

It makes sense to keep faeces smooth. In case of constipation, lactulose, containing laxatives, should be avoided because of their tendency to cause flatulence.

Loss of appetite, weight loss and recommendations

Also refer to chapter: "Rehabilitation and palliation of pancreatic cancer patients".

Fatigue, anxiety, depression as well as problems resulting from therapy can all contribute, in addition to tumour progression, to loss of appetite and weight loss (table 7.2).

Table 7.2 - Possible causes of weight loss in patients with ovary cancer.

Reduced food intake due to :
– Lack of appetite
– Decreased food intake due to vomiting
– Decreased food intake due to pain
– Impaired bowel passage
Impaired utilisation due to:
– Reduced release of nutrients in the gut
– Limited absorption of nutrients
– Reduced synthesis (development of body substance)
Increased energy demand due to:
– Fever
– Increased release of adrenaline and noradrenalin
– Increased release of cytokines
– Cytokine therapy (e.g., tumour necrosis factor)
Loss of energy rich body substance through:
– Fistula secretion
– Tapping of ascites
– Tapping of pleural effusions

Appetite can be influenced by psychopharmacological drugs, especially tricyclic anti-depressants and by hormones. One may attempt hormonal treatment with gestagens, cortisone or androgens. These can improve appetite and lead to weight gain.

While corticoids (e.g., prednisolone 10-30mg/die or dexamethasone 2-4mg a day) have a short-term appetite-stimulating effect of two to four weeks as well as a reconstituting effect, and after this time typical side effects become predominant, the weight-increasing effects of megestrol acetate (160 to 480mg a day) last significantly longer.

Special dietary recommendations are not necessary unless extensive intestinal resections have been performed or short bowel syndrome is present. This recommendation remains true despite observations hinting towards possible tumour preventive benefit of increased consumption of fruit and vegetable (Bingham and Riboli, 2003; IARC, 2003).

Short gut syndrome and recommendations

Also refer to chapter: "Rehabilitation and palliation of patients with colon carcinoma".

Sometimes extensive abdominal operations including resection of the spleen, parts of the pancreas or parts of the stomach are necessary. Extensive gut resections are not infrequent.

Untreatable diarrhoea, fatty faeces, wasting of body fat and muscles, weight loss, excessive gastric acidity, loss of minerals, gall bladder and kidney stones all characterise short gut syndrome. Consequences for the whole organism and loss of weight are unavoidable unless artificial feeding is instituted (Lim and Ho, 2001).

At least in the early stages, substantial loss of fluid and electrolytes necessitate parenteral artificial feeding. After a few weeks enteral tube feeding can be given which can be utilised without residue by the remaining gut.

In the first few months of short bowel syndrome, eating problems are most pronounced. In the later stages there is a certain adaptation and compensation by the remaining gut. Sometimes tube feeding can be dispensed of at this stage. However, lifelong feeding restrictions remain necessary.

Ileostomy and advice for care

The principles and techniques of ileostomy care are similar to those of colostomy (see chapter 11). However, the stools are of a loose consistency and drain continuously from the ileostomy. It is, therefore, necessary that drainage bags, or pouches, must be worn at all times. The size of the opening and the pouch size will vary at first. The stoma has to be checked three weeks after surgery, when swelling has gone away. The final size and type of appliance is selected after approximately three months, when the person's weight and stoma size are stable. Bag changing and other wound care should be done as instructed.

Small bowel contents contain active digestive enzymes, which can cause severe peristomal skin excoriation if leakage occurs. Cutting the wafer to the correct size, correctly applying the pouch, and carefully cleaning and drying the skin around the stoma with every pouch change are the best ways of preventing skin irritation. The collecting pouch must be emptied as needed, usually four to six times a day, by releasing the clamp from the bottom of the pouch and emptying the contents directly into the toilet. The pouch has to be changed every four to six days.

Since the fluid loss through ileostomy is greater than with colostomy, fluid intake must be increased to prevent dehydration. Fluid loss can be a problem in the summer, because perspiration adds to the fluid lost through the ileostomy. There are no dietary restrictions except to avoid foods that are high in fiber, corn and peanuts, but the food should be eaten slowly and chewed well to prevent food blockage. A greater loss of electrolytes and certain vitamins, especially vitamin B12, may also be experienced, thus requiring regular controls.

After ostomy surgery, digestion and absorption of medications, either alone or in combination, may be affected. Some medications can change the color of your stool.

A person receiving an ileostomy has many questions about lifestyle changes. Family relationships, sexual function, and body image are all areas of concern to be discussed with an enterostomal nurse (ET nurse) and in self-help groups. The exchange of information between patients in self-help groups is the best source of advice in many cases. Adjustment to life with an ileostomy and monitoring for complications will be parts of an ongoing process.

Entera/parenteral nutrition and recommendations

For more details refer to chapter: "Rehabilitation and palliation of patients with pancreatic carcinoma"

The food industry offers high caloric protein enriched drinks as aromatised liquid food. These are taken between or in addition to the usual meals. Drinks with 1kcal per mL are best tolerated. They can lead to noticeable weight gain.

If oral feeding is not sufficient, food can be given via a tube inserted into the stomach (PEG) or a percutaneous endoscopic jejunostomy (PEJ) to the short bowel.

It is beneficial that gastric and enteral passage remain intact, unlike in parenteral feeding. The mucous membranes of the gut remain healthy and there are no bacterial super infections. Diarrhoea and immune function of the gut is preserved (Faries et al., 1999).

Preparations for tube feeding depend on location of the tube. For tubes in the stomach or duodenum (PEG) nutrient-defined high molecular diets are suitable. These contain polymer nutrients (intact proteins, polysaccharides and triglycerides) in accordance with physiological criteria of normal food, they are standardised, complete and cover all nutritional requirements.

Chemically-defined (low molecular) diets are used if the tube is situated in the duodenum (PEJ). They need not be digested. They consist of oligopeptides, disaccharides, and medium chain triglycerides. They are free of fibres. Industrial foods should be preferred to home-made foods.

Indication of full parenteral feeding in cases of tumour cachexia is contested. It is indicated in cases of short bowel syndrome and in cases of temporarily limited and localised mechanical obstruction through tumour progression until, e.g., PEG or PEJ tubes are in place. Intensive laboratory surveillance is necessary.

Most frequent complications are catheter infections with or without sepsis and metabolic complications. An arterio-venous port must always be inserted. Frequent biochemical tests are necessary.

Sexual problems and recommendations for prevention and treatment

Cancer treatments that impair ovarian function, have a major impact on female sexual function. Sexual dysfunction has been cited as a major source of distress for cancer survivors in several surveys. Long-term survivors of ovary cancer often complain of decreased libido, sexual arousal and orgasm (Taylor *et al.*, 2007)

Much of the loss of desire for sex in women with ovarian failure is linked to dyspareunia from vaginal atrophy. If hormonal treatment is needed, it is safest to use low-dose oestrogens in the form of vaginal ring or suppositories to treat pain that does not respond to appropriate use of water-based lubricants or vaginal moisturisers. Since little oestrogen escapes into the systemic circulation, these products can often dramatically improve dyspareunia with negligible risk of promoting cancer recurrence. Sexual rehabilitation of cancer in women cannot however be reduced to simple hormonal replacement or mechanical device.

Hormonal changes, psychologic consequences, therapeutic interventions and of course behaviour of the partner influence libido and actual behaviour (Ferell *et al.*, 2003; Schover, 2005). Questions relating to sexual dysfunctions are complex in nature. In particularly problematic situations, psychotherapy can help women cope with difficult changes in sexual functioning.

Fertility problems, pregnancy and recommendations for prevention and treatment

For more details refer to chapter: breast cancer

For young patients with early tumour state and good differentiation of the tumour (Stadium FIGO IA G1), fertility-deserving treatment can be chosen by preservation of uterus and contra-lateral ovary.

There is no evidence to suggest any detrimental effect of a carcinoma on a developing foetus. Depending on the timing and nature of chemotherapy, adverse effects on the foetus must be anticipated however.

It is not justified to advise against pregnancy after fertility-preserving operation of ovarian cancer.

Genetic particularities and recommendations

An estimated 5% of all ovarian cancers are due to inborn germline mutations, more than 90% of all inherited ovarian cancers are due to mutations in the BRCA1 or BRCA2 gene. The average cumulative risks in BRCA1 mutation carriers by the age of 70 are 39% and in BRCA2 mutation carriers 11% for ovarian cancer (Antoniou *et al.*, 2003).

Table 7.3 - Criteria for genetic counselling of relatives.

– Families with at least two patients suffering from breast and/or ovarian carcinoma, one of those below the age of 50 (this age limit does not apply to families with three or more patients)
– Families with one patient with one-sided breast carcinoma at the age of 30 or earlier
– Families with one patient with bilateral breast carcinoma at the age of 40 or earlier
– Families with one patient suffering from ovarian cancer at the age of 40 or earlier
– Families with one patient with both breast and ovarian carcinoma
– Families with a male patient with breast carcinoma

Primary prevention for women with high risk of hereditary ovarian cancer can be offered by oral contraception and ablation. The pill reduces the risk of developing cancer by 60% when used for six years. Prophylactic salpingo-oophorectomy reduces it by more than 90%. High risk families should be offered the opportunity to participate in specific early cancer detection programmes (vaginal exploration and ultrasound for ovarian cancer). They should be informed about prophylactic medication (oral contraceptive pill or surgery oophorectomy) and should be offered individualized psychological support (Kuschel *et al.*, 2000).

Lack of information, education, counselling program

Education and information are important aids in overcoming illness. This involves the patient's understanding of what is happening to her body and why a certain form of therapy has been chosen. Many women want information pertaining to the disease, treatment, and self-care issues. Many patients express that they would like to participate in a counselling programme to discuss psychological issues raised by suffering from ovarian cancer.

The more psychologically distressed the women, the more information they want about coping strategies, and the more serious the illness is, the more shared decision-making is desired (Stewart *et al.*, 2000). However, the majority of women do not wish to make decisions about tumour therapy themselves, but they would like to know why a particular form of therapy has been chosen.

Health education takes place in discussion groups in which psychologists, physicians and social workers all take turns moderating the groups. Education counselling programmes comprise general information on ovarian cancer, its causes, and different therapeutic approaches including alternatives and complementary treatment (table 2.12).Consequences of therapy on sexuality (Black, 2004), prevention of recurrent disease, aftercare, coping with anxiety, how to cope with pain and treatment of relapsing disease will be discussed and information on entitlement to social care, legal aspects and career consequences will be given.

Besides questions relating to nutrition, side effects of therapy and hormonal symptoms, social provisions and psychological strategies to relax and to combat fear are important topics.

It is useful for patients and their families to have access to printed versions of information and advice which they have received in health education sessions (e.g., in the form of differentiated self-help literature which should not be industry-affiliated). This printed material should of course never take the place of consultations with a physician but should rather provide the basis for productive discussions with the attending physician.

Patients are more and more often finding information for themselves, using literature, Internet and other media, on the unfavourable prognosis of their disease. Further explanatory information and, in particular, assistance in dealing with this information is necessary. This may be done in a one-to-one setting or in group discussions. Interested patients and their families should be advised on Internet resources which, in the physician's opinion, are informative, useful and provide well-founded information.

Carriers of BRCA1 and 2 mutations have to be informed about the increased risk of breast cancer and about the necessity of frequent aftercare visits (Vadaparampil et al., 2004). The possible inheritance of predisposing genes in high risk families and the availability of genetic counselling by human geneticists need to be mentioned.

Rehabilitative measures aimed at reducing psychological problems (rehabilitation to combat resignation and depression)

For more information see chapter "Psychological support and self–help groups in cancer rehabilitation and palliation". Long-term survivors of ovarian cancer have been noted to experience high levels of depression and anxiety, chronic fear of disease recurrence, significant sexual dysfunction and identity disturbances. Many women with recurrent disease exhibit significant distress because recurrence signifies to them that their disease is incurable (Sun et al., 2007).

Causes of anxiety disorders and depression can be very complex (Norton et al., 2004). Fear of follow-up diagnostic tests, fear of progression or recurrence, fear of the uncertain future, and also family, economic and social problems are frequent (tables 2.5 and 7.4). Survivors experience chronic fear of recurrence, sexual dysfunction and identity disturbances (Black, 2004). Hormonal changes cause vegetative disturbances with depressive cases, insomnia, distress and nervousness. In cases of disease progression these are often linked to pain, feeding problems and sometimes even problems with short bowel syndrome and stoma implantation (fig. 2.1 and 5.2).

Increased attention, conversations, "taps on the shoulder", and social activities on their own are often not sufficient to solve psychological problems. It may be necessary to involve a psycho-oncologist (see chapter: "Psychological support and self-help groups") (table 2.2).

Table 7.4 - The most important psychosocial factors during aftercare.

- Emotional problems (anger, depression, anxiety, aggression, suicidal thoughts, hopelessness, pessimism, loss of purpose, fatigue, problems with self-esteem and identity)
- Problems with partner and family (communication and relational problems, change of role sexuality)
- Professional problems (strains and changes of the professional situation, restrictions on working capacity, unemployment, early retirement and others)
- Social problems (isolation, incertitude in dealing with friends and acquaintances, changing behaviour during leisure time and other, financial problems, securing adequate care at home)
- Compliance problems (avoidance of diagnostic and therapeutic measures, coping with cancer, with social and occupational problems)

Patients and their family who carry BRCA1/2 gene need special psychological attention (Vadaparampil *et al.*, 2004; Watson *et al.*, 2004). Women with a BRCA1/2 mutation experience significant challenges. These include decision making regarding surgical options and notification to offspring and family along with a sense of isolation which may lead to psychological and emotional distress.

Many women want information about coping strategies (Stewart *et al.*, 2000). There is no standardised approach to coping with the disease; every patient reacts in a different way, needs to be addressed individually and needs support for her specific needs. Some, often those with a firm religious belief, may do very well without any professional psychological help.

Support groups offer an opportunity to share experiences and emotions as well as exchange information. They are also a possible source of emotional support and therefore can contribute to quality of life of patients with ovarian cancer. Knowing that others had similar symptoms and reactions, and that those experiences are normal, is very important for support group participants. A support group may help to cope with the practical and emotional aspects of the disease. Talking with other women with ovarian cancer may also help ease feelings of isolation. Participation in support groups can be an important source of emotional and informational support for patients.

Fatigue

See also chapter: "Psychological support and self-help groups in cancer rehabilitation and palliation".

A remarkably high proportion of ovarian carcinoma survivors suffer from fatigue. Fatigue (extreme tiredness and exhaustion) is probably multi-factorial in origin (tables 2.8, 2.9, 2.10). Somatic factors contributing to fatigue include anemia, weight loss, pain, fever, medication, infections and dysbalance between endogenous cytokine levels and their natural antagonists. Frequently, hormonal changes cause fatigue which can be successfully treated by hormonal replacement.

Depression, cognitive impairment and fatigue can be symptoms of chemotherapy-induced anemia. The positive influence of erythropoetin on fatigue symptoms with low Hb has been proved in a series of international studies. The target haemoglobin level should be 12 g/dl. There is an increased risk for serious cardiovascular events when administered to a target > 12g/dl. If no somatic cause can be found and treated, non-medication measures should be used first (e.g., physiotherapy, ergometric training, conversation therapy, behavioral therapy, diet, change of environment) (Watson, 2004).

Sometimes, fatigue symptoms are linked to the antidepressant medications themselves. Psychotropic drugs have, however, also been used successfully to treat fatigue.

Rehabilitative measures aimed at reducing social problems ("rehabilitation to combat the need for care")

See also chapter: "Social support in rehabilitation and palliation".

One of the aims of rehabilitative measures is to strengthen the patient's own resources and to prevent the risk of the need for care, or at least reduce such a need (tables 3.1, 3.2).

If home care cannot or cannot yet be arranged, the time spent in hospital can be followed up by a temporary stay in an institution for follow-up care. In Germany there are rehabilitation hospitals ("AHB hospital") which are designed especially to meet the needs of patients with gynaecological tumours and in which plans are made for the patients' social assistance, in addition to medical and psychological guidance. Counselling of the patients and their family members is one of the tasks of such a rehabilitation institution. Experienced physicians, psychologists and representatives of self-help groups share their experiences, information and helpful advice. In Germany every cancer patient has a legal claim to a three-five week stay in such an institution. Some of the *maisons de repos* in France have a similar function.

Providing contact addresses (self-help groups, counselling centres, etc.) is helpful.

In addition to psychological support, self-help groups often provide their members with specific knowledge about medications and resources as well as social laws. The concept behind self-help groups is based on the idea that sharing of mutual experiences and situations offer a person strength. Self-help groups for women with cancer exist in most countries. Self-help groups play an important role with regard to the aims of follow-up on the social level; their impact is often limited, however, by the complexity of problems patients are facing.

Securing adequate care at home

If the patient is no longer able to care for himself/herself, support must be organized. In patients with extended ovary cancer, this situation is particularly frequent. Early organization of assistance and support is crucial in patients with poor prognosis and rapidly progressing disease. The planning of further care must be done with the patients' family.

Assistance such as "meals on wheels", household assistance, home nursing care, care assistance, and under certain circumstances nursing home or hospice care need to be arranged.

Rehabilitative measures aimed at reducing occupational problems ("rehabilitation to combat early retirement")

See also chapter: "Vocational Integration in Cancer Rehabilitation"

Asbestosis, talcum and total dust have been hypothesized to influence development of ovarian cancer; these observations, however, are being discussed in a very controversial way (Langseth and Kjaerheim, 2004).

Whether or not the patient is capable of working depends on tumour spread, whether resection was done R0 or R1. It also depends on severity of concurring diseases, whether additional chemotherapy was done. Last but not least, subjective ability to work plays a role. In Germany duration of treatment and incapacity to work are usually estimated at about seven-eight months.

Patients with inoperable ovarian carcinoma and with active tumour are not usually able to work. They should ask for early retirement on grounds of ill health as soon as possible. Exceptions apply for psychological reasons, if the patient is keen on continuing to work. In this case work-facilitating measures are helpful, for example the gradual resumption of work tasks. More often than not, however, these patients soon realise that they are not up to their job once they try to phase back in.

For ovarian cancer patients who have been treated potentially curatively, there are professional limitations, which are mainly due to chemotherapy and hormonal changes.

When judging the chances of professional reintegration it should be kept in mind that the risk of cancer relapse is high during the first or second year, and that side effects of therapy such as platin/taxol-induced polyneuropathy may take months to resolve.

Gradual resumption of work is recommended. The particular advantage of this arrangement is that work load and fitness level of the patient can be matched without financial disadvantages. Unfortunately, this sensible vocational rehabilitation approach is only possible in a few countries and even there often only in large companies and in the civil service.

Palliative measures

Informing the patient in the event of disease progression: Delivering bad news

It is difficult to specify the best time to begin a conversation with a patient about shifting the focus from cure to maintaining quality of life with palliative care. Several issues complicate initiating such conversations with patients (van Grueningen, 2005). The attending physician must inform the patient about disease progression in a personal conversation (table 2.11). Even when prognosis is desperate, positive aspects have to be mentioned (e.g., improved palliative therapies, improved pain management, etc.).

One must always inform about relative risk and consequences of necessary treatments. Even palliative tumour therapies have subjective and objective effects of varying severity, which must be taken into consideration, especially in elderly patients. Toxicity associated with some palliative treatments can be important (Dunton, 2002), and resource implications are considerable (Doyle, 2001).

Answering the question: "How much therapy and which one?" not only requires oncological expertise. Ethical competence and communication skills are just as important. Under no circumstances should therapeutical decisions be made exclusively depending on response in terms of likelihood of remission; goals such as reduction of physical symptoms, emotional stabilisation, and maintenance of daily activities are pre-eminent.

The ability to make appropriate quality of life decisions requires strong, clear communication between doctors, treatment staff, patient and family caregivers. There is no better situation than having well informed, highly skilled doctors working with a motivated, well informed patient and supportive family caregivers.

Localisation and symptoms of recurrences

By the time cancer is diagnosed, it is often already advanced, inoperable, has infiltrated surrounding organs or developed distant metastases, leaving only the possibility of supportive and palliative treatment.

Ovarian carcinoma can spread by intraperitoneal implantation, lymphatic invasion, and hematogenous dissemination. Intraperitoneal relapses grow around the bowel and cause obstruction (table 7.5). These manifest as sub-ileus or ileus. In case of hematogenous spread, peritoneal and pleural cavitis are most often affected, less frequently liver (2%), lung (7%), CNS (2%) and skeleton (1.6%).

Table 7.5 - Localisation of regional recurrences in patients with ovarian cancer.

– Peritoneal carcinosis 80%
– Colon 74%
– Small bowel 56%
– Bursa omentalis 18%
– Stomach 15%

Choice of therapeutic modalities

The assessment of emotional and physical costs must be carefully considered with any patient before deciding further cancer therapies. Decisions regarding how to manage events associated with progressive disease need to be carefully considered in the light of associated risks of morbidity (and mortality) and resulting quality of life. For example, such considerations might include whether patients with bowel obstruction should undergo palliative surgery, receive total parenteral nutrition, or whether women with ascites should undergo repeated paracentesis. Relapse therapy of ovarian cancer virtually equals palliative therapy. The aim of any treatment is primarily symptom alleviation, and prolonging life is only of secondary importance (tables 3.10, 7.6 and 7.7). However, patient expectations are that these palliative treatments will make them live longer and even cure them (Doyle *et al.*, 2001), although objective prolongations of survival are rare with response rates ranging from 27% to 60%.

Table 7.6 - Symptoms hinting towards possible tumour progression.

– **Changing bowel habits:** Abdominal discomfort and bowel problems are often the only symptom of intra-abdominal tumour growth.

– **Colicky pain and persistent para-vertebral pain** with radiation to the back, sometimes with circular radiation, raise the possibility of retro-peritoneal dissemination. Abdominal cramps can be red flag symptoms of peritoneal carcinomatosis with early bowel obstruction.

– **Distension, nausea, vomiting, sudden constipation** are often reported in small bowel obstruction, less frequently in large bowel obstruction.

– **Loss of weight:** weight loss and cachexia despite normal alimentation.

– **Unexplained weight gain** with increased waist circumference: protein deficiency, cardiac insufficiency, but also peritoneal carcinomatosis need to be considered when the waist circumference increases (ascites and/or flatulence).

– **Dyspnea:** (pleuritis carcinomatosa with effusion).

Table 7.7 - Factors that need to be considered (besides potential tumour regression) before initiating palliative tumour therapy.

– To which extent can the patient tolerate chemotherapy.
– To which extent will the patient suffer from side effects of this therapy for the rest of her life.
– To which extent home care is influenced by therapy.
– Can therapy be administered on an outpatient basis, or will admission be necessary for example due to insufficient support at home.
– What influence will concomitant conditions (such as diabetes, renal failure, cardiovascular disease, poor nutritional status) and functional disability have on outcome.
– Will insight, will to survive, coping strategies, and social provision influence the preferred therapeutic option?

Surgical interventions for recurrent ovarian cancer remain controversial. Some studies show that patients with recurrent disease may derive a significant survival benefit from optimal debulking, other studies show therapeutic benefit of secondary surgery only in late recurrences after one year.

For early relapse (disease progression within about 6 months after completion of postoperative chemotherapy) re-operation can only be recommended in case of ileus. Surgery is indicated in case of palliation needs such as colon or ureter obstruction (Classe *et al.*, 2004). Partial resections of the small intestine, hemicolectomy of colon ascendens, transversum, descendens or sigmoideum, in exceptional cases even complete ex-enteration, can be necessary for intra-abdominal relapse. Gastroenterostomy, insertion of PEG or PEJ, stoma and/or artificial nutrition may be indicated.

Irradiation may be indicated for brain metastases, painful bone metastases, ulcerating metastases at the top of the vagina, lymphatic metastases, and pain relief.

On the whole, treatment of ovarian cancer relapse is a domain of **chemotherapy**.

Local and regional problems and palliative therapies

Liver and lung metastasis

Solitary liver metastases are extremely rare. Therefore, neither surgical removal of metastases nor isolated regional chemotherapy or embolisation can be expected to bring about any significant benefit in survival time. Systemic chemotherapy, on the other hand, can alleviate symptoms.

Peritonealcarcinosis (malignant ascites)

It is important to know whether ascites is ex-sudative or trans-sudative in nature. Trans-sudative ascites is most often not due to malignoma (but to cardiac failure, hypoproteinemia caused by either nephrotic syndrome or liver cirrhosis, hypervolaemia, hyperhydration). Ex-sudative ascites is most often due to tumour spread. Cholesterol levels above 45mg/dL, CEA levels above 12ng/mL in the ascites and ascites/serum LDH superior to 1.0 are a strong indicator of malignancy as well as raised serum levels of the tumour-marker Ca12-5.

Malignant ascites is a common complication of advanced ovarian cancer. It causes significant patient morbidity, discomfort and distress to many patients in advanced stages, and it may become a major treatment problem for the physician (Becker *et al.*, 2006). Large amounts of ascites can cause increased abdominal pressure with troublesome symptoms like pain, dyspnea, loss of appetite, anorexia, nausea, reduced mobility and problems with the body image.

Survival after the development of malignant ascites in patients with ovarian cancer is significantly longer than that of other malignancies, with a reported median survival of greater than 300 days (Parsons, 1996).

Spasmolytic medication work best for pain. Although **diuretics** are commonly used, the evidence supporting their use is weak. Up to now, there is no approved reliable method to predict those patients with malignant ascites who will respond to diuretics (Becker *et al.*, 2006). Diuretic therapy and dietary modifications have a limited role as most patients continue to accumulate ascites.

Available data show good, although temporary, relief of symptoms related to the build-up of fluid in about 90% of patients managed by **paracentesis**. Rapid re-accumulation can necessitate frequent procedures, thus subjecting the patient to the risks of bleeding, infections, visceral perforation, and hypotension associated with invasive drainage. Repeated large volume paracentesis without plasma volume expansion may be associated with significantly higher incidence of hypotension and renal impairment (tables 7.8, 7.9).

Table 7.8 - Methods of peritoneal drainage.

– Large volume therapeutic paracentesis
– Peritoneo-gastric shunting
– Peritoneo-urinary shunting
– Peritoneo-venous shunting
– Peritoneal port or catheter placement
– Hemodialysis catheter drainage
– Semi-permanent catheter placement

Table 7.9 - Possible complications of abdominal paracentesis.

– Secondary peritonitis
– Pulmonary emboli
– Hypotension
– Cachexia

Alternatively, permanently implanted drainage catheters and shunting procedures represent another group of treatment options. Shunts offer advantages such as conservation of electrolytes and proteins. Palliative drainage catheters have a lower associated risk of electrolyte imbalance than serial large volume paracenteses, minimize procedural risk associated with either repetitive paracentesis or shunt procedures.

Initially the **peritoneo-venous shunt** was developed for use in patients with intractable ascites as a result of cirrhosis of the liver, but it subsequently became a popular procedure in managing malignant ascites. The objective of using shunts is to achieve symptom relief and prevent the need for distressing paracentesis and the resulting protein and fluid depletion. However there are some absolute and relative contraindications (table 7.10).

Table 7.10 - Contraindications for shunting.

– Ascitic fluid protein content superior to 4,5g/L (higher risk of shunt occlusion)
– Hemorrhagic ascites
– Lobulated ascites
– Portal hypertension
– Coagulation disorders
– Advanced cardiac or renal failure
– Short life expectancy

In all reported studies patients with ovarian and breast cancer who undergo peritoneo-venous shunting have the best response rate whereas the response rate in patients with gastro-intestinal cancers is far worse. Because of poor prognosis, it is agreed by most authors that a shunt should only be used when other treatment options like diuretics have failed and when the life expectancy of the patient is long enough to derive benefit. There is no consensus regarding the time span, some authors suggest an expected survival of more than three months. Shunt insertion is contraindicated in patients with malignant ascites due to gastro-intestinal cancer.

Systemic chemotherapy may be attempted, although experience has shown that it is less effective in cases of peritoneal carcinosis than in other metastasis locations.

Intraperitoneal chemotherapy (table 7.11) can limit ascites production for a short period of time, but tends to have only a local effect – if indeed any – due to cavity formation. If local chemotherapy is done, substances with good response rate in systemic application should be chosen (Sood *et al.*, 2004). Hyperthermic peritoneal chemotherapy may have an added effect on chemotherapy but this is not without risks (Hildebrandt *et al.*, 2004).

Table 7.11 - Cytostatics with intraperitoneal efficiency.

– Bleomycin 60mg
– Carboplatin 300-600mg/m^2
– Cisplatin 90-100mg/m^2
– Mitoxantrone 20-25mg/m^2
– Paclitaxel 135-175mg/m^2
– Mitomycin C 10mg/m^2
– Taxol 60-125mg/m^2

Larger instillation volumes are used than for pleurodese in order to prevent adhesions. If cytostatic are left in the peritoneal cavity instead of eliminating them after several hours application time, there is increased systemic absorption with toxicity.

Therapy-induced symptoms have to be taken into account. For example, chemically-induced peritonitis often limits cytostatic treatment. Especially with platinum derivates possible severe myelo- and nephrotoxicity must be anticipated. Intraperitoneal application of vinblastin can cause severe paralytic ileus; adriamycin may lead to painful peritonitis.

Intraperitoneal radioisotopes with 32Phosphorus, 90Yttrium, 198Au37 or 32CrP38 have been used with some success, with the same limitations as local chemotherapy caused by unequal distribution due to intra-abdominal adhesions. They have little effect when retroperitoneal lymph nodes are affected.

Some improvements in ascites have been noted in response to immunotherapy with intraperitoneal alpha or beta interferon, tumour necrosis factor TNF or with administration form like corynebacterium parvum or OK-432.

Bowel obstruction

Bowel obstruction may be caused by a narrowing of the intestine from inflammation or damage to the bowel, tumours, scar tissue, hernias, twisting of the bowel, or pressure on the bowel from outside the intestinal tract. It can also be caused by factors that interfere with the function of muscles, nerves, and blood flow to the bowel. Most bowel obstructions occur in the small intestine and are usually caused by scar tissue or hernias. The others occur in the colon and are usually caused by tumours, twisting of the bowel, or diverticulitis. Symptoms will vary depending on whether the small or large intestine is involved.

The most common cancers that cause bowel obstructions are cancers of the colon, stomach, and ovary. Patients who have had abdominal surgery or radiation are at a higher risk of developing a bowel obstruction. Bowel obstructions are most common during the advanced stages of cancer. Chronic sub-ileus is usually caused by mechanical obstruction. Even when surgery is not an option any more, colorectal stenting can lead to long symptom free periods. Expandible metallic stents have been found to be highly effective when there is a single site of intestinal obstruction that is readily approachable by endoscope (that is, either in the proximal small bowel, or in the distal colon). Patients with multiple sites of obstruction caused by peritoneal and intestinal carcinomatosis are less likely to benefit from this intervention. In these cases often only conservative measures and supportive therapy are indicated. The distinction between full and partial obstruction is important in order to achieve good symptom control.

The main questions to answer in the management of intestinal obstructions are to determine whether there is a single or multiple sites of obstruction, at what stage of the disease progression the obstruction has occurred, whether the patient will derive benefit from a surgical approach or stenting, whether the tumour is refractory to chemotherapy, and whether the patient should be offered PEG and supportive care.

The sites of intestinal obstruction are mainly small or large intestine, or combined small and large intestine.

Although surgical options (i.e., tumour resection, bypass and colostomies) should always be considered, their value is limited in patients who suffer from continued growth with few remaining cancer treatment opportunities. Operation risks are considerable (Jatoi et al., 2004; Pothuri et al., 2004).

Most patients have constant pain and nausea due to intestinal distention; thus, anti-emetics and analgesics are indicated.

Haloperidol is considered the appropriate anti-emetic for malignant bowel obstruction. Corticoids have anti-emetic and anti-inflammatory effects as well. Octreotide (sandostain) has been shown not only to palliate the symptoms of intestinal obstruction but also to directly slowly and evenly reverse the associated downward spiral. It inhibits multiple secretagogues (thus reducing intestinal fluid secretion and decreasing peristalsis).

Gastric venting, or decompression of fluids and gas proximal to the obstruction, plays an important palliative role. However, the longer the nasogastric tube remains, the higher is the risk for morbidity, including nose and throat pain, abscess formation, erosion of nasal cartilage, and social isolation. Therefore theses tubes should only remain for a few days, and some consideration should be given to placement of a gastrostomy tube to take over the task of gastric venting when long-term need is anticipated.

Increased morbidity, the propagation of a false sense of hope among patients and family members, and unjustified expense have all served as strong reasons against parenteral nutrition as routine initiation.

In order to prevent ileus in partial malignant bowel obstruction, the stool should be kept soft.

Hydronephrosis

Hydronephrosis is a common complication of advanced ovarian carcinoma. The presence of this complication at the start of chemotherapy has a negative impact on survival. Ureter obstruction and hydronephrosis are usually due to tumour compression rather than infiltration. If there is ureter infiltration, distal ureter resection with de novo implantation is indicated (Psoas Hitch technique).

One should always be aware of the altered kinetics of some drugs in case of impaired renal function. In particular the dose of opioids needs to be adjusted to the degree of renal function disorder in order to avoid tolerability problems. Buprenorphine, which is mainly excreted via the faeces, can be administered to patients with renal impairment up to renal failure without the need for dose adaptation.

Pleuritis carcinomatosa, malignant effusion and advice for treatment

Intervention only makes sense if there are symptoms. Small collections that do not cause symptoms should be observed.

The accumulation of fluid in the pleural space is often associated with dyspnea, cough, and chest pain. Options include thoracentesis, chest-tube placement, video-assisted thoracoscopy (VATS) and pleurodesis (Covey, 2005). The pleural cavity needs to be thoroughly drained during pleurodesis, before instigating fibrosing substances. If there is a large residual effusion at the time a sclerosing agent is administered, the likelihood of success is low, and the possibility of turning a simple effusion into a multi-loculated collection requiring further interventions is high.

Chemical pleurodesis is achieved by instilling a sclerosing agent into the pleural space to incite an inflammatory reaction, which ultimately causes the visceral pleura to adhere to the parietal pleura, thereby eliminating the pleural space in which fluid can accumulate. Any cytotoxic effect will only affect the uppermost cellular layers. Disadvantages of local instillation therapy are possible pain on inspiration, and reformation of encapsulated collections, that are more difficult to access.

Most commonly used substances with success rates between 54% and 98% are bleomycine, tetracycline, mitoxantrone, fibrin and talkum. When tetracycline is used (10-20mg/kg body weight in 50mL solution), local and possibly systemic preventative pain medication is necessary.

Surgical pleurodesis with adhesion of both pleurae is sometimes the only option to treat particularly persistent breathlessness.

Bone metastasis

They are relatively rare. With localized pain, pain radiation therapy is indicated. Periphery-acting pain medications frequently have only short-term effects, if any at all. For this reason they should be administered very early together with long-term morphine preparations.

Systemic palliative therapies

Chemotherapies

Patients often confuse treatment "response" with "cure" and consequently do not fully comprehend the intent of clinical trials or palliative chemotherapy.

Many centres recommend chemotherapy only if the tumour measures more than 5cm, if there are symptoms, or if symptoms are being anticipated (Gore, 2001). Initial response to platinum-based first line therapy is important to decide on second line treatment. For this reason, platinum-responders and platinum-non-responders are distinguished.

Patients with platinum-resistant tumours do not benefit from another course of platinum-based chemotherapy. "Platinum-resistance" is defined as tumour progression after platinum-based initial therapy with less than six months relapse free interval. In these cases, prognosis is poor. Other chemotherapies may be tried. Etoposid, paclitaxel, docetaxel, topotecan, treosulfan, hexamathylmelamin, ifosfamid, liposomal doxorubicin, gemcitabin and others all have response rates around 20% (Ledermann and Wheeler, 2004). Combinations and high dose therapies are less successful. They are more toxic, impair quality of life and should therefore be avoided (Dunton, 2002). Quality of life data should be considered when choosing the chemotherapy regime.

Relapsing patients with platinum-sensitive tumours (remission after six months after primary, platinum-based treatment) will respond with 50% probability to a second cycle of platinum-based therapy. The longer the remission, the higher the success rate. Combination of paclitaxel or docetaxel with carboplatin further improves response rates.

Hormonal therapies

For patients who refuse chemotherapy or where side effects are prohibitive, hormonal therapy with anti-oestrogens, gestagens, GnRH-Analoga or androgens are an alternative. Response rates are superior to 20%.

Besides their disease stabilisation effect gestagens are also useful for tumour induced anorexia/cachexia. Megestrol acetate provides superior anorexia palliation among advanced cancer patients compared with dronabinol alone (Jatoi et al., 2002).

Immunotherapies

Numerous therapy forms are offered by various producers. They are supposed to improve non-specific immune functions and activate the body's own immune defenses against the tumour (**immunostimulants or immune modulators**). All these therapy options are based on widely speculative assumptions, do not appear very plausible from a theoretical standpoint and are not recognized by standard medicine. Their therapeutic effects on tumour are – if any – only minimal. Monoclonal antibodies and biological target therapies are opening up new therapeutic hopes due to their high tumour specificity; they differ from chemotherapy and radiation therapy by their completely different mode of action. Unfortunately, these therapy options, as with other innovative therapy forms, are still in the experimental stages; one cannot yet give information on actual pros and cons. Therefore these therapy options are only possible within the context of controlled randomized therapy studies.

Special features of pain therapy

See also chapter: "Pain management in cancer rehabilitation and palliation".

Long-acting opioids are preferable, and medications such as sustained-release patches might offer advantages because of their non-oral method of administration.

In addition to analgesics, tricyclic antidepressants (for example, amytryptilin long-acting initial dose 25mg/die with a maintenance dose of 50 to 75mg/die after five to seven days) and/or benzodiazepines, for an anxiolytic effect, can contribute to pain alleviation. Anxiety has an influence on pain intensity. Due to their sedative effects, these medications are best administered in the evening.

Colicky pain represents a different pain mechanism, which must be treated differently from continuous pain to achieve adequate analgesia. The colicky pain in malignant bowel obstruction is thought to be due to luminal spasms in conjunction with peristalsis converging on the site of obstruction. Agents with anti-cholinergic activity decrease smooth muscle tone and reduce peristalsis. Activation of muscarine receptors results in an additional beneficial decrease in intestinal fluid secretions (butyl-scopolamin).

Psychological pain management approaches capitalize on the interactions between mental symptoms and pain, and may help some cancer patients more than analgesics.

Chronic pain patients frequently suffer from insomnia, anxiety, hopelessness and despair. They are prone to depression. All these symptoms lower the pain threshold and result in more severe pain and a higher analgesic requirement. Psychosocial support should therefore always be considered as an adjunct pharmacotherapy.

Low dose of cortisone has pain relieving and anabolic effects and may sometimes have a positive effect on the patient's psychological state.

Complementary and alternative therapies

There is some support for the use of several modalities as potential complements to conventional cancer care, particularly for the quality of life issues associated with chronic cancer. For example, pain is a major problem for many cancer patients. There is much support for the use of hypnosis in managing pain associated with medical procedures and some support for its use in managing chronic cancer pain. There is less evidence to support the use of modalities such as acupuncture, meditation and massage for management of chronic pain. However, there are some compelling data to support the use of acupuncture for nausea and vomiting associated with cancer treatments, and some data suggest that qigong, neuro-emotional techniques, meditation techniques, and massage can decrease levels of pain and improve sense of well-being.

So far no scientific study has proved any tumour-inhibiting effects of mistletoe preparations. The assertion that the patient's quality of life can be improved through its use is very difficult to confirm. Yet these mistletoe preparations are not only used by those practising alternative and nature-oriented forms of medicine, but also by some oncologists. The reason for this is hardly the belief in its effectiveness, but rather the possibility of being able to offer the patient a further therapy option.

Experience has shown not only that "faith can move mountains", but that it can also improve the quality of life. One should not shatter these patients' faith in a particular therapy form with evidence-based arguments.

Ensuring the quality of rehabilitative and palliative measures

Rehabilitation in ovary cancer patients can only be achieved through the work of a qualified rehabilitation team (fig. 1.4). Special experience and a specialised infrastructure are essential. Due to the experience necessary, the rehabilitative institution should care for at least thirty ovary cancer patients per year. Verifiability of the quality of rehabilitation and palliative therapies must be guaranteed.

In rehabilitation and palliation it is not the team alone, but also the patient who takes on the task of assessing many treatment measures (Wan et al., 1997), although expectations of a successful palliative treatment are often very different in patients (Doyle et al., 2001). Many patients accept tumour therapy for reasons that are possibly quite different from those of the physicians who recommend it.

The evaluation of rehabilitative measures in tumour patients is directed not at survival time, but rather at quality of life criteria. This involves primarily subjective and objective parameters such as improvement of pain, appetite, weight, mobility, overcoming fears (table 7.12).

The evaluation of rehabilitative and supportive measures is much more difficult than checking the outcome of intervention procedures generally used in potentially curative follow-up care (length of recurrence free period, detection of early recurrence) and, of course, also the evaluation of the outcomes of curative measures taken in the context of primary therapy (for example, remission rates and remission length). Most of the existing trials place emphasis on response rate, which per se is not a direct measure of patient benefit. Justification for using such treatments for palliation would require that they offer some improvement in the quality of life (Doyle et al., 2001).

Quality of life questionnaires of the European Organization for Research and Treatment of Cancer (such as EORTC QLQ C-30) and the functional assessment of cancer therapy ovarian (Fact-O) can be used (Barat and Franchignoni, 2004). Both are internationally validated questionnaires and have been used in multiple studies. They are composed of multi-item scales and yes/no questions assessing physical, role functioning, cognitive, emotional, and social effects. The EORTC QLQ C-30 also includes symptom measures and a global health and QL scale. The ovary version of the FACT offers additional questions more specific to ovarian cancer.

Table 7.12 - Possible therapeutic aims and their effectiveness parameters in the rehabilitation of ovary carcinoma patients.

Therapeutic aims	Effectiveness parameters
Reduction of disorders resulting from surgery/chemotherapy/radiation therapy	WHO-toxicity scale, neurological examination including the sensory, motor, and autonomous system CTC-classification, examination of organ function. Questionnaires: FLIC, SIRO
Reduction of hormonal disturbances	Reduction of symptoms (e.g., hot flashes, fatigue, depressions, insomnia, etc.)
Pain relief	Pain diary, reduction of analgesic drugs, pain sensitivity scales. Questionnaires: Pain Disability Index (PDI), EORTC QLQ- C30, SE36, SDS, RSCL
Improvement of nutritional status	Symptoms, weight measurements, EORTC-questionnaire: FACT-CT
Sexuality, genetic counselling	Questionnaires
Improvement of physical fitness, activities of daily living	Ergometry, WHO- und EORTC-Performance-Status, walking distances, muscle force, vigorimeter. Questionnaires: (EORTC) LC-13, LC-13, FACT-Ct, FACT-An, KPS
Family member counselling	Questionnaires
Information on curative follow-up and rehabilitation/palliative measures	Questionnaires, tests
Reduction of anxiety, depression	Rating scales. Questionnaires: STAI, BDI, BSI, HADS-D, PAF, POMS
Coping with illness	Questionnaires : FKV, FKV-LIS, BEFO, TSK, FIBECK
Clarification and improvement of vocational fitness	Resumption of work, length of time of inability to work
Reduction of necessity of nursing care	Reduction of level of care. Questionnaires: Barthel Index, ADL, FIM
Relief of physical and psychological symptoms in the palliative situation	Questionnaire: POS

Abbreviations
PDI = Pain Disability Index; POMS = Profile Of Mood Status; POS= Palliative Care Outcome Scale; RSCL = Rotterdam-Symptom Checklist; SDS = Symptom Distress Scale; SF-36 = Medical Outcome Study Short Form-36; SIRO = Stress Index Radio Oncology; STAI = Spiegelberger Trait Anxiety Inventory; FACT-AN = Functional Assessment of Cancer Therapy Anemia; FIM = Funktional Independence Measure; FIBECK = Freiburger Inventar zur Bewältigung einer chronischen Erkrankung; HDS = Hospital Anxiety and Depression Scale; KPS = Karnofsky Performance Status; ADL = Activities of Daily Life; ECOG = European Cooperative Oncology Group-Scale

Different outcome scales in palliative care of cancer patients have been developed (Aspinal *et al.*, 2002; Bausewein *et al.*, 2005). The scales cover physical and psychological symptoms, spiritual considerations, practical concerns, emotional concerns of the patient and family, and psychosocial needs of the patient and family. The Palliative Care Outcome Scale (POS) is a multidimensional instrument covering these physical, psychosocial, spiritual, organizational, and practical concerns.

Rehabilitative care can be offered either on inpatient or outpatient basis. Carcinoma sufferers who have undergone surgery and chemotherapy are often weakened. For this reason, patients in Germany – as opposed to most other countries – are usually offered inpatient rehabilitation in specialised hospitals following primary therapy.

Basically, improvement in quality of life aimed at in rehabilitation is achieved when less nursing care is necessary ("rehabilitation to combat the need of care"), when the patient can be vocationally reintegrated ("rehabilitation to combat early retirement"), when he/she feels secure ("rehabilitation to combat resignation and depression") and when the patient's physical handicaps and functional limitations are at a minimum ("rehabilitation to combat disability").

Bibliography

- Antoniou, Pharoah AP, Narodet S *et al.* (2003) Average Risks of Breast and Ovarian Cancer Associated with BRCA1 or BRCA2 Mutations Detected in Case Series Unselected for Family History: A Combined Analysis of 22 Studies..Am J Hum Genet 72: 1117-30
- Aspinal F, Hughes R, Higginson I *et al.* (2002) A user's guide to the palliative care outcome scale. Palliative care & policy publications. Kings College, London
- Barat M, Franchignoni F (2004) Assessment in physical medicine and rehabilitation. Maugeri Foundation books PI-ME Press Pavia
- Bausewein C, Fegg M, Radbruch L *et al.* (2005) Validation and clinical application of the German version of the palliative care outcome. J Pain Symptom Manage 30: 51-62
- Bingham S, Riboli E (2004) Diet and Cancer. The European Prospective Investigation in Cancer and Nutrition. Nat Rev Cancer 4(3): 206-15
- Becker G, Galandi D, Blum HE (2006) Malignant ascites: Systematic review and guideline for treatment. Eur J Cancer 42: 589-97
- Bundesarbeitsgemeinschaft für Rehabilitation (2003) Rahmenempfehlungen zur ambulanten onkologischen Rehabilitation. Schriftenreihe der Bundesarbeitsgemeinschaft für Rehabilitation (BAR), Frankfurt
- Carmack Taylor C (2004) Predictors of sexual functioning in ovarian cancer patients, J Clin Oncol 22: 881-9
- Chanan-Khan A, Srinivasan S, Czucman M (2004) Prevention and management of cardiotoxicity from antineoplastic therapy. J Support Oncol 2: 251-66
- Classe JM, Catala L, Marchal F *et al.* (2004) Locoregional recurrence of ovarian cancer: The place of surgery. Bull Cancer 91, 11: 827-32
- Covey A (2005) Management of malignant pleural effusions and ascites. J Support Oncol 3: 169-76
- Dunton JC (2002) Management of treatment-related toxicity in advanced ovarian cancer. Oncologist 7: 11-9

- Doyle C, Crump M, Pintilie M *et al.* (2001) Does palliative chemotherapy palliate? Evaluation of expectations, outcomes, and costs in women receiving chemotherapy for advanced ovarian cancer
- Dubois A, Schlaich M *et al.* (1999) Evaluation of neurotoxicity induced by paclitaxel second-line chemotherapy. Support Care cancer 7: 354
- Faries MB, Romeau JL (1999) Use of gastrostomy- and combined gastrojejunostomy tubes for enteral feeding. World J Surg 23: 603-7
- Gore M (2001) Relapses epithelial ovarian cancer. ASCO educational book 37th annual meeting, 2001, 468-76
- Grueningen van V, Daly B (2005) Futility: clinical decisions at the end-of-life in women with ovarian cancer. Gynecol Oncol 97: 638-44
- IARC (2003) Handbook of cancer prevention, No 8: Fruits and vegetables. International Agency for Research on Cancer (IARC-WHO)
- Jatoi A, Windschitl H, Loprinzi C *et al.* (2002) Dronabinol Versus Megestrol Acetate Versus Combination Therapy for Cancer-Associated Anorexia. J Clin Oncol, 20, 2: 567-73
- Jatoi A, Podratz KC *et al.* (2004) Pathophysiology and palliation of inoperable bowel obstruction in patients with ovarian cancer. J Support Oncol 2: 323-37
- Junker A, Kretschmar A, Bohm U *et al.* (2004) Treatment of patients with intestinal cancer. Increased neurotoxicity after oxaliplatin and related liver metastasis. Med. Monatsschr Pharm 27, 10: 349-52
- Kuschel B, Lux M, Goecke T *et al.* (2000) Prevention and therapy for BRCA1/2 mutation carriers and women at high risk for breast and ovarian cancer. European Journal of Cancer Prevention 9, 3: 139-50
- Langseth H, Kjaerheim K (2004) Ovarian cancer and occupational exposure among pulp and paper employees in Norway. Scand J Work Environ Health 30, 5: 356-61
- Ledermann JA, Wheeler S (2004) How should we manage patients with "platinum sensitive" recurrent ovarian cancer? Cancer Invest 22, 2: 2-10
- Levy MH, Cohen SD (2005) Sedation for the relief of refractory symptoms in the imminently dying: A fine intentional line. Semin Oncol 32: 237-46
- Lim JF, Ho YH (2001) Total colectomy with ileorectal anastomosis leads to appreciable loss in quality of life. Techniques in coloproctology 5, 2: 79-83
- Mielke S, Sparreboom A, Mross K (2006) Peripheral neuropathy: A persisting challenge in paclitaxel-based regimens. Eur J Cancer 42: 24-30
- Norton TR, Manne SL, Rubin S *et al.* (2004) Prevalence and predictors of psychological distress among women with ovarian cancer. J Clin Oncol 1, 22, 5: 919-26
- Parsons SL, Lang M, Steele R (1996) Malignant ascites. Eur J Surg Oncol 22: 237-9
- Paice J (2003) Mechanisms and mamagement of neuropathic pain in cancer. J support Oncol 1, 2: 107-14
- Pothuri B, Guirguis A, Gerdes H *et al.* (2004) The use of colorectal stents for palliation of large bowel obstruction due to recurrent gynaecologic cancer. Gynecol Oncol 95 (3): 513-7
- Pothuri B, Meyer L, Gerardi M *et al.* (2004) Reoperation for palliation of recurrent malignant bowel obstruction in ovarian carcinoma. Gynecol Oncol 95, 1: 193-5
- Schover L (2005) Sexuality and fertility after cancer. The American society of Hematology
- Sood AK, Lush R, Geisler JP *et al.* (2004) Sequential intraperitoneal topotecan and oral chemotherapy in recurrent platinum-resistant ovarian carcinoma. Clin Cancer Res 15, 10: 6080-5

– Stewart D, Cheung A, Dancey J *et al.* (2000) Information needs and decisional preferences among women with ovarian cancer. Gynecol Oncol 77, 3: 357-61
– Sun C, Ramirez P, Bodurka D (2007) Quality of life for patients with epithelial ovarian cancer. Nat Clin Pract Oncol 4, 1: 18-29
– Vadaparampil ST, Wey JP, Kinney AY (2004) Psychosocial aspects of genetic counselling and testing. Semin Oncol Nurs 20, 3: 186-95
– Wan GJ, Counte MA, Cella DF (1997) The influence of personal expectations on cancer patients' reports of health related quality of life. Psycho-oncology 6: 1-11
– Watson M, Forster C, Eccles D *et al.* (2004) Psychosocial impact of breast/ovarian (BRCA1/2) cancer-predictive genetic testing in a genetic testing in a U.K. multi-centre clinical cohort.
– Watson T, Mock V (2004) Exercise as an intervention for cancer related fatigue. Phys Ther 84: 736-43
– World Health Organization (2001) International classification of functioning, disabilities and health. www. who.int/classification/ICF

Rehabilitation and palliation of patients with gastric cancer

Aims of rehabilitation and palliation: Definition as distinct from curative tumour follow-up care

Measures taken in order to lengthen survival time (potentially curative follow-up care – prophylaxis, early detection and therapy of disease recurrence), as well as those measures concerned with improving quality of life (rehabilitative and palliative follow-up care) represent the focus in the follow-up care of patients with gastric cancer (fig. 1.1).

With **potentially curative follow-up care**, the main emphasis is placed on controlling the disease. The use of these follow-up care measures is however more than controversial. Thus, the value of adjuvant therapy, administered prophylactically to prevent recurrence, is viewed critically. Routine diagnostics for detecting disease recurrence have curative therapeutic consequences only in rare cases, and therapies designed to treat recurrences tend to be palliative rather than curative in nature.

The value of **palliative and rehabilitative follow-up care** is unambiguous, as opposed to the term of potentially curative follow-up care. In contrast to curative therapy, it is not the controlling of the disease which represents the focus of all efforts, but rather, it is the minimization of tumour mass and therapy-related disability which constitutes the aim of therapeutic procedures. The negative effects of disease and therapy in physical, psychological, social and vocational areas are to be eliminated or at least mitigated (tables 1.5, 1.6, 1.12, 1.14 and fig. 2).

It is not so much the length of survival time as the quality of the remaining time which is to be influenced positively by means of rehabilitative and palliative measures. The requirements for the necessary therapeutic methods during rehabilitation are primarily dependent on the limitations of quality of life and not, as with curative therapy, on the extent, risk of recurrence and prognosis of the disease.

Rehabilitative measures

Rehabilitation can be considered for patients undergoing potentially curative as well as palliative treatment. It consists of somatic, psychological, social and vocational assistance. An acceptable amount of information on the disease status is a prerequisite before initiating rehabilitative measures (table 8.1). Without this information, valuable time is wasted in performing additional research, thus threatening the success of rehabilitation. Dietary consultation would be difficult, psychological care would be unsatisfying and a social-medical assessment, with the introduction of social and occupational aids, would have questionable relevance.

Table 8.1 - Minimum amount of information prior to rehabilitation in gastric cancer patients.

– Extent of tumour including grading tumour resection (whether R0, R1 or R2 resection?)
– Surgical procedures (for example, with or without stomach substitute or interposed colon segment?)
– Curative or palliative therapeutic approaches?
– Progression of tumour growth, location and extent of tumour metastases?
– Psychosocial information (for example, information on the degree to which the patient is informed, on any existing problems with coping and compliance, on support offered by family members, on social and occupational problems, etc.)

Before carrying out rehabilitative measures (tables 1.12, 1.13) a rehabilitative assessment must take place, with rehabilitation planning and documentation of the goals to be achieved (tables 1.6, 1.7, 1.8, 1.10). Here, the consequences of stomach surgery constitute the main focus (table 8.2, 8.3).

Table 8.2 - Rehabilitative problems in gastric cancer patients.

– Effects of partial or total gastrectomy (postgastrectomy symptoms)
– Effects of chemotherapy (for example, polyneuropathy, cardiac disturbances)
– Alterations in pharmacokinetics
– Anemia
– Osteopathy
– Lack of information/need for information
– Psychological strain/anxiety disorders
– Social difficulties
– Dependence on nursing care
– Inability to perform work/pursue profession

Table 8.3 - Physical impairments after gastric resection.

– Nutritional problems (weight loss, malabsorption, malassimilation)
– Reflux problems (oesophagitis, reflux gastritis)
– Dumping syndrome (early, late dumping)
– Anemia (hypochrom, hyperchromic anamia)
– Diarrhea
– Osteopathies

Rehabilitative measures aiming at reducing physical problems ("rehabilitation in order to combat disability")

Physical impairments are often faced in the presence of extensive comorbidities and polypharmaceutical therapies in older patients.

Nutrition deficiencies and dietary advice

A connection between certain eating habits and increased risk of gastric cancer is very likely (Riboli, 2002). Recommendations resulting from this knowledge do not, however, apply to the specific risk of recurring illness. Development of recurrent disease and the further course of illness take place in conditions different from those present in the case of primary tumours. Therefore, dietary counselling is not to be performed according to the standards of a general "diet for cancer prevention," but, rather, it is the individual's symptoms and complaints – postgastrectomy symptoms – which comprise the basis for nutritional advice.

A typical example of inadequate dietary counselling is the often-heard general advice to eat small frequent meals, without any other limitation. Such recommendations cannot possibly meet the needs of patients displaying a diverse assortment of complaints, depending on their respective anatomical situations. General dietary recommendations (table 8.4) are often simply inadequate.

Abnormal transit, insufficient general nutrition and micronutrient deficiencies are the most common problems. The main resulting symptoms are early and late dumping syndromes, reflux œsophagitis, weight loss, anemia and osteopathy. Dietary measures, in rare cases, repeated surgery, and in particular adequate follow-up of metabolic and nutritional parameters with regular substitution, are the chief therapeutic necessities (Schölmerich, 2004). The patients' complaints are varied, which is not so much due to individual sensitivity as to the implemented surgical procedure.

Thus, patients who have undergone partial resection have, as a rule, different and fewer nutritional difficulties than those who have undergone total gastrectomy. Patients with anastomosis carcinoma have comparatively fewer problems due to pre-existing adaptation to the smaller gastric reservoir. In the case of an upper partial resection, difficulties which arise will be different from those following the Billroth I or II resection. Patients having undergone gastrectomy may also display different symptoms or complaints depending on the surgical technique employed.

Table 8.4 - General recommendations following total stomach resection.

– Eat slowly
– Chew well
– Eat six-ten meals a day (in the first six months following surgery)
– Eat foods with low volume and high energy
– Drink liquids between mealtimes and not during mealtimes (in the first six months following surgery)
– Avoid foods which are very hot or cold, are heavily smoked or cured or grilled
– Avoid very sweet or very salty foods
– Avoid carbonated drinks
– Use hygienic utensils and dishes
– Take in at least 50 kcal/kg body weight
– Eat complex carbohydrates rather than simple sugars
– Eat foods rich in vitamin C and calcium
– Eat easy-to-digest proteins
– Eat foods and prepared foods low in fat (about 30% fat and in some cases medium-length triglycerides)
– Raise the head of the bed 10 to 15cm (use a wedge pillow), do not eat lying down. (exception: dumping problems)

Weight loss and advice

Weight loss is among the most common complaints (Schölmerich, 2004). Quality of life and reintegration into the social and occupational environment are negatively affected by this symptom. The patient's ensuing condition of weakness can help contribute to the development of other illnesses.

In many patients who have undergone gastric resection, weight loss has already occurred before the surgery. Weight loss is virtually unavoidable following gastrectomy. It is more extreme after total gastrectomy than after partial gastrectomy. In the case of the latter, weight gain is often reestablished at a later point during the postoperative course: In some cases, normal weight is even achieved. Following total gastrectomy, weight gain is greatly delayed, if present at all. The former normal weight is attained only in exceptional cases in patients who have undergone gastrectomy.

Several factors are responsible for weight loss (table 8.5) and are to be considered when giving nutritional advice.

Nutritional therapeutic guidance and counselling are of great importance for keeping weight loss at a minimum. Consequent dietary counselling with an emphasis on the highest possible caloric intake and weight gain is, however, dangerous. Instead, foods must have the proper composition with regard to protein, fat, carbohydrates, vitamins and minerals. The average energy intake should be at least 35-50kcal/kg body weight: Here, the increased requirements for calcium, iron and vitamins are to be taken into consideration.

Increased fat intake would lead to weight loss rather than weight gain, due to the asynchronous release of pancreatic enzymes and food passage which together are responsible for inadequate fat metabolism (pancreocibal asynchrony). Lipids render food utilization more difficult: For this reason, fat intake should be kept as low as possible directly following surgery. Steatorrhea should always be ruled out in cases of weight loss; probatory administration of pancreatin preparations is advised.

As a result of weight loss, dental prostheses often no longer fit properly, cause pain and interfere with food intake. All gastrectomy patients should therefore undergo refitting for dental prostheses.

Table 8.5 - Possible causes of weight loss in potentially curatively resected gastric carcinoma patients.

– Decreased food intake due to lack of appetite
– Decreased food intake due to fear of pain
– Malassimilation
– One-sided and incorrect nutrition
– Relative (secondary) pancreatic insufficiency (with pancreocibal asynchron)
– Colonization of the small intestine by harmful bacteria (with afferent loop syndrome)
– Dysphagia following truncal vagotomy

Gastric emptying syndrome and advice

Disturbances in motility or even gastric atonia can occur, primarily in the early postoperative phase. Motor activity, secretion and resorption of the gastro-intestinal tract have not yet become accustomed to the surgically altered situation. A differential diagnosis which should always be considered is a possible stenosis in the region of the anastomosis and in the proximal jejunum. This can be organic or functional in nature and can arise in the early as well as in the later postoperative phases. Occlusion of the gastric outlet due to edema is also not uncommon during the first few months following surgery.

Before therapy takes place, it must be ascertained whether a mechanical obstruction is present, whether the peritoneum is affected or if extended primary atonia is present. In the case of mechanical obstruction, the obstacle must be removed by endoscopic or, if necessary, by surgical means. In the case of extended primary atonia, mobility-influencing means should be employed; with peritoneal carcinosis, therapy attempts should be made using cytostatic agents.

Dumping syndrome and advice

The term "dumping syndrome" encompasses two symptom complexes which differ as to symptoms, etiology and timing of occurrence:
– So-called early dumping syndrome, also referred to as postalimentary early syndrome;
– Late dumping syndrome, a better name is reactive postalimentary hypoglycemia.

Both syndromes occur more frequently in patients who have undergone gastrectomy than those with partial gastrectomy; their frequency and intensity are influenced in addition by the postoperative time interval. After partial resection has taken place, the size of the residual stomach and the width of the anastomosis are of significance.

The smaller the residual stomach, the higher the risk of **early dumping**. A drop in blood pressure, due to the physiologically unnatural rapid pouring of liquids into the small intestine which is filled with chyme, is responsible for the symptoms of early dumping (table 8.6).

Table 8.6 - Symptoms associated with early dumping.

– Feeling of being full/abdominal pain
– Drop in blood pressure
– Profuse sweating
– Tachycardia
– Heat flashes
– Nausea
– Fainting
– Diarrhea

Dietetic measures are of critical importance (table 8.7). In the case of early dumping they are directed towards the accelerated gastric emptying and/or towards the excessively high osmotic action of the food ingested. In patients with extreme symptoms it is advised in some cases to take meals lying down or to lie down immediately following meals in order to prevent the rapid transport of chyme into the small intestine. Patients should not drink during or immediately following a meal. Early dumping is nearly always associated with inadequate mixing of chyme with pancreatic enzymes (relative pancreatic insufficiency), for which reason the administration of pancreatic enzymes is obligatory.

Table 8.7 - Recommendations for gastric resection patients for avoiding dumping symptoms.

Warnings	Recommendations
No liquids during or immediately following meals	Consumption of liquids before or between meals
No hasty mealtimes	Eating slowly, chewing thoroughly
No physical exercise after the meals	Periods of rest after meals
No voluminous meals	Meals taken in a position with head elevated
No easlily broken down carbohydrates	Six to eight small meals
No highly carbonated water and tea	Drinks and foods at normal temperatures
No concentrated sugar	In cases of lactose intolerance no milk, cheese, yogurt
No salty, hot and spicy food	

Late dumping and advice

A drop in blood sugar level due to a reactive temporary hyperinsulinism and participation of other hormones such as GIP or enteroglucagon are being discussed as causes of late dumping. Initially there is rapid filling of the small intestine with large, primarily easily absorbed quantities of carbohydrates and consecutive unphysiological hyperglycemia with increased release of insulin. Symptoms are similar to those of early dumping. A "craving for sugar" is relatively rare.

With late dumping, an improvement in the symptoms is achieved by avoiding the ingestion of easily absorbed carbohydrates. At any rate, their relative quantity in relation to the whole meal should be reduced. In theory, eating fibers such as pectin or guar is helpful, as this delays glucose absorption. In practice, however, fiber and acarbose are often not well tolerated by gastrectomy patients. It is helpful to eat a snack one hour after a meal in order to prevent a situation of hypoglycemia.

Pancreatin substitution in a non-acid-protected form (granulate) is indicated in cases of early dumping as well as late dumping due to the late or inadequately occurring exocrine pancreatic enzyme secretion and a too brief period of time spent by nutrients in the small intestine. Dumping-specific symptoms will most likely not be positively influenced by these measures. However, the nutrition-utilization disturbances and deficiencies which necessarily arise due to the pancreocibal asynchrony may be ameliorated.

Afferent loop syndrome and advice

Complaints are observed only in B2 resection patients. Two syndromes are to be distinguished: Afferent loop syndrome type I and blind loop syndrome type II. Therapy entails elimination of the cause. It is often necessary to convert a Billroth II to Billroth I or to make a Braun's anastomosis.

Reflux oesophagitis and advice

Many gastrectomy patients report difficulty swallowing, pain on swallowing and heartburn. Even in the absence of symptoms, this should be considered when observing nutrition and everyday activities and behaviour, since a clinically occult reflux problem nearly always exists. Total gastrectomy patients are at greater risk than partially resected patients.

While stomach acid-related reflux (acid reflux oesophagitis) can be present (but does not necessarily have to be) in partial gastrectomy patients, reflux following total gastrectomy is invariably caused by reflux of bile and intestinal fluids containing digestive juices (alkaline reflux oesophagitis). After a proximal resection, acid reflux oesophagitis is quite common. Chronification of reflux oesophagitis leads to fibrosis, scarring and later to stenosis of the oesophagus; food passage becomes more and more difficult and finally, in advanced stages, impossible. The cause of the reflux symptoms lies in the loss of the important anti-reflux barriers, the oesophagus sphincter and pylorus; however, the manometrically quantifiable disturbance in motility of the remaining portion of the oesophagus is also significant.

A third form of reflux oesophagitis caused by the backward flow of gastric secretions and/or contents of the duodenum, including bile and pancreatic secretions, which is etiologically and above all therapeutically distinct from the other forms, is due to stenosis or duodenal atonia. This condition may be associated with organic as well as functional causes.

Observing dietetic recommendations and non-medicinal general measures (table 4.7) make up the basis of treatment of all three forms of reflux oesophagitis. H2 inhibitors do not help, unless it is a case of symptoms following proximal partial resection. Eating pureed rice mixed with a small amount of water and a packet of acid-binding antacid will ease acute pain.

The mixture gives rise to the formation of a protective film covering the mucus membrane. Pharmaceuticals that enhance gastric motility (i.e., metoclopramide) are useful when the oesophagitis is a result of slowed food transport. Metoclopamide should be taken approximately 20 minutes before mealtimes.

If stenosis is the cause of the problem, then such medication is contraindicated. Then, a dilatation must be performed. If the oesophago-gastric closure mechanism is no longer effective, as for example is the case following a proximal resection or gastrectomy, then raising the head of the bed (wedge pillow) at least 10 to 15cm can alleviate the symptoms in many patients, even if it is the sole measure taken.

For the prevention of alkaline reflux in gastrectomy patients, the unimpeded drainage of duodenal secretions is of critical importance. This can be attained either by means of a Roux-en-y anastomosis or an interposed jejunum segment which is at least 40cm long in which the reflux exhausts itself. Since the introduction of the Roux-en-Y reconstruction technique with the drainage of duodenal contents, alkaline reflux oesophagitis as a late complication of gastrectomy has become considerably less common. The length of the inactivated loop of jejunum, or the length of the interposed segment, and thus the distance between the papilla of Vateri and the oesophagus, plays a major role.

Reflux gastritis and advice

Surgical removal of the pylorus necessarily increases the risk of reflux of aggressive duodenal contents into the residual stomach. This type of reflux gastritis typically involves morning nausea, sometimes vomiting of bitter, clear yellow liquid. During the course of the day the symptoms generally become milder. Taking as many small meals as possible alleviates the symptoms. It is also recommended that a snack be taken during the night. If symptoms persist, an attempt can be made with motility-enhancing preparations (for example, metoclopramide) or bile acid neutralizing medications (for example, cholestyramin).

Maldigestion, malabsorption and advice

Following total gastrectomy, most patients develop maldigestion and weight loss which may improve spontaneously after a certain period of adaptation. Many symptoms, not least of all extreme weight loss, are a result of the maldigestion. Flatulence is usually a result of incomplete breakdown of nutrients. Diarrhea and sour-smelling stools are an indication of incomplete fat digestion.

After a total gastrectomy, patients lose lipids in the stool in about 9 to 24% of the cases, nitrogen loss as a measure of protein absorption disturbances is 6 to 26%, which corresponds to a total calorie loss of 65 to a maximum of 500kcal. This, among other causes, explains the extreme weight loss so often observed in gastrectomy patients.

Numerous works make reference to malabsorption of separate nutrients. Besides the colonization of the small intestine by harmful bacteria and rapid passage of food components, exocrine pancreatic function disorders also represent a possible pathological mechanism which contributes to disturbed digestive function (Friess *et al.*, 1996). This is a relative functional disorder, as the pancreatic function is actually intact; however, the mechanisms leading to the release of pancreatin are disturbed.

In order to compensate for this relative pancreatic functional disorder, and with the aim of improving digestion of lipids and thus general nutrient utilization, pancreatic enzymes – in a non-acid-protected form (granulate) – should always be taken at the beginning of meals for at least the first few months following gastrectomy. Capsules run the risk of not being absorbed. As a rule, it makes sense to substitute pancreatic enzymes for at least the first six to eight postoperative months; subsequent to this, clinical symptoms and laboratory diagnostics determine the further course.

A simple means of achieving pancreatic enzyme secretion and mixing of chyme at the right time is the "Mestrom lipid cocktail" (Mestrom, 1998). Approximately five minutes before taking a meal the gastrectomy patient is to chew on a piece of zwieback toast spread thinly with butter.

Alterations in pharmacokinetics and advice

As a result of the removal of the stomach it is clear that acid blockers can no longer work following gastrectomy. It is more difficult to answer the question of possible alterations with respect to resorption of drugs and pharmacokinetics following partial and/or total gastrectomy. There are amazingly few studies pertaining to this subject. In individual cases the drug level has to be measured in the blood.

The often decreased duration of food passage would also seem to be associated with altered resorption of certain drugs. Due to the reduced or completely absent acid secretion following total or partial gastric resection, the resorption of drugs is either reduced (for example, with weak acids) or increased (for example, in the case of unstable acidic substances). This and the altered time spent by orally administered substances can affect the absorption and interaction of drugs. It has been established that oral antibiotics which normally display a rapid rise in the blood level should be avoided (Nell, 1991). The absence of acid should be taken into account when administering the various pancreatin preparations.

Weight loss and the altered resorption of medications and pharmacokinetics and the altered insulin level resulting from pancreocibal asynchrony often necessitate a readjustment of diabetes therapy. Patients with type 2 diabetes are not infrequently able to do without oral antidiabetics after surgery. With type 1 diabetes, the blood sugar level can fluctuate dramatically. More frequent blood sugar measurements are necessary; an intensified insulin chart is recommended and in young patients, an insulin pump.

Diarrhea and advice

Several factors are to be considered as the cause of frequently occurring diarrhea in partial resection as well as in total gastrectomy patients. They are: dumping syndrome, lactose intolerance, food intolerance, the absent acid barrier, reflex hyperperistalsis and inadequate lipid breakdown due to pancreocibal asynchrony. The rate of passage is always accelerated when lipids or proteins delay emptying.

Frequency and severity of diarrhea correlate with the length of the postoperative time interval. Proper dietary guidance is often the best contribution to prophylaxis and therapy. Following a low-fat regimen and taking pancreatic enzyme preparations are recommended when pancreocibal asynchrony is the cause. An improvement can be achieved by means of a diet low in lactose if secondary lactose intolerance is present. This condition quite often does not manifest itself until after gastric resection and is due to the shortened transit time of chyme in the small intestine.

A common cause of postoperative diarrhea is the removal of the vagal nerve. This type of diarrhea is quite common in the first weeks following surgery, but it then usually disappears spontaneously as more time passes after the surgery. If dietary means of controlling diarrhea have been exhausted and the condition persists, codeine drops, loperamide or other motility-reducing preparations may be indicated.

Anemia and advice

One of the most common causes for subjective and physical weakness is anemia (table 8.8). It can be tumour-associated, it can occur as a result of chemotherapy or radiation therapy, or in connection with bone marrow infiltration, hemolysis or can be nutrition-dependent. Considerable improvement in the patients' physical status may be achieved by raising the hemoglobin level. A target hemoglobin level of at least 12-13g/dL should be set.

Table 8.8 - Functional consequences of anemia.

– Physical functioning
– Cognitive functioning
– Social functioning
– Emotional functioning
– Role functioning
– Fatigue

In recipients of gastric cancer surgery, there is often hypochromic anemia present, due to blood loss. In this case iron should be administered intravenously. Blood transfusions are only necessary in cases of acute and severe symptoms.

The administration of erythropoetin is indicated for chemotherapy or radiation therapy-related anemia. Treatment should be continued as long as Hb levels are inferior to 12 g/dL. Iron should be given additionally when transferrin saturation is inferior to 20%, ferritin is inferior to 100 micrograms and the proportion of hypochromic erythrocytes superior to 20%. Erythropoetin is indeed effective in cases of anemia due to bone marrow infiltration as well; however, cytostatic or radiation therapies would generally be the preferred treatment in this case.

Hyperchromic anemia may arise in gastric surgery patients. Its appearance depends on the extent of resection, the level of preoperative B12 reserves, the condition of atrophy of the residual gastric mucosa as well as on whether or not an anastomosis is present. In partially resected patients this may occur only if atrophic gastritis was present preoperatively (which is relatively common) or if the residual stomach is very small. The reserve capacity of a healthy adult's stomach for B12 is three to five years; this is however much shorter in the majority of gastric cancer patients. One reason for this is the fact that patients with gastric cancer often suffered from atrophic gastritis long time before atrophic gastritis. Substitution of vitamin B12 is to be carried out for the rest of the patient's life at approximately three month intervals. Taking vitamin B12 orally is completely ineffective. Regular blood checks are required.

Hypochromic anemia is generally the result of chronic blood loss due to the tumour or as a result of surgery. In several cases, patients have already had chronic oozing of blood from the stomach as well as hypochromic anemia before surgery; others have had vitamin B12 deficiency and at least latent hyperchromic anemia due to atrophic gastritis (Roviello *et al.*, 2004). Following successful surgery, the situation gradually improves with time leading to spontaneous recovery. Substitution of iron is only necessary in the case of iron deficiency, if iron reserves are depleted and if malabsorption of dietary iron has been proven to exist at the same time. Previous determination of serum iron, serum ferritin and endoscopic examination in order to rule out bleeding are therefore indispensable. In most patients, normalization of the low serum iron levels occurs quite soon without requiring iron substitution.

Osteopathy and advice

It has been generally known for several years, that illnesses of the skeletal system may occur as a long-term complication following gastric resection. The pathophysiology leading to this is complex (Heiskanen *et al.*, 2001). While the calcium salt content of the radius is reduced after a period of ten years in gastric partial resection patients by a percentage of 25%, this percentage is 56% following gastrectomy. Women are at higher risk than men. The cause of osteomalacia is vitamin D deficiency which is due to the disturbed absorption of lipids and thus of fat-soluble vitamins. In addition, frequently-occurring milk and dairy product intolerance with consequent calcium deficiency also play a role.

Proper dietary guidance and counselling make a major contribution towards prevention of this condition. Milk and dairy products are especially high in calcium. As many gastrectomy patients develop clinically relevant lactase insufficiency and do not tolerate milk products, calcium should come from other sources such as cheese, whole milk yogurt, buttermilk or kefir. Milk tolerance can be improved by administering lactase.

In addition to this, the intramuscular injection of vitamin D is recommended for all gastrectomy patients at six-month intervals. It is to be assumed that osteomalacia can be prevented through the substitution of pancreatic enzymes and the consequent improved absorption of fat-soluble vitamins. Daily substitution using calcium tablets containing 800 to 1,500 milligrams as well as 500 units of vitamin D represent an alternative to vitamin D injections.

Polyneuropathy and advice

See also chapter on ovarian carcinoma.

Some of the neoadjuvant, additive or adjuvant forms of chemotherapy give rise to neuropathy which greatly affects the quality of life of patients afflicted with this condition. Unambiguous proof of effectiveness of vitamin B preparations has not yet been provided either for the therapy or for the prophylaxis of this chemotherapy-induced neuropathy. Electrotherapy (Stanger baths) can bring about at least temporary improvement in symptoms. Anticonvulsants such as gabapentine and carbamazepine often alleviate pain; however, they also have adverse effects. Polyneuropathy can also occur independently of chemotherapy, due to thiamine deficiency from poor nutrition. Sensorimotor disorders are for the most part similar to those displayed in cases of beriberi (Koike *et al.*, 2004). In this case, substitution with vitamin B complex can be helpful.

Immobility and physiotherapy

When compared to dietetics, substitution therapy and supportive measures, physical therapy tends to play only a minor role in gastric cancer patients. It can, however, contribute to physical recovery. It constitutes part of the total concept within the context of inpatient gastric cancer follow-up treatment.

Adhesions of scars with subcutaneous tissue can be prevented through massage of the scars according to the techniques of connective tissue massage. Use of ultrasound treatment can exert a favourable influence on scar development. With physical therapy, elements of weight training are incorporated, step by step, into the patient's mobilization training. It is begun with isometric strength exercises, continuing with gradually increasing auxotonic or isotonic muscle exercises primarily for the extremities and concluding with the introduction of coordination exercises into the physical therapy plan as the patient continues to gain strength and recover his/her health.

Tension in the abdominal muscles with the accompanying risk of reflux of the small intestine's contents into the œsophagus should be avoided during any gymnastic exercises. Following gastrectomy, massages are best carried out in a sitting position; when lying down, the patient should have his/her upper body slightly elevated.

Necessity of information and patient education (discussion groups and health education)

Explanation and information are important aids in helping to cope with the disease. This involves the patient's understanding of what is happening in his/her body and why a certain form of therapy has been suggested. The majority of patients do not wish to make decisions about tumour therapy themselves, but would like to know the reasons for pursuing a certain treatment strategy.

In gastric cancer patients, health training is of special importance. The intensive inclusion of patients in the planning of their health training has been shown to increase motivation (tables 2.12 and 8.9). It is the aim of health training to explain possibilities and limitations of standard medicine, to protect patients from harmful alternative therapy forms, as well as to convey to them the usefulness and necessity of follow-up exams.

Table 8.9 - Topics in health education for gastric cancer patients.

Prophylactic measures
– Adjuvant therapy (when and why is it needed, which therapy)
– Prevention or reduction of chemotherapy / hormone / radiation therapy side effects
– Significance of follow-up examinations
– Recurrence (prophylaxis, signs and therapy in cases of recurrence)
– Prognosis
– Significance of immune resistance

Nutrition
– Weight loss (causes and prevention)
– Most common nutritional disorders
– Postgastrectomy complaints
– Different forms of nutrition for the individual postgastrectomy symptoms
– Is there a "cancer diet"?
– Healthy diet

Psychological aids
– Opportunities for relaxation, overcoming fears, depression, fatigue
– References to psychological assistance
– Dealing with family members

Social aids
– Information pertaining to legal protection measures for cancer patients
– Information pertaining to financial reductions
– Insurance, life insurance, granting of loans, loan payment
– Information on self-help groups, hospice, palliative wards

Vocational counselling and aids
– Occupational consequences
– Avoidance of certain types of work-related strain
– Measures and aids for successful vocational reintegration

Family members should also be allowed to participate. Health education takes place in groups in which psychologists, dietary advisors, physicians and social workers all take turns moderating the groups. An educational program separate from the health education program should be set up for gastrectomy patients and their family members under the guidance of a physician or dietary advisor experienced in the field of nutritional therapy. It has also been proven to be helpful for those patients who have undergone surgery recently to meet with others who have had the same surgery several years earlier.

It is useful for patients and their family members also to have access to printed versions of the information and advice which they have received in health education sessions (for example, in the form of differentiated and industry-unaffiliated self-help literature) (Delbrück, 2005). This printed material should of course never take the place of medical consultations, but rather, it should provide the basis of productive discussions with the attending physician.

Patients are more and more often finding information themselves, using literature, the Internet and other media, on the unfavourable prognosis of their disease. It is often difficult for the laymen to recognize whether the information available is serious. It is useful if the physician can recommend certain Internet sites that he/she considers to be serious, informative and helpful. Further, explanatory information and – in particular – assistance in dealing with this information are necessary. These may be given to patients in health education within the context of a one-on-one meeting or in a group discussion. The interested patient and his/her family members should be referred to Internet addresses which in the physician's opinion are informative, useful and serious.

Rehabilitative measures aiming at reducing psychological problems ("rehabilitation to combat resignation and depression")

See also chapter: "Psychological support in cancer rehabilitation and palliation".

Necessity of psychological support

Besides the tumour illness, which threatens the patient's life, the fear of social and occupational handicaps and postgastrectomy symptoms with their nutritional problems in particular are often the cause of depression. They may be alleviated by proper dietary counselling.

Specialized psychotherapeutic guidance provided by the pycho-oncologist may also be necessary in individual cases, as help is less and less often provided by the patient's family members, who themselves quite frequently require psychosocial support. Depression, cognitive impairments and fatigue can be symptoms of anemia.

The positive influence of erythropoietin on these symptoms with low Hb has been proved.

Depressions

Certain "disturbances in the state of health" such as resignation, depression, self-isolation, lack of motivation and loss of personal contacts are observed particularly frequently. Encouragement of compliance, coping and activation are chief tasks of psycho-oncological guidance. The basic attitude of resignation of affected persons must be overcome.

It is important that it is conveyed to the patient that he or she, as a responsible person and citizen, has a place in society as a whole and in the immediate social surroundings. The positive emotional feelings of having a place in the family and in society and still being able to take on responsibility and give happiness to others are of utmost importance.

Fears

Fears of progress and the uncertain future are frequent. It is the task of the physician and the psycho-oncologist to deal with these fears (table 2.4 and 2.5). Medicinal support may be considered, but it cannot replace cognitive therapy.

Fatigue syndrome

See also chapter : "Psychological support in cancer rehabilitation and palliation".

When patients have symptoms suggestive of a fatigue syndrome, one should consider physical causes primarily rather than psychological causes (table 2.8). Thus, the physician and the dietary consultant play a larger role than the pycho-oncologist in the treatment of this condition. If anemia is the cause, a physiological increase of hemoglobin with erythropoetin can lead to improvement. Some centres successfully use megestrol acetate for the treatment of both emaciation and fatigue symptoms.

Rehabilitative measures aiming at reducing social problems ("rehabilitation to combat the need for care")

See also chapter: "Social support in rehabilitation and palliation".

Need of social support

The aim of these measures is to strengthen the patient's own resources and prevent the risk of a need for care, or at least reduce such a need (tables 3.2 and 3.12). By these means, the patient's risk of requiring nursing care is to be eliminated or at least reduced. If independent care is no longer possible, appropriate nursing care must be provided.

It is often the case that some people (usually older) already have difficulty maintaining their household due to their advanced age; self-care at home is further endangered in many cases because of additional illness and therapy-related strain.

Different forms of care assistance such as "meals on wheels", household assistance, nursing assistance, home nursing care and in some cases living in a nursing home or hospice program (table 1.15) have to be organized with the participation of family members. It is necessary to provide contact addresses (self-help groups, counselling locations, etc.).

Organization of outside assistance

If home care cannot or cannot yet be guaranteed, a temporary stay in a clinic for follow-up care can be provided. In Germany, there are rehabilitation clinics which are specialized to meet the needs of patients with gastro-intestinal tumours and which, besides providing accompanying medical follow-up care, also help to plan for further social assistance (AHB clinics). In France some *"maisons de repos"*, and in Italy the bridge clinics, have similar functions.

A subsequent **stay in a rehabilitation hospital** (AHB-hospital), directly following the standard hospital stay, is recommended for all patients in Germany. In Germany and France, these institutions have emerged from earlier tuberculosis institution situated in picturesque and out-of-the-way regions. Unfortunately, this distance from populated areas tends to defeat the socialization aims of rehabilitation programs.

In Germany, there is a special mandatory disability insurance which is set up to meet the financial demands in the case of a patient's needing nursing care. A patient is granted financial aid provided by an **insurance for nursing care** only when the need for care has existed for at least six months.

Procuring information about questions concerning medical care, nursing care, socio-legal issues, and practical issues: legally defined privileges for cancer patients

Assistance in social care is available in most countries. Cancer patients in most European countries are subject to legal privileges, ranging from tax reductions, financial grants, free use of public transport and a vocational protection against wrongful dismissal (see also chapter "Social support in cancer rehabilitation and palliation"). In addition to psychological support, **self-help groups** often provide their members with specific knowledge about medications and resources as well as social laws.

Rehabilitative measures aiming at reducing vocational problems ("rehabilitation to combat early retirement")

See also chapter: "Vocational integration in cancer rehabilitation".

Harmful occupational substances

Until now, there are no known correlations between certain harmful occupational substances and gastric cancer. Working *per se* has no influence on the risk of disease recurrence or prognosis (Zakharian *et al.*, 1994), although gastric cancer is observed particularly frequently in certain occupational groups (Aragones *et al.*, 2002).

Restrictions of working capacity

Assessment of the capacity to work depends on postgastrectomy symptoms, whether a R0 or R1 resection has been performed, accompanying disease(s) and on certain occupational strains. Patients with inoperable tumours and/or present tumour activity are deemed incapable of performing work. They should complete their applications for compensation for this state of disability as soon as possible, as this can be expected to take several months to be processed.

Workloads to be avoided

For "cured" gastric cancer patients there are numerous occupational limitations which result from postgastrectomy symptoms (table 8.10). Vocational reintegration can be expected to take place more easily for patients following B1 partial resection than for gastrectomy patients (Zakharian *et al.*, 1994). Limitations in ability to work, carry out a profession or occupation apply especially to those jobs which are associated with physical exertion (Delbrück and Locossou, 1990).

For many patients following total gastrectomy, but also for partially resected patients, many activities requiring physical exertion are no longer possible, often due to weight loss and weakness alone. White collar workers on the other hand can more easily return to their respective occupations, although gastrectomy patients must be expected to have more difficulties with concentration (Zakharian, 1994). Total gastrectomy patients are not allowed to carry out activities involving frequently alternating, standing or bending positions due to the risk of reflux. The necessity of frequent mealtimes further limits the spectrum of potential occupations for gastrectomy patients.

Cancer patients with a total gastrectomy generally do not demonstrate a significant improvement in their level of physical fitness, even in the long term. For that reason, one should apply prudently for disability retirement, especially in cases of older patients who are within the age range for employment and who have occupations involving physical exertion.

In **gastrectomy patients under 50 years of age** with prognostically favourable forms of the illness, an attempt to change the workplace should be made if the former occupation involved physically strenuous activities. If a change of workplace is not possible, vocational reorientation should also be considered in young patients (below 43 years of age) with a favourable prognosis. Occupations involving only a small amount of physical exertion in service branches are to be favoured.

Table 8.10 - Occupational strains which cured gastric carcinoma patients should avoid following total gastrectomy (R0).

Limitations	Reason for limitation
Work requiring frequent bending over	Risk of reflux œsophagitis
Physically challenging work, no lifting or carrying heavy burdens	Low body weight, risk of reflux œsophagitis
Jobs performed at great heights with the possibility of vertigo (for example, roofers)	Dumping symptoms with symptoms due to low blood sugar
Work requiring long-term concentration	Dumping symptoms with symptoms due to low blood sugar
Activities in the first six postoperative months	Relatively slow adaptation to altered food transit in the gastro-intestinal tract
Activities associated with strong odors or caustic fumes	Provocation of vomiting, nausea and diarrhea
Night work and work in shifts not allowed	Lower stress tolerance
Work in which frequent breaks, not normally scheduled in the job, are possible	More frequent mealtimes necessary
Work as truck driver unsuitable	Frequent breaks not normally scheduled in the job are necessary, psychological and physical stress, risk of dumping syndrome with difficulty concentrating

In partial resection patients, later adaptation can take place accompanied by an increase in physical performance. In this case, it is recommended that one waits approximately one year to make a socio-medical assessment in order to make a more accurate and realistic assessment of the patient's performance ability. A step-by-step approach to resumption of work is advised.

How to return to work

There are many questions to be answered: Which workplace-conserving measures are to be taken – including reintegration assistance, occupational and vocational support and vocational reorientation, as well as change of vocation – who is financially responsible, in which cases does a vocational reorientation make sense and can it be accomplished? These questions are ideally answered for the cancer patient during his/her subsequent stay in an oncological rehabilitation clinic which – at least in Germany – works closely with retirement insurance and vocational advisors.

These rehabilitation clinics are obligated to counsel every cancer patient within working age and to provide vocational assistance if necessary. It is further required to issue a detailed statement in patient's final medical report which makes recommendations regarding the ability of the gastric cancer patient to pursue his/her former occupation or if he/she is able to work at all, at which point he/she will be able to be fully or only partially employed, and which further means of vocational assistance should be considered/implemented.

Palliative measures

Informing the patient about disease progression. Delivering bad news

Despite the unfavourable prognosis in the case of tumour recurrence, there are more points in favour than against patient information. This does not mean, however, that the patient should be forced to confront the full implications of his or her illness. Information without the simultaneous offering of prospects and assistance is never constructive. Many fears associated with the illness originate from the fact that the affected person does not know how the situation should be assessed or what he/she should expect. It is better in any case for the patient to be informed by the attending physician than by prayer healers, moneymakers, or by random information found on the Internet (table 2.11). Even when prognosis is desperate, positive aspects have to be mentioned (e.g., references to progress in palliative therapy, better pain control, provision of constant medical/psychological service, better supportive care). Patients without a good foundation of knowledge tend to look for alternative medicine and to consult quack-doctors.

The assessment of emotional and physical costs must be carefully considered with any patient before deciding further cancer therapies.

Choice of treatment modalities

The physician has to inform the patient about all therapies at disposition, no matter if curative, supportive or palliative.

Cancer-unrelated limitations and concomitant illnesses (for example, diabetes, renal insufficiency, cardiovascular illnesses, altered pharmacokinetics due to age-related and/or therapy-related changes in organs, poor nutritional status and functional limitations) present limitations (Extermann, 2007). Psychological barriers such as denial of illness, loss of will to live, inadequate coping and poor social support pose obstacles to the therapeutic modalities recommended in the guidelines of many national and international specialist associations. The specific qualities of the individual patient are to be considered in palliative therapy (Schwarz, 2004).

At the time of definitive diagnosis, a malignant tumour is often already advanced, inoperable, and has infiltrated surrounding organs or developed distant metastases, leaving only the possibility of supportive and palliative modes of therapy. In the few cases where surgical treatment may represent potentially curative therapy, the risk of recurrence is very high. Only the few cases of tumour recurrence which appears at the proximal resection border may be approached surgically with potentially curative intentions.

All other types of recurrence are inaccessible to potentially curative therapy. The decision for palliative tumour therapy should be discussed with the patient (table 3.10, 6.32). Even palliative tumour therapies have subjective and objective side effects of varying severity, which must be taken into consideration, especially in elderly patients. Pros and cons of possible tumour therapy as well as possible therapy alternatives must be discussed with the patient and, if necessary, determined in cooperation with the participating specialist divisions (oncology, gastroenterology, radiology, visceral surgery).

For patients with inoperable and therefore incurable disease, the aims of treatment are to reduce the tumour burden, improve symptoms and modestly extend median survival time. Surgery can effectively palliate symptoms in patients with advanced malignancy and thereby maintain quality of life. However, the goal of surgical palliation should be weighed against the associated risks. The decision to operate can be challenging even for the most experienced surgeon.

The average age of gastric carcinoma patients is more than 65 years. Pharmacokinetics and pharmadynamics in this age group often do not allow the standard chemotherapy (Hurria et al., 2007). Many of the recommended standard chemotherapeutic treatment modalities have been tested in studies on considerably younger patients, whereby a good general condition with no concomitant illness was a prerequisite for acceptance into the study. The prolongation of survival time achieved in these studies are therefore not representative of the majority of gastric carcinoma patients. In addition, the primary aim of all therapy modalities should not lie in extending survival time, but rather in the rapid and lasting improvement of attendant clinical circumstances.

It not only requires excellent background knowledge in oncology, but also competence in ethics and communication when answering the questions pertaining to therapeutic alternatives and how much therapy makes sense in a palliative situation.

Local and regional problems.
Recommendations for palliative therapies

Locoregional recurrences are possible in three locations: intraluminal, in the region of the anastomosis, extraluminal, in the region of the tumour bed and in the area of lymphatic drainage. The tumour can infiltrate the liver, pancreas, spleen and transverse colon per continuitatem. In females, spread of metastases to the ovaries (Krukenberg tumour) is not uncommon.

Along the lymphatic pathways, not only the lymph nodes of the greater and lesser omentum, but also the lymph nodes around the celiac trunk and thus the retroperitoneum tend to be affected. In the case of hematogenous seeding, liver and lungs are primarily affected when the tumour is of the intestinal type; with the diffuse type, the peritoneum is more often affected. Further common locations associated with hematogenous metastases are the skeletal system and, less commonly, the brain.

Bleeding and stenosis

Endoscopic procedures are applied in particular for eliminating local complications such as bleeding and stenosis. The Nd:YAG laser is most commonly used. Its effectiveness is superior to 95%, particularly in the case of diffuse bleeding; for tumour obstruction it is superior to 80%. With local bleeding the APC beamer is used. Secondary measures are however often necessary following the laser procedure.

Malignant dysphagia

Placements of self-expandable metal stents or plastic tubes are established palliative treatment options. As an alternative and/or complementary therapy, radiologic techniques (external beam radiation/brachytherapia) and locally endoscopic techniques (laser, APC-beamer, PDT) are often used. In the long term, there appears to be a marginal benefit for metal stents when compared with plastic tubes. However, metal stents seem to be safer and associated with a prolonged improvement of the dysphagia score (Eickhoff *et al.*, 2005).

Liver metastases

In extremely rare cases there is a solitary liver metastasis; for this reason a significant increase in survival time cannot be expected, either from metastases surgery or isolated regional chemotherapy or embolization. Combined systemic chemotherapy can have an alleviating effect on symptoms. Low-dose liver irradiation (pain radiation) can lead to rapid alleviation of symptoms associated with capsule pain. Low doses of cortisone have pain-relieving and anabolic effects and may sometimes have a positive effect on the patient's psychological state.

Peritoneal carcinosis (malignant ascites)

For more details see chapter on ovarian cancer.

Neither surgical nor radiation therapy intervention has a life-extending or quality of life improving effect. The development of malignant ascites can markedly reduce a patient's quality of life. Associated nausea, anorexia, dyspnea, and pain can cause significant morbidity.

Diuretic therapy and dietary modification have a limited role as most patients continue to accumulate ascites. Serial paracenteses is a better option. Symptoms like discomfort, dyspnea, nausea and vomiting seem to be significantly relieved by drainage of up to 5L of fluid. However, rapid reaccumulation can necessitate frequent procedures, thus subjecting the patient to the risks of bleeding, infection, visceral perforation, and hypotension associated with invasive drainage.

Because of poor prognosis, it is agreed by most authors that a shunt should only be used when other treatment options have failed and when the life expectancy of the patient is long enough to derive benefit.

About the time span there is no consensus, some authors suggest an expected survival of more than three months. In general shunt insertion is contraindicated in patients with malignant ascites due to gastro-intestinal cancer (Becker *et al.*, 2006).

Systemic chemotherapy may be attempted, although experience has shown that this is less effective in cases of peritoneal carcinosis than in other metastastic locations. Intraperitoneal chemotherapy can limit ascites production for a short period of time, but tends to have only a local effect – if any – due to formation of separate cavities. Hyperthermic peritoneal chemotherapy may have an added effect on chemotherapy but is not without risks (Hildebrandt *et al.*, 2004; Garofalo *et al.*, 2006). Spasmolytic medications work best for pain. In order to prevent an ileus, the stool should be kept soft.

Systemic palliative therapies

Chemotherapy

Compared to sole employment of best supportive care, chemotherapy for adenocarcinoma contributes to a short but significant increase in survival time of a few weeks and improvement in quality of life (Wohrer *et al.*, 2004; Wöhner *et al.*, 2004).

With gastric lymphoma, chemotherapy is especially effective and brings about a clear increase in survival time besides alleviating pain. Likewise, in cases of GIST tumours with tyrosine kinase inhibitors, baffling remissions are often still attained, with long-lasting disappearance of symptoms.

Quality of life data should be considered when choosing the chemotherapy regime. Due to the fact that symptoms from metastases (with an adenocarcinoma as the primary tumour) appear quite early, it is becoming more common to recommend chemotherapy at an asymptomatic stage. Liver and pulmonary metastases generally respond well, peritoneal carcinosis responds poorly to chemotherapy. 5-fluorouracil with or without additional folinate, etoposide, the taxanes, mitomycin C, oxaliplatinum, irinotecan and cisplatin are relatively effective. Administered as monosubstances they induce remission rates of 20%.

The probability that remission after polychemotherapy takes place is considerably higher but the toxicity also increases. It is very doubtful if intensive chemotherapy is of benefit in gastric cancer. In patients whose general condition is severely limited (Karnofsky inferior to 60%), the use of this subjectively and objectively strenuous form of therapy is to be discussed for each individual case.

Treatment has to be tailored to the patient. Besides the response and remission rates, tolerance and the difference in pharmacokinetics and pharmacodynamics in the older patient should also be considered when selecting a certain therapy regime. Elderly patients should be assessed and treated differently than younger patients (tables 6.32, 8.11) (Hurria *et al.*, 2007). Toxicity associated with some palliative treatments can be significant, and resource implications are considerable. Most of the existing trials place emphasis on response rates, which *per se* are not a direct measure of patient benefit. For justification of the use of such treatment for palliation it would be required that they offer some benefit in the quality of life for those patients treated.

Table 8.11 - Causes for the frequent reduced tolerance of cytostatics in the elderly.

– Slower intestinal motility: altered absorption
– Achlorhydria: altered absorption
– Altered hepatic metabolism
– Altered biliary and renal elimination
– Altered distribution and storage of lipophilic cytostatics in fat and muscle tissue
– Reduced hematopoetic reserve
– Altered nutritional status
– Altered cardiac and pulmonary functional capacity
– Frequent comorbidity
– Psyche
– Varying levels of compliance

Nutrition

In order to minimize the danger and damage to the patient by exposing him/her to the risk of invasive procedures, the form of therapy should be chosen according to the following hierarchy: oral > enteral > parenteral. The indication for total parenteral nutrition should be defined narrowly, as a great number of patients can be given nutrition adequately and safely via the enteral route, either following successful stenting or after placement of a PEG/PEJ.

Nutrition in the case of obstruction of gastro-intestinal transit

Nutrition intake can be guaranteed for a limited period of time by means of bouginage, or in some cases laser, insertion of a tube, gastroduodenal stenting, in emergencies also possible by means of bypass surgery, percutaneous endoscopic gastrostomy (PEG) or feeding by jejunum tube (FCJ = fine needle catheter jejunostomy) (Dormann, 2004; Miner et al., 2004; Nash 2002). Around 25% of patients can eat normally after placement of a stent and a further 30-40% is able to take in soft foods. These measures are, of course, only effective for a limited time. Secondary endoscopic procedures are often necessary; but they can no longer halt tumour cachexia because disease progression is unabatable.

Characteristics of pain therapy

See also chapter: " Pain management in cancer rehabilitation and palliation".
If pain is due to the tumour, early administration of central analgesics is to be considered; peripheral analgesics are often associated with considerable side effects in gastric resection patients (table 5.32). With liver capsule pain, low-dose corticoids can simultaneously alleviate pain and exert positive effects on the psyche as well as the appetite. Long-lasting forms of morphine should be given preference in this case (table 5.20 Transdermal forms such as fentanyl (Durogesic®smut) or buprenorphin

(Transtec®) have the added advantage that they cause few adverse effects. They offer a greater advantage because of their non oral method of administration (table 5.23).

Measures for quality assurance

As with acute therapy, certain guidelines and quality assurance procedures should also apply to rehabilitation and palliation (Delbrück, 1997; Barat and Franchignoni, 2004). Whether – and if not, then why – the goal has not been achieved must be documented.

Unfortunately, there are only few guidelines on this subject in rehabilitation and palliation of gastric cancer patients. There are guidelines for gastric cancer therapy (AACR, 2002) but none regarding rehabilitative needs of these patients and how to secure quality of the different rehabilitative and palliative measures.

To guarantee quality of rehabilitation and palliation you have to ensure quality of structures, quality of rehabilitative and palliative measures and to evaluate the outcome.

Quality of structural features

Therapies needed in rehabilitation and palliation should be provided by specialized rehabilitation services with a team of patient care specialists (fig. 1.4). Nutritionists play an important role in this team.

Gastric cancer rehabilitation services include critical components of assessment, physical reconditioning, skill training, and psychosocial support. They may include vocational evaluation and counselling.

A gastric cancer rehabilitation service necessitates special rehabilitative equipment as well as qualified and experienced personnel. Due to the experience necessary, the rehabilitative institution should care for at least sixty gastric cancer patients per year. The team should be coordinated by a physician experienced in rehabilitation and palliation with demonstrable oncological and gastoenterological knowledge.

In Germany, over 50% of gastric cancer patients who have undergone surgery go on to spend three-five weeks in inpatient rehabilitation (AHB) in an oncology-oriented rehabilitation clinic following surgery. In theory, rehabilitative care is also possible on an outpatient basis; however, inpatient care is generally preferred in Germany. The reason for this is that gastric carcinoma patients are nearly always too physically weak to profit from treatment on an outpatient basis.

There are well-defined structural guidelines for these rehabilitation institutions in which patients with gastric carcinoma may receive follow-up care, either as inpatients or outpatients (Bundesarbeitsgemeinschaft für Rehabilitation, 2003). If quality control checks reveal that a rehabilitation clinic is not following the guidelines sufficiently, it loses its license and thus its basis for existence. If the requirements stated in the guidelines are not fulfilled, the clinic loses its financial basis for existence.

Quality of medical and therapeutic processes

Evaluation of rehabilitation and palliation measures is not based on survival time, but rather on criteria for quality of life. There are numerous self- and other-based evaluation scales which document this and which can be used for assessment of course of treatment and evaluation. Subjective parameters (for example, improvement of pain, appetite, mobility, overcoming fears, coping with illness or patient satisfaction) as well as objective parameters (for example, management of weight loss, improvement in nutritional status, correction of anemia, etc.) are employed for this purpose.

Outcome assessment and evaluation

The evaluation of rehabilitative and supportive measures is much more difficult than checking the outcome of intervention procedures generally used in potentially curative follow-up care (length of recurrence-free period, detection of early recurrence). In order to quantify the positive results of palliative oncological and rehabilitative oncological intervention, certain parameters may be implemented. They are listed in table 8.12.

Quality of life questionnaires of the European Organization for Research and Treatment of Cancer such as EORTC QLQ C-30) and the functional assessment of cancer therapy (Fact-) are internationally validated questionnaires and have been used on multiple studies. They are composed of multi-item scales and yes/no questions assessing physical, role functioning, cognitive, emotional, and social effects.

In the palliative care of cancer patients, different outcome scales have been developed (Aspinal et al., 2002; Bausewein et al., 2005). The scales cover physical and psychological symptoms, spiritual considerations, practical concerns, emotional concerns and psychosocial needs of the patient and family. The Palliative Care Outcome Scale (POS) is a multidimensional instrument covering these physical, psychosocial, spiritual, organizational, and practical concerns.

Table 8.12 - Possible therapeutic aims and their parameters for effectiveness in the rehabilitation of gastric carcinoma patients.

Therapeutic aim	Effectiveness parameter
Reduction of disturbances resulting from surgery/chemotherapy/radiation therapy	WHO toxicity scale, CTC classification, examination of organ function, FLIC
Clarification and improvement of subjective postgastrectomy symptoms	Symptoms, questionnaires
Improvement of nutritional status	Weight measurements, measurements of total protein, albumin concentration, biometric impedance analysis. EORTC-questionnaire: Fact-CT
Stabilization of medication due to altered kinetics	Drug monitoring, 24-hour blood glucose profile
Clarification and alleviation of malassimilation/maldigestion	Fat in stools/stool weight
Improvement of physical condition	Ergometry, Karnofsky index, WHO and EORTC performance status, walking distances, vigorimeter, muscle force (hand-held dynamometry, exercise capacity, symptom limited bicycle ergometry. Questionnaires: EORTC-QLQ-C30, Fact-G, SIP, SF-36, Nottingham Health profile
Counselling for family members	Questionnaires
Information on illness, follow-up care, signs of disease recurrence, therapy options for disease recurrence, information on illness-compromising behaviour	Questionnaires, test papers
Alleviation of anxiety, depression	Rating scales. Questionnaires STAI, POMS, BDI, BSI, HADS-D, PAF
Coping with illness	Questionnaires: FKV, FKV-LIS, BEFO, TSK, FIBECK
Clarification and improvement of vocational capacity/productivity	Establishment of vocation, length of period of disability
Reduction of need for nursing care	Reduction of required level of nursing care, Questionnaires: Barthel index, FIM, ADL

Abbreviations of questionnaires

ADL = Activities of Daily Life; DDC = Daily Diary Card; EORTC-QLQ = European Organization for Research and Treatment of Cancer Quality of Life Questionnaire; ECOG = European Cooperative Oncology Group-Scale; Fact-An = Functional Assessment of Cancer Therapy Anemia; FACT-Ct = Functional Assessment of Anorexia and Cachexia; FIBECK = Freiburger Inventar zur Bewältigung einer chronischen Erkrankung; FIM = Functional Independence Measure; FLI-C = Functional Living Index-Cancer; HADS-D = Hospital Anxiety and Depression Scale; KPS = Karnofsky Performance scale; LCSS = Lung Cancer Symptom Scale; PDI = Pain Disabilty Index; POMS = Profile of Mood Status; RSCL = Rotterdam-Symptom Checklist; SF-36 = SF-36 Health Survey; SIP = Sickness Impact Profile; SIRO = Stress Index Radio Oncology; STAI = Spiegelberger Trait Anxiety Inventory

Measurements of quality of life

The EORTC QLQ C-30 also includes symptom measures and a global health and QL scale. Basically, improvement in the quality of life, which is an important objective during rehabilitation, is attained when less nursing care is necessary ("rehabilitation to combat the need of care"), when the patient can be vocationally reintegrated ("rehabilitation to combat early retirement"), when he/she feels secure and knows that his/her fate is in somebody's hands, in a positive sense ("rehabilitation to combat resignation and depression") and when the patient's physical handicaps and functional limitations are at a minimum ("rehabilitation to combat disability").

Bibliographie

- Aragones N, Pollan M, Gustavsson P (2002) Stomach cancer and occupation in Sweden: 1971-1989. Occup Environ Med 59, 5: 329-37
- Bundesarbeitsgemeinschaft für Rehabilitation (2003) Rahmenempfehlungen zur ambulanten onkologischen Rehabilitation. Schriftenreihe der Bundesarbeitsgemeinschaft für Rehabilitation. BAR, Frankfurt
- Barat M, Frannchignoni F (2004) Assessment in physical medecine and rehabilitation. Maugeri Foundation Books, PI-ME Press Pavia 16
- Becker G, Galandi D, Blum HE (2006) Malignant ascites: Systematic review and guideline for treatment. Eur J cancer 42: 589-97
- Delbrück H (editor) (1997) Standards und Qualitätskriterien in der onkologischen Rehabilitation. W Zuckschwerdt Verlag, München
- Delbrück H (2005) Magenkrebs. Rat und Hilfe für Betroffene und Angehörige. Kohlhammer Verlag, Stuttgart 3. Auflage
- Delbrück H, Locossou R (1990) Necessities, possibilities and difficulties of vocational rehabilitation in patients with early stomach carcinoma – experiences in 89 patients. Rehabilitation 29, 2: 121-4
- Dormann A, Meisner S, Verin N et al. (2004) Self-expanding metal stents for gastroduodenal malignancies: Systematic review of their clinical effectiveness. Endoscopy 36, 6: 543-50
- Eickhoff A, Knoll M, Jakobs R et al. (2005) Self-expanding metal stents versus plastic protheses in the palliation of malignant dysphagia. J Clin Gastroenterol 39, 10: 877-85
- Extermann M (2007) Interaction between comorbidity and cancer. Cancer Control 14, 1: 13-22
- Friess H, Bohm J, Muller MW et al. (1996) Maldigestion after total gastrectomy is associated with pancreatic insufficiency Am J Gastroenterol 91, 2: 341-7
- Garofalo A, Valle M, Garcia J (2006) Laparoscopic intraperitoneal hyperthermic chemotherapy for palliation of debilitating malignant ascites. Eur J Surg Oncol 32, 6: 682-5
- Heiskanen JT, Kroger H, Paakkonen M et al. (2001) Bone mineral metaboslism after total gastrectomy. Bone 28, 1: 123-7
- Hildebandt, B, Rau B, Gellermann J et al. (2004) Hyperthermic intraperitoneal chemotherapy in patients with peritoneal carcinosis. J Clin Oncol 22, 8: 1527-9

- Hurria A, Lichtman S (2007) Pharmacokinetics of chemotherapy in the older patient. Cancer control 14 1: 32-43
- Koike H, Ijima M, Mori K *et al.* (2004) Postgastrectomy polyneuropathy with thiamine deficiency is identical to beriberi neuropathy. Nutrition 20, 11-12: 961-6
- Mestrom (1998) Essen und Trinken nach Magenoperation. Ars bonae curae Verlag, Sprockhövel
- Miner TJ, Jaques DP, Karpeh MS *et al.* (2004) Defining palliative surgery in patients receiving non curative resections for gastric cancer. J Am Coll Surg 198, 6: 1013-21
- Nash C, Gerdes H (2002) Methods of palliation of esophageal and gastric cancer Surg Oncol Clin N Am 11, 2: 459-83
- Nell G (1991) Auswirkungen der partiellen und totalen Gastrektomie auf die Resorption und Interaktion von Arzneimitteln. In: Delbrück H (ed) Krebsnachsorge und Rehabilitation, Magenkarzinom. Zuckschwerdt, München
- Ribolie, Lambert A (eds) (2002) Nutrition and lifestyle: Opportunities for cancer prevention. IARC Sci Publ. No 156: 151-4
- Roviell F, Fotia G, Marelli D *et al.* (2004) Iron deficiency anemia after subtotal gastrectomy for gastric cancer. Hepatogastroenterology 51, 59: 1510-14
- Schölmerich J (2004) Postgastrectomy syndromes – diagnosis and treatment. Best Pract Res Clin Gastroenterol 18, 5: 917-33
- Schwarz RE (2004) Defining palliation in patients undergoing gastrectomy for gastric cancer. J Am Coll Surg 199, 6: 1001-2
- Vickery CW, Blazeby JM, Conroy T *et al.* (2000) Development of an EORTC module to improve quality of life assessment in patients with gastric cancer. Br J Surg 87: 362
- Wöhner *et al.* (2004) Palliation chemotherapies for advanced gastric cancer. Ann Oncol 15: 1585-95
- Wohrer SS, Raderer M, Hejna M (2004) Palliative chemotherapy for advanced gastric cancer. Ann Oncol 15, 11: 1585-95
- Zakharian AG, Stoliarov VI, Kolosov AE (1994) Vocational rehabilitation of patients after radical surgery for stomach cancer. Khirurgia (mosk) 2 11-2

Rehabilitation and palliation of patients with pancreatic cancer

Aims of rehabilitation and palliation: Definition as distinct from curative tumour follow-up care

The chief aim of all medical, **potentially curative follow-up care measures** (recurrence prophylaxis, early detection and therapy of disease recurrence) is to lengthen survival time (fig. 1.3). The actual tumour illness thus represents the focus of curative follow-up care.

With **rehabilitation and palliation**, on the other hand, it is not the influencing of the illness, but rather the reduction of disabilities due to the tumour and therapy as well as improvement of quality of life, which constitute the aims of therapeutic procedures (fig. 1.2). It is the intention to alleviate the negative effects of the cancer disease and therapy, not only physically, but also psychologically, socially and vocationally (tables 1.4, 1.5 and 9.1). The ICF (International Classification of Functionality, Disability and Health), and not the ICD (International Classification of Diseases), the standard classification system used in curative oncology, is the basis for assessment, therapy and quality assurance (Barat and Franchignoni, 2004). It is thus considerably more comprehensive than the ICD, as it includes psychological aspects in addition to biological ailments. It has replaced the ICIDH (International Classification of Impairments, Disabilities and Handicaps) system, and has served since 2001 as a comprehensive and unifying language for all nations and fields for describing the functional condition of health, disability, social impairment and relevant environmental factors for the patient to be rehabilitated (WHO, 2001; Barat and Franchignoni, 2004).

It is not so much the survival time as the quality of the time remaining which is to be positively influenced (fig. 1.1). The therapy measures used for this purpose are varied. They are employed as a result of the all-encompassing aims of the many occupational groups (fig. 1.4). Besides the physician with experience in rehabilitative oncology as well as gastroenterology, the nutrition expert, the psychologist, the pain therapist and the social worker all play major roles. The need of certain therapeutic measures which may become necessary during rehabilitation depends on the severity of tumour or therapy consequences and not, as in potentially curative follow-up care, on severity and prognosis of the actual cancer illness.

Table 9.1 - Rehabilitative problems in pancreatic carcinoma patients.

– Effects of partial or total pancreas resection (classic or pylorus-preserving Whipple procedure)
– Adverse effects of chemotherapy, effects of radiation therapy
– Effects of exocrine and endocrine pancreatic insufficiency
– Disturbances at the site of the biliodigestive anastomosis
– Weight loss
– Enteral and parenteral nutrition, tube feeding
– Lack of information/need for information
– Psychological strain, anxiety disorders
– Need for nursing care
– Inability to work/pursue profession

In theory, the aims of curative follow-up care can be differentiated simply and clearly from those of rehabilitation and palliation. In practice, however, there is much overlapping. This involves in particular tumour recurrence therapy and palliative measures. Potentially curative therapy for recurrences does not only serve to prolong survival time, but also to alleviate symptoms.

The fact that disease recurrence may not be eliminated even when it has, by means of routine diagnostics, been detected at an asymptomatic stage or very "early" (Shore, 2004), calls the value of routine follow-up diagnostics into question. The value of prophylactic forms of therapy (adjuvant chemotherapy and radiation therapy) is controversial, and therapy of disease recurrence brings about only – if any at all – marginal gains in survival time (Neoptolemos, 2003). As long as potentially curative measures (recurrence prophylaxis, early detection and therapy of recurrence) have failed to show a significant survival benefit, rehabilitative and palliative measures in the follow-up care of pancreatic carcinoma patients will remain the main focus.

Rehabilitative measures in follow-up care

Rehabilitative measures can be considered for patients undergoing potentially curative as well as palliative treatment.

A certain minimum amount of information on disease status is prerequisite before initiating rehabilitative measures (tables 1.6, 1.7, 1.8, 1.9 and 9.2).

Table 9.2 - Minimum informations required before initiating rehabilitative measures.

– Localization of the tumour (for example pancreas head, body, tail)
– Extent of tumour (for example pTNM)
– Which surgical procedure has been used (for example, Whipple procedure with or without preservation of stomach)?
– Has chemotherapy or radiation therapy taken place (for example, which cytostatic agents at what dosages and with what results)?
– Curative or palliative therapy approach (for example R0, R1 or R2 resection of the tumour)?
– Psychosocial information (for example, about statements given pertaining to degree of patient information, about any problems with coping or compliance, amount of support given by family members, about social and occupational problems, etc.)

Rehabilitative measures aimed at reducing physical problems ("rehabilitation in order to combat disability")

The spectrum of possible somatic handicaps ranges from metabolic disorders, malnutrition and undernutrition, gastro-intestinal symptoms to pain (table 9.1). Radical extraction of the entire pancreas and additional chemotherapy or radiation therapy give rise to more numerous disorders than does sole resection of the pancreas head or tail. Performing the pylorus-preserving pancreatoduodenectomy can minimize many complications following the Whipple procedure (Ogata, 2002). The type and extent of rehabilitative measures necessary are determined by accompanying illnesses, prognosis, age and motivation.

Problems after total pancreatectomy and recommendations

Insulin-dependent diabetes always results, as insulin and glucagon-producing cells are no longer present.

Patients who have undergone pancreatectomy are highly sensitive to insulin. Regulation of blood sugar is extremely unstable, since not only the blood sugar-lowering insulin is absent, but also the blood sugar-raising substance glucagon. Fluctuating blood sugar levels are also caused by the varying amounts of carbohydrates absorbed in the presence of digestive disturbances. In contrast to other patients with type I diabetes, high postprandial blood glucose levels drop within the first forty minutes following food intake. This is due to the partial gastric resection which has been performed in the Whipple procedure. At night there is a marked tendency to develop hypoglycemia (table 9.3).

Table 9.3 - Causes of hypoglycemia.

- Too much insulin injected
- Too few (or none at all) carbohydrates consumed
- Excessive physical activity
- Excessive alcohol consumption
- Hormonal disorders
- Altered carbohydrate resorption (for example, in postoperative condition)
- Interaction with other drugs
- Psychological disorders

Even minimal amounts of insulin lead to a prompt and lasting drop in the blood glucose level. Only relatively few insulin units are necessary. The insulin requirement is low, on average 27I.U. per day (0.30-0.50IU/kg body weight).

As a rule, a slightly elevated blood glucose level in patients who have undergone total pancreatectomy should be deemed acceptable, since the danger of hypoglycemia is greater than that of hyperglycemia. Long-term vascular, renal or ophthalmological complications from diabetes are observed only rarely in spite of the frequency of elevated blood sugar levels.

In cases of infection and stress, correction of the insulin dosages must often be amended, as the risk of decompensation of blood glucose is especially high at these times. It is very important that pancreatectomy patients become familiar with the symptoms of hypoglycemia and hyperglycemia and can determine their blood glucose level themselves, as well as therapeutic consequences related to the different levels. Mastery of intensified insulin therapy is required for the patient. The amount of insulin has to be readjusted constantly.

Besides functional endocrine disorders, consequences of the **exocrine enzyme deficiency** also necessarily occur (table 9.4). These can however be kept at a minimum through the regular administration of pancreatic enzyme preparations and injection of fat-soluble vitamins.

Table 9.4 - Necessary substitution therapy for total pancreatectomy patients.

- Insulin substitution
- Complete substitution of pancreatic enzymes
- Substitution of visible fats in foods with medium-chain triglycerides
- Monthly injections of fat-soluble vitamins
- Monthly injections of vitamin B12
- Calcium, magnesium and iron (as necessary)

As lipids are not sufficiently absorbed, and as some vitamins can only be absorbed and metabolized in the intestine in the presence of lipids, there is the danger of vitamin deficiency disorders, unless the fat-soluble vitamins A, D, E and K are substituted regularly by intramuscular injection.

Important nutrients such as calcium, magnesium or iron can be lost by the organism. Consequences for bone metabolism as a result of the vitamin D and calcium deficit are a threat and must be compensated if necessary. Leg cramps occur frequently due to magnesium deficiency. As is the case with the Whipple procedure, two thirds of the stomach, the duodenum, and the gallbladder are removed and the bile duct is reattached to another loop of small intestine in connection with total pancreatectomy. Some symptoms can be explained by this fact.

Problems after partial pancreatectomy with removal of pancreas head (Whipple procedure) and recommendations

With the classic Whipple procedure, not only the pancreas head and a more or less large portion of the pancreas body, but also two-thirds of the stomach are removed. With the modified Whipple procedure, on the other hand, the stomach with its pyloric sphincter is preserved (Ogata, 2002). The outlet of the pancreatic duct and the bile ducts are moved from the duodenum and reattached at another location in the small intestine (jejunum). This altered anatomy is the cause of many functional disturbances.

Some complaints are due to the **lack of digestive enzymes** (table 9.5). Pancreatic insufficiency can be absolute as well as relative. It is absolute when enzyme production in the residual pancreas is insufficient; it is relative when, in spite of sufficient enzyme production, the chyme is not properly mixed with the digestive enzymes. The reason for such a relative insufficiency is the asynchronous entry of chyme into the small intestine following the Whipple procedure. Because of the removal of the pyloric sphincter, chyme arrives in the small intestine so early that the pancreas cannot keep up with enzyme production and secretion, and the proper mixing of the chyme with enzymes does not take place.

Table 9.5 - Symptoms associated with digestive enzyme deficiency.

– Bloating
– Diarrhea
– Fatty stool (fatty deposits on the stool)
– Sour or "biting" odor of stool
– Voluminous and yellowish-white stool
– Pain
– Weight loss

A further cause of reactive enzyme deficiency is the loss of the duodenum. This leads to a decreased secretion of the hormones secretin and pancreozymin, which play a role in the regulation of the exocrine pancreatic enzymes. It is only after a certain lapse of time that the upper small intestine takes over this function of the duodenum: All the more reason to prescribe pancreatic enzymes, at least for the first months following the Whipple procedure.

For the long term, **vitamin deficiency** is a risk, especially of the fat-soluble vitamins. The reason for this is disturbances in the digestion of lipids. Of the fat-soluble vitamins (vitamins A, D, E and K), injections of vitamin D at least should be given regularly (approximately every six months).

Due to the partial removal of the stomach, some patients may develop vitamin B12 deficiency. Disturbances in blood production and nerve pain become threats to the patient. Vitamin B12 must therefore be substituted at regular intervals, in addition to the fat-soluble vitamins. Following the "modified", that is, the pylorus-preserving Whipple procedure, this is not necessary.

The enzymes produced in the pancreas are not only responsible for digestion of fats and proteins, but they also support the breaking down of carbohydrates. This is one of the reasons why patients who have undergone pancreas surgery often report **bloating** and pain. In these patients, the food ingested travels in an undigested state to the large intestine, where it is broken down by bacteria, leading to increased production of gases. In order to combat the problem the patient is advised to chew well, eat several small meals and take enzyme preparations.

The partial gastric resection generally performed in the Whipple procedure can be the cause of **early and/or late dumping syndrome**. The cause of early dumping is the shorter amount of time spent by chyme in the stomach and a sudden flow of the chyme out of the residual stomach into the small intestine and accompanying stretching of the affected intestinal segments. Late dumping is caused by a disturbance in the regulation of the secretion of insulin. Symptoms arise such as fainting and profuse sweating. When nutritional guidelines are followed closely, symptoms due to early as well as late dumping syndromes can be almost completely prevented.

Not only the exocrine, but also the endocrine pancreatic functions may be impaired. The patient can develop **diabetes**. Whether or not diabetes develops after the Whipple procedure depends on how much of the pancreatic gland, that is, how many islet cells have been removed, as well as to what extent the endocrine regulation is impaired. In the absence of the regulation mechanism, a patient can develop a manifest case of diabetes after losing even a few islet cells. Oral antidiabetics have virtually no effect. In this case, insulin substitution is always necessary.

Patients who have undergone the Whipple procedure tend to **develop inflammation and anastomosis ulcers** at the site of sutures joining the residual stomach and the small intestine. Prophylactic use of acid blockers can be helpful. The reason for the increased risk of developing ulcers are the acids, which are harmful to the mucosa, and bile which flow freely into the residual stomach in the absence of the pylorus. Patients who have had the pylorus-preserving procedure are at risk for developing ulcers as well.

A further reason for the prophylactic use of acid blockers is that the pancreatic enzymes have optimum effectiveness at a pH of 6 to 7. Since Whipple patients have had the pyloric sphincter removed, and the acidic stomach contents pass quickly and freely into the small intestine, the pancreas often cannot keep up with enzyme production and the mixing of chyme with pancreatic and bile juices is inadequate.

Sometimes a **gastric emptying disorder** develops due to a narrowing in the region of the junction between stomach and small intestine. Contraction of tissue due to scars, or edema at the site of the sutures may be the causes. Functional causes are also possible. Belching, feeling of fullness following meals and vomiting are typical symptoms, in which case such a narrowing should be considered as the cause. This complication can be treated endoscopically. As differentials, however, one must also consider the possibility of stenosis of the anastomosis region and the proximal jejunum which is frequently due to tumours.

Gastric atonia is common. This condition can be associated with symptoms similar to those of gastric emptying syndrome. Patients should be advised to eat slowly, to chew food thoroughly and to avoid fatty foods. Frequent but small meals are necessary.

Postoperative gastric emptying disorders are more common after the pylorus-preserving Whipple procedure (approximately 30 to 50%) than after the standard Whipple procedure (approximately 10%). Medications which stimulate gastric motor activity (for example, metoclopramide drops) can alleviate symptoms. They do not help in the case of obstruction; in fact, they are contraindicated.

Due to the translocation of the bile ducts and removal of the papilla, penetration of intestinal microbes into the bile ducts is facilitated; there they can cause **ascending cholangitis**. Intermittent fever with chills, upper abdominal pain and jaundice are typical symptoms. Patients with cholangitis must receive antibiotic treatment immediately.

Problems following removal of the pancreas tail and recommendations

The risk of developing insulin-dependent diabetes is higher after removal of the pancreas tail, as the islet cells, responsible for producing insulin, are located primarily in the pancreas tail.

The spleen is often also removed, making necessary a pneumococcal vaccination (Pneumovac®) as well as yearly influenza vaccinations. The vaccinations last longer if they are administered before the surgery takes place; this, however, is only possible in the rarest of cases.

Following spleen removal, thrombocytosis develops, with the accompanying threat of thrombosis. Aspirin given at this time can be helpful. Within three months, however, the thrombocyte count generally returns to normal.

Exocrine pancreatic insufficiency and recommendations

Following total extraction of the pancreas, the patient has to take digestive enzymes for the rest of his/her life. With the Whipple procedure, on the other hand, enzyme substitution depends on symptoms present (table 9.5) and on the results of functional tests. Elastase levels – a relatively sensitive marker for exocrine pancreatic function – are usually low during the first six months following the Whipple surgery. During this time at least, pancreatic enzymes should be substituted. The substitution of pancreatic enzymes is also necessary beyond this time period in the case of diarrhea and when the daily stool lipid loss is over 15g/die.

As a rule, the substitution of pancreatic enzyme preparations is not required when the stool is dark in color, when diarrhea is not present and there is no weight loss.

Pancreatic enzyme preparations should be given shortly before a meal, ideally together with the first bite. If the pancreatic enzyme preparations are taken after this point, they are less effective.

The doses vary according to the level of residual function of the pancreas. Each preparation should contain as much lipase as possible in order to limit the total number of packets or capsules necessary every day. Suitable products are pancreatin preparations containing at least 10,000F.I.P. units of lipase.

Diarrhea and recommendations

Several causes must be considered. Diarrhea is often the consequence of excessive fat consumption or inadequate fat digestion. After reducing fat intake and/or additional use of pancreatic enzyme preparations, the condition improves promptly. In some cases, a too rapid transition to MCT fats or excessively coarse fiber in the diet can also be causes.

Sometimes a sudden emptying of chyme into the small intestine (dumping) occurs, leading to the reflex of increased activity in the lower parts of the intestine (gastrocolic reflex).

A further reason can be milk and milk product intolerance: Symptoms which, as they also are in the case of gastric resection, are not uncommon. Recipients of the Whipple procedure often cannot tolerate fresh milk in particular.

Avoiding milk or taking lactase alleviates symptoms. Lactic acid enzymes are available on the market (Lactrase®) which, in cases of milk intolerance, can be stirred into milk, cream, ice cream, joghurt and cheese.

Another cause can be the removal of or damage to the vagal nerve during surgery. The tendency, especially in the first months following surgery, for diarrhea to occur for this reason, generally disappears spontaneously. Codeine drops or Imodium ® alleviate symptoms.

Occasionally, colonization of the intestine takes places by harmful bacterial. In this case tetracycline should be taken. Transformation surgery should by performed if necessary.

Peritoneal carcinosis should always be considered as a possible cause as well. This condition manifests itself through paradoxical diarrhea. Calmative intestinal medications (for example, Imodium®), sometimes also spasmolytic agents, may alleviate symptoms.

Disorders of the biliodigestive anastomosis and recommendations

An anastomosis can sometimes contract. Bile drainage then becomes more difficult, causing jaundice.

In some cases the opposite happens, that is, a dilation occurs. If, as a result, air enters the bile ducts (aerobilia), this is less serious than when residual food particles or even virulent microbes penetrate into the bile ducts. The latter are the cause of cholangitis, an infection which must receive immediate antibiotic treatment. Without treatment, the risk of developing a liver abscess is high.

In patients with colic-like pain, problems in the region of the bile ducts should always be considered as the possible cause. Prompt diagnostic clarification is absolutely essential!

Disturbances following placement of an internal bile drainage system (bilioduodenal prosthesis/stent) and recommendations

This is a common complication. When patients report that their stool is grayish-white and their urine is dark, the prosthesis must undergo immediate endoscopic replacement. Sudden phases of fever are usually associated with occlusion and consequent cholestasis.

Flatulence and recommendations

Inadequate mixing of chyme with digestive enzymes is generally the cause of flatulence. Insufficiently digested food travels to the large intestine, giving rise to colonization by atypical microbes which ferment the contents, causing flatulence.

Taking digestive enzymes, eating more frequent and smaller meals and chewing thoroughly prevent flatulence and diminish abdominal pain. It is important to avoid gas-producing foods.

Lactulose-containing laxatives can sometimes be the cause of flatulence.

Loss of appetite and recommendations

Fatigue, anxiety, depression as well as resulting therapy problems can all contribute, in addition to tumour progression, to loss of appetite.

Many appetite-stimulating drops derive their effectiveness from alcohol. Alcohol stimulates the production of stomach acid. Patients with pancreatic illnesses should be restrictive with these alcohol-containing drops. Their effectiveness also requires the stomach's functions to be intact; this is generally no longer the case following the Whipple procedure. Teas containing bitter substances such as vermouth, bitter clover, yarrow, sage and spices have a stimulating effect on the appetite.

Aversion to foods can sometimes be overcome by changing the flavor of foods. This is readily done by introducing different flavoring substances. Flavorings can be obtained in pharmacies and drugstores. Acceptance of different food supplements available on the market can be improved by adding these flavorings.

If all dietary measures have remained unsuccessful, one may attempt treatment using hormones (gestagens, cortisone or androgens). These can improve the appetite and lead to weight gain. While corticoids (for example, prednisone 10 to 30mg/die or dexamethasone 2 to 4mg/die) have a short-term appetite-stimulating effect of two to four weeks as well as a reconstituting effect, and after this time have primarily the typical adverse effects associated with cortisone, the weight-increasing effects of megestrol acetate (160 to 480mg/die) last significantly longer.

Cortisone however influences glucose metabolism and should be used only with great caution in patients who have undergone pancreas resection, and especially in patients with manifest or latent diabetes.

With gestagens, it should be noted that these cause water retention in the tissues and thus a "false" weight gain. Development of thrombosis is also facilitated by gestagens. Pancreas cancer patients have an intrinsic risk of thrombosis.

The appetite can be influenced by means of psychopharmaca – especially tricyclic antidepressants. The appetite increasing effects of some hormones (for example, gestagens) are also based on their positive effects on the psyche.

The pharmaceutical industry is developing specialized medications aimed at combating tumour-related appetite loss, which involve "immunonutrition" or "organ protection", or are supposed to inactivate the hypothalamic satiation centre. In the United States, some physicians swear by the cannabinoids' ability to increase patients' appetites. Up to now advantages of cannabinoids versus megestral acetate are not proven (Jatoi et al., 2002). In Europe, appetite-stimulating hormones are preferred.

Family members sometimes can do more good by talking as little as possible about upcoming meals with the patient in order to avoid anxiety concerning the next meal and the appearance of sub-threshold nausea. "Sick people should never be forced to eat!" Set mealtimes are not necessary. The patient should always be able to eat when he/she feels like it.

Weight loss and recommendations

Weight loss is among the most common complaints. Many pancreatic cancer patients have experienced dramatic weight loss already before surgery. Following surgery, in some cases following radiation or chemotherapy, and not least of all tumour progression, further weight loss is observed (table 9.6). Cachexia in pancreatic cancer patients does not however merely result from appetite loss and maldigestion, but also from hypercatabolism due to an acute phase reaction sustained by the tumour. TNF-alpha and PIF are molecules which are the focus of current clinical research.

Table 9.6 - Most common causes of non-tumour related weight loss in recipients of pancreatic cancer and gastric cancer surgery.

– Reduced food intake
– Enzyme production in the residual pancreas too low
– Relative enzyme deficiency due to accelerated passage through the small intestine in the case of pancreocibal asynchrony
– Disturbances in biliary metabolism
– Bacterial colonization of the small intestine
– Improper nutrition
– Psychological causes, fear associated with eating
– Pain

Nutritional therapeutic guidance and counselling play a major role in limiting weight loss.

Thalidomide influences weight loss and cachexia in inoperable pancreatic cancer patients by inhibiting TNF-alpha (Gordon et al., 2005). Up to now advantages of cannabinoids (Dronabinol®) are not proven (Jatoi et al., 2002).

Enteral nutrition and recommendations

In the case that diabetes is not present, a slightly altered standard diet is recommended. Meals should be low in fat. Nutritional requirements of recipients of the Whipple procedure are for the most part the same as those for gastric surgery patients (table 9.7). Following pylorus-preserving pancreatoduodenectomy, restrictions may be reduced; after this, nutritional status and quality of life are quite good (McLeod 1999).

Table 9.7 - General nutritional recommendations following the Whipple procedure.

– Eat slowly
– Chew food well
– Choose low fat, easily digestible and well-tolerated foods
– Take several small meals daily instead of three main meals
– Avoid foods which are too hot, too cold, spicy, cured and grilled or excessively sweet or salty
– Choose low fat foods
– Avoid alcohol entirely

The food industry produces high-calorie, protein-enriched drinks in the form of flavored liquid nutrition (astronaut food) which one can either take between or in addition to meals. Drinks containing 1kcal/mL are best tolerated. These can bring about noticeable weight gain. Unfortunately, many patients report that they do not tolerate this "astronaut food". There are many reasons for this (table 9.8).

Table 9.8 - Causes of astronaut food intolerance.

– Diarrhea occurs frequently when too much of the astronaut drink is consumed at once or when it is drunk too quickly.
– Some patients, especially recipients of the Whipple procedure with partial gastric resection, develop diarrhea and dumping symptoms after consumption of hyperosmolaric supplements. In this case, supplements can be diluted to half-strength with tea. There are also supplements with different osmolarity values.
– Sometimes a lack of fiber causes diarrhea. In this case, fiber-rich supplements can be taken.
– Whipple surgery recipients in particular do not tolerate very well the fats present in the supplements and diarrhea is the result. With these patients, liquid and tube nutrition with a high percentage of MCTs should be administered. There are special supplements with high amounts of MCTs.
– If the temperature of tube-administered nutrition is too low, it should be heated before giving it to the patient.

If oral nourishment is no longer possible (for example, with gastric outlet stenosis) for ensuring adequate nutrition, it can be administered by means of a **tube** as a percutaneous endoscopic jejunostomy (PEJ) into the small intestine.

The advantage of this form of nourishment as opposed to **parenteral nutrition** lies in the fact that with artificial enteral nutrition, the natural food passage through the gastroenteral tract remains intact. The intestinal mucosa thus remains intact and bacterial colonization does not develop. The barrier and immune functions of the intestine thus remain intact as well.

Tube feeding poses fewer problems, is associated with fewer complications and is less costly than parenteral nutrition. It is important for the tube food preparations always to be fresh. Opened bottles must be refrigerated and even then can only be kept for a maximum of one day. The prepared food is to be given at room temperature. The amount should be increased gradually; otherwise it can cause diarrhea. Diarrhea is in fact one of the most common complications (table 9.9).

Table 9.9 - Possible causes of diarrhea in recipients of tube nutrition.

– Too rapid administration of food preparation
– Hypoalbumenia
– Bacterial contamination of the food preparation
– The particular combination of food contents
– Accompanying medications
– Antibiotic therapy

The incidence of diarrhea in patients receiving enteral nutrition who also take antibiotics is considerably higher than in patients receiving oral nutrition who also take antibiotics; this suggests a synergistic effect of both therapy options with regard to the triggering of diarrhea. In such cases of diarrhea it is helpful to switch from the formula diet to a product with a high percentage of water-soluble fiber, as this can contribute to compensation of an intraluminal lack of substrate. Up to 30% of antibiotic-related cases of diarrhea are attributed to clostridium difficile. Medications which can often cause diarrhea in recipients of enteral nutrition include antacids containing magnesium, digoxin, methyldopa, electrolyte concentrates and sorbitol-containing drugs. Sorbitol is often added to enhance flavor and is present in many liquid medications.

Typical errors in diet (for example, too rapid administration of food, too little fluid intake) and nutrition-dependent complications (for example, constipation, diarrhea, feeling of fullness, etc.) can be avoided. If the catheter is blocked, it sometimes helps to flush with Coca-Cola®.

Table 9.10 - Causes of contamination of enteral nutrition solutions.

– Insufficient cleaning of materials
– Supplements which are required for preparation or modification of formula diets
– Insufficient storage or transport conditions
– Storage of opened bottles containing tube nutrition and prepared powder foods at room temperature
– Inadequate hygienic hand disinfection
– Incorrect use of application system
– Use of application system for more than 24 hours
– Retrograde contamination by ascending microbes

Need of parenteral nutrition and recommendations

Parenteral nutrition is always considered when enteral nutrition is no longer possible, or insufficient or if the food in the gastro-intestinal tract cannot be digested or metabolized adequately. Reasons for parenteral nutrition may be due to short intestine syndrome or a temporary mechanical hindrance of gastrointestinal transit until the moment PEJ tube is inserted. A nutritional deficit can be corrected much more quickly by means of parenteral nutrition than with enteral nutrition; the reestablishment of acceptable physical condition and cellular and humoral immunity can take place.

The administration of parenteral nutrition requires intensive monitoring; it does not however require hospital admission. The presence of a port system is mandatory. Parenteral nutrition from home always depends on the close interaction among hospital and general physicians with a commercial service-provider.

Necessity of information and patient education (discussion groups/health training/conversation groups) and recommendations

Education and information are important aids in helping to cope with the disease and the side effects of therapy. Important topics include the patient's understanding of what is happening inside his/her body and why a certain therapy option has been chosen. The majority of patients do not wish to make decisions about tumour therapy themselves, but they would like to know the reasons for pursuing a certain treatment strategy. It is the aim of health training to inform the patients of the possibilities and limitations of standard medicine, to protect them from harmful alternative forms of therapy and to convey to them the significance of medical surveillance (table 9.12). One-to-one and group counselling sessions are effective for this purpose; in the latter patients' family members may also participate.

Besides questions concerning nutrition, special training for diabetics and postoperative disorders, issues such as social support and psychological assistance for relaxation and coping with anxiety constitute the focus of group meetings. General information is given on pancreatic cancer, its causes, the different therapy options, prevention of recurrence, follow-up examinations, coping with fears and pain as well as information on social rights and assistance, including occupational consequences of the illness (tables 9.11, 9.12). Family members should be offered the opportunity to participate in these group meetings.

Table 9.11 - Aims of diabetes counselling

– Designing and conveying the contents of the training program
– Teaching using specific aids
– "Diabetes check"
– Individual counselling for questions pertaining to living with diabetes (occupation, travelling, sports, etc.)
– Counselling for adjusting insulin dosages
– Cooperation with conceptualization of therapeutic strategies for patients
– Cooperation in socio-medical decisions

Table 9.12 - Topics in health training in patients with pancreatic

Prophylactic measures
– Characteristics of therapy options (when, why and which one)
– Prevention or reduction of chemotherapy, hormone or radiation therapy side effects
– Significance of follow-up examinations
– Signs of recurrent illness, recurrence prophylaxis, therapy in cases of recurrence
– Possible pain therapy
– Prognosis
– Significance of immune functions

Nutrition
– Causes of weight loss
– Prevention of further weight loss
– Most common dietary disturbances
– Specific features of diets
– Is there a "cancer diet"?
– Healthy diets

Psychological assistance
– Opportunities for relaxation – coping with fears and depression – fatigue symptoms
– References to psychological aids
– Dealing with family members

Social assistance
– Information pertaining to legal protection for cancer patients
– Information pertaining to financial aid/special rates or reductions
– Insurance – life insurance – credit granting – paying off debts
– Information on self-help groups – hospice programs – palliative wards

Vocational counselling and assistance
– Occupational consequences
– Avoidance of certain stressful or strenuous situations at work
– Steps to take and assistance aimed at successful vocational reintegration

The dietary advisor, the psychologist, the social worker and the physician should take turns in moderating the group.

Patients and their family members should also have access to printed versions of the information and advice that they have received in health education sessions (for example, in the form of differentiated and industry-unaffiliated reference literature). This printed material should of course never take the place of medical consultations, but they should rather provide the basis of productive discussions with the attending physician.

The Internet is becoming more and more of an additional source of information for patients as well as their family members. It is often difficult for the layperson to recognize whether the information available is serious. It is useful if the physician, on his/her own initiative, recommends certain websites that he/she considers to be well balanced, informative and helpful

Rehabilitative measures aimed at reducing psychological problems ("rehabilitation to combat resignation and depression")

For a more in-depth description see chapter on psychological support in cancer rehabilitation and palliation.

In some cases, the psychological problems occur in connection with pain, eating difficulties, weight loss, affecting social and occupational areas of the patients' lives; they are resolved when the symptoms disappear.

Many patients harbor fears that their disease will progress and that they will lose control during the further course of illness and/or have to relinquish their autonomy and integrity.

Depression

It is quite often depression and the fear of an uncertain future with which the patients are confronted. Additional counselling by a psychologist (psycho-oncologist) with experience working with tumour patients is very helpful in these situations (table 2.2).

Assistance in coping with illness, alleviating fears and depression and strengthening compliance are the main areas which are dealt with in psycho-oncology. There are different types of coping strategies for patients dealing with the imminence or threat of death made real by the disease (table 2.6). Here, behaviour patterns which represent an active form of confrontation should be encouraged.

Denial of illness and distancing oneself from past events have no place within the context of modern concepts of rehabilitation. It still remains unclear however which illness coping strategy is to be considered effective and in which cases of coping behaviour psychological assistance is indicated. There is no standardized procedure; indeed there should not be one, as each affected individual responds differently, is to be dealt with differently and requires different forms of assistance. Some patients – it is particularly those with strong religious beliefs who very often fall into this category – do well without any professional psychological assistance.

Fears

Stress-free discussions in a calm environment, taking the time to listen and to convey a sense of trust all comprise the essential elements of anxiety therapy. The better the psychosocial guidance, the more influential the discussions can be in offsetting the patients' fears. The participation of the psycho-oncologist, the family and, in some cases the social worker, is of great significance (tables 2.3, 2.5).

If anxiety is associated with medical problems, alleviation of fears can sometimes be achieved through education, information and counselling. If anxiety is accompanied by pain, psychotherapy is only possible after the pain has been treated satisfactorily.

Anxiety can be influenced by means of anxiolytic drugs, primarily benzodiazepines. Benzodiazepines are preferred to other medications as they are well tolerated, have few adverse effects and possess a wide therapeutic breadth. Substances with short-term effects such as lorazepam, midazolam and oxazepam have established themselves as the drugs of choice. If anxiety symptoms already reappear before the next dose has been administered, a transition to benzodiazepines with long-term effects should be made (for example, diazepam or clonazepam).

Neuroleptic drugs have anxiolytic qualities as well. Haloperidol in particular should be mentioned here: It is chosen in situations in which patients also experience confusion or hallucinations. Tricyclic antidepressants are considered primarily when anxiety is associated with depression. These however can take up to two weeks to take effect. If it has been decided to discontinue administrating these drugs, this should take place gradually within a period of two-three days in order to prevent withdrawal symptoms.

Confusion, disorientation and/or hallucinations tend to occur most commonly during the terminal phase. Neuroleptics are suitable for symptomatic therapy, with delirium syndrome (for example, haloperidol), benzodiazepines with extreme anxiety as well as with agitation and restlessness (for example, lorazepam, midazolam).

Fatigue

See also chapter: "Psychological support in cancer rehabilitation and palliation".

Fatigue (table 2.8) is present to a greater or lesser degree in nearly all pancreatic carcinoma patients. It manifests itself as drowsiness, exhaustion and a lack of motivation, and its presence is multifactorial. Besides depression and pain, other factors such as sleeping disorders, anemia, malnutrition and adverse effects of the therapy can all contribute to this condition (table 2.9). Medication responsible for this can be anxiolytic drugs and antidepressants which may also represent the cause of the fatigue symptoms. Opiates can induce fatigue symptoms as well. In exceptional cases, a patient may profit from pharmacotherapy using psychostimulants, but more patients can be helped through behavioural modification counselling.

If anemia is the cause, a physiological increase of hemoglobin with erythropoetin can lead to improvement. Some centres successfully use megestrol acetate for the treatment of both emaciation and fatigue symptoms.

Self-help groups

It is beneficial for patients to share their own experiences among themselves, learn from each other and give mutual help and support. Patients who have undergone pancreas surgery should therefore join self-help groups. In some countries there are special self-help groups for recipients of pancreas surgery. Here, social, legislative, specialized assistance and advice from the patients' own experiences can be shared. In this way mutual support can be given. These self-help groups should be viewed by the attending physician as partners and not as competitors. Only those groups should be recommended which do not destroy the patients' trust in scientifically-oriented oncology and which are willing to cooperate with methods in standard medicine.

Rehabilitative measures aimed at reducing social problems ("rehabilitation to combat the need of care"

For a more in-depth description, see chapter "Social support in cancer rehabilitation and palliation".

The aim of these measures is to strengthen the patient's own resources and prevent the risk of a need for care, or at least reduce such a need.

If the patient is no longer able to care for himself/herself, outside care must be arranged. In patients with pancreatic cancer, this situation presents itself especially frequently (Shore, 2004). The early organization of outside assistance and social support is therefore crucial in these patients, who are generally older with, as is generally known, rapidly progressing illness.

The planning of further care must take place with the patients' family members. Forms of assistance such as "meals on wheels", household assistance, home nursing care, care assistance and in some circumstances the arrangement of nursing home care or hospice have to be arranged. Providing contact addresses (self-help groups, counselling centres, etc.) is helpful.

The first contacts to be made to achieve this end are social workers in the hospital, rehabilitation clinics, cancer counselling centres, insurance companies as well as charity organizations (table 3.12). Self-help groups play a role not to be underestimated within the context of the aims of follow-up treatment on the social level; these are however often only of limited value due to the complexity of the problems with which the patient is confronted.

If home care is not, or has not yet been, arranged, the time spent in the hospital can be followed by a temporary stay in an institution for follow-up care. In Germany, there are rehabilitation hospitals ("AHB hospitals") which are designed especially to meet the needs of patients with gastrointestinal tumours and in which plans are made for the patients' social assistance, in addition to medical and psychological guidance. Counselling of patients and their family members is one of the tasks of such rehabilitation centres. Experienced physicians, psychologists and representatives of self-help groups share their experiences, information and helpful advice. In Germany, every cancer patient has a legal claim to a three-five week stay in such an institution. Some of the *maisons de repos* in France have a similar function.

Hospice programs – palliative wards

See also chapter: "Social and vocational assistance".

Hospice programs and palliative wards play an important role (table 1.15). Here efforts are focused on care, supportive care, including adequate pain therapy and psychological guidance, rather than oncological counselling. It is not unusual however that patients and their family members express apprehension when the subject of a transfer to a hospice ward is raised. The idea of being "given up" by physicians and no longer being able to fight for survival is apparently a difficult thing to accept in our western culture.

Rehabilitative measures aimed at reducing vocational problems ("rehabilitation to combat early retirement")

See also chapter: "Vocational integration in cancer rehabilitation".

Need of vocational support

Every cancer patient of working age must be advised on eventual effects of cancer and cancer therapies restrictions of working capacity, workloads to be avoided and measures for the protection and maintenance of workplaces.

Restrictions of working capacity

According to our current state of knowledge, work does not affect tumour growth, risk of recurrence or prognosis.

Assessment of vocational fitness and the capacity to work depends on tumour location, whether R0 or R1 resection has taken place, on the extent of pancreas resection, on accompanying illnesses, on whether or not adjuvant therapy has been given, on the physical condition of the patient and, not least of all, on the coping.

Patients with inoperable pancreatic carcinoma or with tumour recurrence are generally not fit for work. They should submit applications for work incapacity pension as soon as possible. Exceptions can be made – for psychological reasons – when the patient expresses a strong desire to resume working. In this case work-facilitating measures are helpful, for example the gradual resumption of work tasks. During these "work trials" most patients will become aware that they are no longer able to complete the tasks they were once able to master.

Harmful occupational substances

Association between certain harmful occupational substances and pancreatic cancer have not been conclusively demonstrated, although pancreatic cancer appears to occur more frequently in certain occupations (Alguacil *et al.*, 2003) and possible links to exposure to pesticides have been discussed (Silverman *et al.*, 2001).

Workloads to be avoided

For potentially curatively treated and "cured" pancreatic cancer patients (R0 resection) there are numerous occupational limitations which are due primarily to postoperative physical weakness. Physically strenuous activities are no longer possible following total pancreatectomy and even following the Whipple procedure. Sitting or desk jobs are on the other hand still possible (Rosemeyer, 1996).

How to return to work

The issues of which workplace-conserving measures, including reassimilation assistance, work and career promotion, as well as change in workplace come into question who takes financial responsibility, when vocational reorientation makes sense and is practicable, where detailed information is available are all best addressed in the oncological rehabilitation clinic and, if necessary, by the rehabilitation advisor of the patients' respective pension schemes.

Palliative measures

Informing the patient about disease progression delivering bad news

Despite the unfavourable prognosis of tumour recurrence, there are more points in favour of than against patient information. This does not mean, however, that the patient should be forced to confront the full implications of his or her illness (tables 2.11, 9.13). Detailed information is also required for every type of tumour therapy.

Many fears associated with the illness originate from the fact that the affected person does not know how the situation should be assessed or what he/she should expect. It is better in any case for the patient to be informed by the attending physician than by prayer healers, moneymakers, or by random figures found on the Internet. Information without the simultaneous offering of prospects and assistance is never constructive.

Patient information consists principally of the providing of information; however, it is the accompanying emotional support given which is crucial for dealing with information. Unfortunately, some physicians discuss these essential matters with the affected persons and their family members only when specifically requested to do so. The ability to make appropriate quality of life decisions requires strong, clear communication between the doctors, treatment staff, patient and family caregivers. There is no better situation than having well informed, highly skilled doctors working with a motivated, well informed patient and supportive family caregivers.

Table 9.13 - Key tasks in communication with patients (Maguire *et al.*, 2002).

- Eliciting the patient's main problems, the patient's perceptions of these, and the physical, emotional, and social impact of the patient's problems on the patient and family
- Tailoring information to what the patient wants to know; checking his or her understanding
- Eliciting the patient's reactions to the information given and his or her main concerns
- Determining how much the patient wants to participate in decision making (when treatment options are available)
- Discussing treatment options so that the patient understands the implications
- Maximising the chance that the patient will follow agreed decisions regarding treatment and advice about changes in lifestyle

It is helpful to announce the educational discussion beforehand and to decide in advance whether the patient would like to include family members or other persons close to him/her. If other persons are to be included, the patient has to give his/her prior consent.

During the meeting, the seriousness and the implications of the clinical findings should indeed be conveyed to the patient; however, the prognosis should never be discussed in terms of remaining time left for the patient. Even pancreatic cancer can take an unexpected turn. In cases of hopeless prognosis, positive aspects should always be mentioned as well (for example, references to advances in palliative therapy, better pain therapy available today, the availability of constant medical and psychological guidance, etc.).

It is important to indicate that one is always available for discussions with the patient, to listen and to make certain that the patient has understood, to listen and to find out what the patient has understood and what meaning the contents of the discussion have for him/her. A patient's wish – which often can be gathered from observing the patient's behaviour – to push the problem aside, either temporarily or for the longer term, should be respected.

Often doctors ignore patient's perceptions of their physical, emotional and social impact of the problems. They pay little attention to checking how well patients have understood what they have been told. Less than half of psychological morbidity in patients is recognized.

Doctors often may not realize how often patients withhold important information from them or the reasons for this (table 9.14.)

Table 9.14 - Reasons for patients not disclosing problems (Maguire *et al.*, 2002).

- Belief that nothing can be done
- Reluctance to burden the doctor
- Desire not to seem pathetic or ungrateful
- Concern that it is not legitimate to mention them
- Doctors' blocking behaviour
- Worry that their fears of what is wrong with them will be confirmed

Symptoms and localization of recurrences

At the time of diagnosis in the patients, who are generally older, the illness has usually reached a locally advanced and no longer operable stage, thus presenting a palliative situation (table 9.15) (Shore, 2004).

Table 9.15 - Most common complaints associated with recurrence of pancreatic carcinoma.

– Jaundice
– Weight loss
– Thrombosis
– Pain
– Ascites
– Disturbances in gastro-intestinal transit

Choice of treatment modalities

By the time cancer is diagnosed it is often already advanced, inoperable, has infiltrated surrounding organs or developed distant metastasis, leaving only the possibility of supportive and palliative treatment. Metastasis usually occurs either at the site of resection or in the liver (Smeenk, 2004). The basis for palliative tumour therapy which is then performed is in these instances best supportive care (table 3.10). The value of these palliative tumour therapy forms must never be assessed using remission criteria alone, but rather, must contain quality of life criteria (table 9.18). The aims of treatment are to reduce the tumour burden, improve symptoms and modestly extend median survival. Survival time may be a quantifiable and reproducible criterion for demonstrating effectiveness of primary therapy, but it is only one of many success criteria within the context of palliative therapy.

The question of whether or not to have tumour therapy, and if so, then which tumour therapy to choose, should be decided on the basis of the patient's wishes, his/her functional status, psychosocial aspects, etc. With regards to the question of which tumour therapy forms are to be chosen in the case of progression of illness, one must always consider whether and how the affected patient would profit from the therapy, and whether and how cancer and/or therapy-related morbidity would affect him/her. Other factors to be considered are concomitant illnesses (for example, diabetes, renal insufficiency, cardiovascular illnesses, poor nutritional status and functional limitations), the awareness of one's own illness, the will to live, coping behaviour and social support as well as the type of therapy strategy to be chosen. Answering the question "How much, and which therapy?" not only requires an oncological basis of knowledge, but also competence and skill in the fields of ethics and communication. Many of the chemotherapy and radiation therapy standards recommended for pancreatic carcinoma recurrence are based on the results of therapy studies conducted on younger patients who are in good general condition. Conclusions drawn in connection with these unrealistic studies do not necessarily apply to patients with pancreatic cancer, who are generally older. In geriatric patients, drug pharmacokinetics and pharmacodynamics may be altered. It is essential to be aware of any pharmacological peculiarities which might be present and to take them into consideration

Local and regional problems and palliative therapies

Radiation therapy, in some cases supplemented by chemotherapy (Oya, 2004), has top priority in treating pain associated with locoregional tumour spread. It should be considered together with systemic pain therapy. Combined radio-chemotherapy is deemed superior to the sole use of radiation or chemotherapy (Hocht *et al.*, 2004; Epelbaum, 2002; Sindelar, 1999); this can however be associated with severe adverse effects. Surgical procedures are limited primarily to drainages, bypasses and reestablishment of gastro-intestinal passage and tend not to have the aim of reducing tumour size (Dunn, 2002). Interventional endoscopy plays a dominant role in palliative treatment of pancreatic carcinoma (Sanders *et al.*, 2007). It is more comfortable for the patient and brings about significant improvement of quality of life. With the development of biliary stents, minimally invasive procedures have replaced surgical techniques.

Local recurrence, lymph node metastases

The pancreas resection bed is the site of most recurrences.

External-beam radiation, radio-chemotherapy, radiation therapy using gemcitabine or other drugs as sensitizors, intra-operative radiation or brachytherapy can alleviate symptoms; they have however little impact on long-term survival due to the development of metastases outside the fields of radiation (Sindelar, 1999; Epelbaum, 2000).

Liver metastases

The liver is the most common site of metastases. In extremely rare cases this is a solitary liver metastasis, for which reason neither surgical treatment of metastases nor isolated regional chemotherapy or embolization can be expected to bring about a significant increase in survival time. Systemic combined chemotherapy can on the other hand alleviate symptoms; in case of pain, adequate pain therapy is indicated.

Peritoneal carcinosis

As a rule, neither surgical nor radiation therapeutic intervention comes into question.

Chemotherapy may be attempted, although this is less effective in cases of peritoneal carcinosis than in other metastases locations. Intraperitoneal chemotherapy can in some instances limit ascites production for short periods of time; it has only – if any at all – a local and temporary effect due to the formation of cavities. Symptomatic ascites can be relieved by puncture or drainage. Pain is best treated with spasmolytic drugs; to prevent ileus, the stool should be kept soft.

A gastroenterostomy, a PEJ or colostomy may be indicated for symptoms of obstruction. Parenteral nutrition can extend life. Insertion of a stomach tube may be indicated.

In a subileus situation, a conservative therapy attempt using high-dose corticosteroids (for example, 36mg dexamethasone per day) is to be made, even at the terminal stage, with subsequent enteral, or if necessary, additional parenteral administration of prokinetic/cholinergic drugs.

Gastric outlet stenosis

Before nutritional therapy is initiated, gastroenteral continuity status is to be investigated. Gastric outlet stenosis, due to tumour infiltration of the duodenum, is a common occurrence. Some centres establish the indication for gastroenteranastomosis (gastroenterostomy, gastrojejunostomy) even before symptoms appear in cases of extensive tumour damage and high risk situations. Percutaneous endoscopic gastrostomy or radiological interventional gastrostomy (PEG or PEJ) should be applied only in inoperable patients or in cases of diffuse peritoneal carcinosis.

Bypass surgery is not always necessary or possible. By means of directed laser therapy, the stenosis in the gastro-intestinal tract can sometimes be dilated and gastroenteral passage can be made possible through implantation of duodenal stents.

With radiation therapy in the gastric bed and para-aortic fields, there is often a delayed reaction of vomiting and nausea. Here, NK-1 antagonists (aprepitant) are quite effective, whereas a combination of 5-HT3 antagonists and dexamethasone is most effective when combatting acute emesis brought on by chemotherapy.

Duodenal obstruction

The issue of duodenal obstruction is controversial, involving a debate as to whether or not routine gastric bypass should be performed at the same time as surgical biliary bypass. Approximately 15-20% of patients undergoing biliary bypass will develop subsequent duodenal obstruction. A portion of patients undergoing gastric bypass procedures will develop delayed gastric emptying, with significant morbidity associated with this procedure. Therefore, it seems sensible to reserve gastric bypass for those with definite obstruction or evidence of impending problems, especially given the availability of endoscopically-inserted metal duodenal stents (Holt, 2004; Sanders *et al.*, 2007).

Obstructive jaundice

Obstructive jaundice is usually due to compression or infiltration of ductus hepaticocholedochus (Bergasa, 2006). Pruritus, occurring as a result of biliary obstruction, is often troublesome.

Through the placement of a **biliodigestive anastomosis** (cholecysto-choledocho-duodeno-jejunostomy or choledocho-jejunostomy) or a stent (either **metal or plastic**), the extremely burdensome symptoms of pruritus and jaundice can be alleviated and the appetite increased. Endoscopically-placed stents remain the mainstay for the palliation treatment of malignant billary obstruction (Chah, 2005; Sanders et al, 2007). The disadvantage of surgical bypass is the risk of short-term complications; the drawbacks of stent implantation are long-term complications such as recurring cholangitis. The complication rate following endoscopic stent implantation is lower than following percutaneous therapy.

The use of metal screen stents, also called mesh or wall stent, has become established. The procedure of percutaneous transhepatic cholangiodrainage should be employed only if endoscopic procedures have failed or in anatomically difficult situations, as well as following partial gastric resection or gastrectomy, especially involving Roux-en-Y anastomosis.

A variety of techniques for surgical biliary drainage are available, although the original procedure of cholecysto-jejunostomy has been superseded due to long-term patency rates. Operative drainage is associated with higher morbidity and mortality rates than stenting and should be reserved for those patients found to be inoperable during surgery and in the rare instance in which stenting by either route has failed, bearing in mind the mortality rate of open drainage of 19-24%.

Table 9.16 - Medicaments against pruritus in pancreatic cancer.

– Antihistaminics	– Cholestyramin
– Androgens	– Rifampicin

Osseous metastases

In most cases, metastases are present at the same time in other organs as well. With localized pain, pain radiation therapy is indicated. Periphery-acting pain medications frequently have only short-term effects, if any at all, for which reason they should be administered very early together with long-term morphine preparations. Enteral administration of bisphosphonates can alleviate pain in some cases.

Systemic palliative therapies

Heparinization

Thromboembolic occurrences tend to complicate the course of illness of patients with pancreatic cancer especially frequently. Low molecular weight heparin is suitable for therapeutic and prophylactic purposes.

Chemotherapy

Gemcitabine, 5-fluorouracil + folinate, etoposide, epirubicine, paclitaxel, irinotecane, topotecane, platinum and oxaliplatinum alone or in combination with radiation therapy or erlotinib (Oya, 2004; Neoptolemos, 2003) all have limited effectiveness in advanced pancreatic carcinoma. The advantages of polychemotherapy as opposed to monotherapy are not unequivocal. Gemcitabine and erlotinib have a small but significant benefit on survival (Morre *et al.*, 2007). On average, chemotherapy brings about a noticeable decrease in tumour size in approximately 10% of patients. The survival benefit is small; however, marked alleviation of symptoms is achieved in around 20-30% of patients. Thus, chemotherapy should more often be applied only after symptoms have appeared and not at an asymptomatic stage. Quality of life data should be considered when choosing the chemotherapy regimen.

Combined radiation-chemotherapy has been deemed more effective than chemo- or radiotherapy alone. The combination with gemcitabine is especially favoured; this combination of agents is however considerably more toxic than monotherapy.

Alternative therapy forms

Numerous therapy forms are offered by various industries to which are ascribed the qualities of improving unspecific immune functions and activating the body's own immune defenses against the tumour (**immunostimulants or immune modulators**). Examples of such substances are mistletoe extract, enzyme and thymus preparations, snake venom, oxygen multistep therapy, phototherapy, symbiosis control, microbiological therapy, vitamins, among many others. All these therapy options are based on widely speculative assumptions, do not appear very plausible from a theoretical standpoint and are not recognized by standard medicine. Their therapeutic effects on tumour are – if any – only minimal.

So far there has been no scientific study that might have proven the tumour-inhibiting effects of mistletoe preparations. The assertion that the patient's quality of life can be improved through its use is very difficult to confirm. Yet these mistletoe preparations are not only used by those practicing alternative and nature-oriented forms of medicine, but also by some oncologists. The reason for this is less the belief in its effectiveness, than the possibility of being able to offer the patient a further therapy option.

Parenteral nutrition/cachexia

Patients and their family members have to receive intensive instruction in order to take over the care of infusion systems. Fluids and the necessary amino acid, carbohydrate, protein, calorie, fat and electrolyte contents must be adjusted to meet the patients' constantly changing nutritional requirements. Catheter infections with and without sepsis, metabolic complications and an oversupply of fluids in patients with cardiac or renal insufficiency are the most common complications and must be avoided.

It was formerly standard procedure to use high percentages of carbohydrates as the source of energy; now the percentage of carbohydrates used is 60 to 70% and that of fats is 30 to 40%. A noticeable decrease in tumour cachexia can be achieved by enriching parenteral nutrition with omega-3 fatty acids.

The traditional view considered cancer cachexia as the result of decreased food intake and increased energy consumption of the tumour (Tisdale, 2002). This view of cachexia as resulting from an energy imbalance, led to aggressive total parenteral nutrition studies in an attempt to provide the energy required to overcome this perceived nutritional deficit. Increasing energy intake by means of enteral or parenteral feeding has not been successful in increasing either total weight or lean body mass, and does not improve functional status, quality of life, or survival. Some trials have shown thalidomide attenuates weight loss and leads to a reduction in loss of lean body mass in patients with cachexia secondary to pancreatic cancer. However, these trials were unable to demonstrate that the attenuation in loss of body weight led to an improvement in quality of life (Gordon *et al.*, 2005).

Although anorexia frequently accompanies cachexia, the drop in caloric intake alone cannot account for the body-composition changes seen in cachexia, and, moreover, cachexia can occur even in the absence of anorexia. The indication for parenteral nutrition in a palliative situation is not without controversy. Cachexia is not due solely to a nutrient deficit or to tumour/host competition for essential nutrients, but to complex metabolic changes in tissues arising from tumour catabolic factors, which may be enhanced by pro-inflammatory cytokines.

Special features of pain therapy

See also chapter: "Pain management in cancer rehabilitation and palliation".

Pancreatic carcinoma is especially feared due to its lack of warning signals, its poor prognosis, its resistance to chemotherapy and radiation therapy and its extreme and uneasily treatable pain symptoms. Specialized knowledge of pain therapy is required in the follow-up treatment of this type of tumour, in order to make the terminal stage more bearable for the patients (table 5.10).

In addition to standard analgesic regimens, a variety of nerve ablative techniques are available. **Causal tumour therapy** also can be considered (table 5.2). Besides external and internal radiation therapy (table 5.15), a wide range of chemotherapies is available. These forms of treatment are, however, not very effective.

Visceral pain is most common. This originates from compression, inflammation and ulceration of the abdominal organs. In most cases nociceptive pain is present, especially when necrotic or autolytic processes are the cause. Experience has shown that this type of pain responds well to a combination of NSAIDs and opioids. The pain can however also be originating from the sympathetic nervous system. With exclusively visceral pain, local analgesic therapy is of great significance. Neurodestructive procedures, for example, celiac plexus neurolysis, may be beneficial (Shafman *et al.*, 1990). Thoracoscopic division of the splanchnic nerves can have significant analgesic effects when medicinal analgesia has become inefficient.

Neurogenic pain is common. This originates through infiltration, damage to or irritation of the nervous system. It is characterized by shooting, cutting or piercing pain symptoms. They can also at times manifest themselves as constant burning or "drilling" pains. Antidepressants combined with opioids and, if necessary, anticonvulsants are then indicated. Neurodestructive analgesic therapy (neurolysis, chordotomy, myelotomy, DREZ lesion, dorsal root entry zone coagulation and thermolesion of the gasserian ganglion) may be considered in cases of severe acute smptoms (for example, disorders of bladder/rectal function) or long-term complications (de-afferencing pain).

The scale plan provided by the WHO for analgesic medication therapy (World Health Organization, 1990) applies, with minor modifications, to pancreatic carcinoma as well (fig. 5.5). According to this, therapy is initiated for mild pain using non-opioid level I analgesics with consideration of any contraindications (for example, ulcer, coagulation disorders, renal insufficiency, hepatopathy) and possible interactions with drugs already in use. The simultaneous administration of two different non-steroidal antirheumatics (NSAR) is not practiced due to the increase in toxicity (table 5.32).

Continuation of medication using non-opioid analgesics, as well as the pain type-appropriate accompaniment with co-analgesics is recommended. Level IV includes opiates which are administered either parenterally or near the spinal cord, local anaesthetics, neurolysis and neurosurgical procedures (tables 5.21, 9.17).

Table 9.17 - Special features of analgesic drug therapy in pancreatic cancer patients.

– Periphery-oriented pain medication is often associated with considerable adverse affects in gastric resection recipients (and following the Whipple procedure). Due to the risk of damage to gastric or small intestine mucosa, ulcers and bleeding, proton pump inhibitors should be given in addition to NSAR preparations. H2 blockers are – contrary to earlier recommendations – not appropriate. These do alleviate gastrointestinal symptoms, but do not avoid ulcers and the much-feared cases of bleeding. In the terminal phase morphine 5-10mg s.c.

– Additional administration of corticoids is indicated in patients with liver capsule pain, painful lymphedema and compression pain. The corticosteroids should initially be given at high doses (hydrocortisone 80 to 120mg), and subsequently at lower doses (hydrocortisone 20 to30 mg). Corticoids have additional positive effects on the psyche and the appetite.

– Neuropathic pain often respond inadequately to therapy using non-opioids or opioid analgesics. An attempt should be made using antidepressants, and with "shooting" pains, anticonvulsants (for example, carbamazepine 200mg/die initially and 400-600mg/die maintenance dose, or gabapentine 1.2-2-4g).

– With pain due to retroperitoneal involvement extending into the nerve plexus, long-term pain alleviation can be achieved by performing CT-directed instillation of alcohol into the plexus.

– Percutaneous radiation therapy is to be considered in cases of osseous metastases. With severe bone pain due to osteolysis, the parental administration of bisphosphonates is indicated.

– For cramping pains, analgesics with spasmolytic effects (for example, metamizole, pentazocine, N-butyl scopolamine, nitro-preparations) are particularly helpful. Oral administration of butyl scopolamine has otherwise no effect; it only has an effect on the gastro-intestinal tract.

– With muscle pain, tetrazepam (200-400mg) works quite well; with muscle spasms, baclofen (60-100mg).

– For nausea and vomiting, anxiety and sleeplessness, neuroleptics are effective (for example, haloperidol 3 x 0.5 to 1mg = 3 x 5 to 10 drops/die or in the terminal phase haloperidol 2.5-5mg s.c. or levomepromazin 5-10mg s.c.). Levomepromazin or dimenhydrinate 100mg s. c. are quite effective against nausea and vomiting.

– For anxiety in the terminal phase: midazolam 2.5-10mg s.c.

The use of opioids has especially become established in the pain therapy of pancreatic carcinoma. When switching from one opioid analgesic to another, differences in dosages are to be noted. For such a switch, the 50% rule applies: This is the calculated equi analgesic daily dose which is reduced by 30-50% and then titrated against the pain. The recommended conversion factors for opioids are only approximations which can be reduced below or exceeded in individual cases.

If oral administration of analgesics is not possible, long-acting morphine preparations can also be applied sublingually by way of the oral mucosa, rectally by way of tube nutrition or transdermally by means of skin patches (table 5.23). The advantage of transdermal application of fentanyl (Durogesic®) and buprenorphine (Transtec®) is the facility of its use. Transdermal therapy makes sense for cases of stable tumour pain. In the terminal phase, a switch from long-acting morphine to parenteral therapy may become necessary. Differences in bioavailability must then be noted. Subcutaneous application is, technically speaking, the simplest and easiest method; here the length of time the canula can stay in place varies from individual to individual. If an intravenous infusion is being administered for any reason, morphine may also be applied intravenously.

Peridural/intrathecal therapy is a potential therapy alternative for patients with opioid-sensitive pain but who experience intolerable side effects (tables 5.37, 5.38, 5.39).

Placement of a portal system with an external pump is to be recommended for peridural/intrathecal therapy for a period of weeks to months. The complete implantation of a pump system should take place only for an estimated therapy length of at least three months.

In addition to analgesics, tricyclic antidepressants (for example, amytryptilin long-acting initial dose 25mg/die with a maintenance dose of 50 to 75mg/die after five to seven days) and/or benzodiazepines, for an anxiolytic effect, can contribute to pain alleviation (tables 5.34, 5.35). Anxiety has an influence on pain intensity. Due to their sedative effects, these medications are best administered in the evening. Clomipramine on the other hand (initial dose 25mg/die with a maintenance dose of 75 to 100mg/die) can be given in the morning due to its activating effect. The additional administration of low-dose corticoids (for example, 30mg hydrocortisone/die) can produce a pain-alleviating effect and at the same time have a stimulating effect on both psyche and appetite. Systemic corticoid medication can also be indicated under the aspect of pain therapy. This especially holds true for neurogenic pain and diffuse pain symptoms associated with paraneoplastic syndrome.

A variety of drugs can be used for sedation, many of which are used in lowered does or by different routes of administration in palliative care. Routine sedation is commonly provided by increasing the doses of opioids, benzodiazepines and neuroleptics that the patient is already taking at non-sedating doses. Extraordinary sedation with continuous infusions of midazolam, thiopental, and propofol can relieve refractory symptoms in most patients in their final days of life (Levy and Cohen, 2005).

Psychotherapy is recommended for patients whose pain is associated with a somatoform, anxiety, or depressive disorder. Anxiolytic drugs have anti-anxiety effects. Benzodiazepines are indicated in subjects with anxiety and/or insomnia. In chronic pain states, somatic pain may be accompanied by other disease-related syndromes like cases dyspnoea, restlessness, anxiety, insomnia. Psychosocial problems exacerbating the pain circumstances have a major impact. That is the reason why "chronic pain" qualifies as a biopsychosocial entity (fig. 5.2).

Complementary and alternative medicine

Cancer patients use a wide variety of non-pharmacological treatments regardless of effectiveness. The physician-patient relationship would benefit from the physician being able to discuss specific complementary treatments with patients, rather than avoid the topic or dismiss such treatments as elusive or not part of conventional cancer care.

For pancreatic cancer patients in particular, experience has shown not only that "faith can move mountains", but that it can also improve the quality of life. One should not shatter these patients' faith in a particular therapy form with evidence-based arguments. There is some support for the use of several modalities as potential complements to conventional cancer care, particularly for the quality of life issues associated with chronic cancer.

Quality assurance and rehabilitative measures

As with acute therapy, certain guidelines should also apply to follow-up care, including rehabilitation and palliation. There are unfortunately few guidelines on this subject. To guarantee quality of rehabilitation and palliation you have to ensure quality of structures, quality of rehabilitative and palliative measures and to evaluate the outcome.

Quality of structural features

Therapies needed in rehabilitation and palliation should be provided by specialized rehabilitation services with a team of patient care specialists. Pancreatic rehabilitation services include critical components of assessment, physical reconditioning, skill training, and psychosocial support. They may include vocational evaluation and counselling.

In Germany, there are structural guidelines for rehabilitation institutions that provide treatment for ambulant or hospitalized patients with gastro-intestinal cancers (Bundesarbeitsgemeinschaft für Rehabilitation, 2003).

Rehabilitative achievements in pancreatic cancer patients can only be made through the work of a qualified rehabilitation team (fig. 1.4). In order for this to be realized, special experience and a specialized infrastructure are essential. Due to the experience necessary, the rehabilitative institution should care for at least thirty pancreatic cancer patients per year. Verifiability of the quality of rehabilitation and palliative therapies must be guaranteed.

Quality of medical and therapeutic processes

The team should be coordinated by a physician experienced in rehabilitation and palliation with demonstrable oncological knowledge. All members of the rehabilitation team should participate in the patient's assessment. Nutritionists play an important role in this team. The collaboration of psycho-oncologists is very useful. Social workers are essential because of the social aids that are often needed. Cooperation and the exchange of information with the previously and subsequently treating physicians are important.

The initial evaluation should include the medical history, diagnostic tests, current symptoms and complaints, physical assessment, psychological, social, or vocational needs, nutritional status, exercise tolerance, determination of educational needs, the ability to carry out activities of daily living and the patient's interests and compliance.

The rehabilitation program must be tailored to meet the needs of the individual patient, addressing age-specific and cultural variables, and should contain patient-determined goals, as well as goals established by the individual team. Both patients and families participate in this training administered by health care professionals.

Outcome assessment and evaluation

The evaluation of rehabilitative measures in tumour patients is directed not at survival time, but rather at quality of life criteria. This involves primarily subjective parameters such as improvement of pain, nutrition, appetite, mobility, overcoming fears, etc. and not such parameters as are found in association with primary therapy (response, remission and length of remission) (table 9.18), Another difference is that in rehabilitation and palliation it is not the physician alone, but also the patient who take on the task of assessing many treatment measures.

Outcome assessment in most clinical trials is affected by a purely medical understanding of the disease. This is reflected in the predominant use of physical, in particular oncologic symptoms, as the content of outcome measures. The assessment of other health aspects like psychological symptoms, interpersonal or social consequences of the disease, seems to be similarly, if not more, important and should be considered in quality control of rehabilitation (table 9.18).

Activities of daily life play an important role in rehabilitation. Widely used measures to assess activities of daily life are the functional independence measure or the Barthel index (Mahoney and Barthel, 1965).

Different outcome scales in palliative care of cancer patients have been developed (Aspinal et al., 2002; Bausewein et al., 2005). The scales cover physical and psychological symptoms, spiritual considerations, practical issues, emotional concerns of the patient and family, and psychosocial needs of the patient and family. The Palliative Care Outcome Scale (POS) is a multidimensional instrument covering these physical, psychosocial, spiritual, organizational, and practical concerns.

Table 9.18 - Possible therapeutic aims and their effectiveness parameters in the rehabilitation of pancreatic carcinoma patients.

Reduction of disorders resulting from surgery/chemotherapy/radiation therapy	WHO toxicity scale, CTC classification, assessment of organ function. Questionnaire: FLIC, SIRO
Pain relief	Pain diary, reduction of analgesic drugs, pain sensitivity scales. Questionnaires: PDI, EORTC QLQ- C30, SE36, SDS, RSCL
Improvement of nutritional status	Weighing, determination of total protein, albumin concentration, biometric impedance analysis, FACT-CT
Improvement of metabolic status in diabetics	Blood sugar daily profiles, HbA1, diabetes journal
Clarification and alleviation of malassimilation /maldigestion symptoms	Stool fats/stool weight
Improvement of physical fitness	Ergometry, Karnofsky index, WHO and EORTC performance status, walking distances, muscle force (hand-held dynamometry), exercise capacity (symptom limited bicycle ergometry, vigorimeter. Questionnaires, QLQ-C30, CCM, FACT-Ct, FACT-G, FACT-An, SIP, SF-36, Nottingham Health profile
Family member counselling	Questionnaires
Information on illness, follow-up care, signs of recurrence, therapy in case of recurrence, behaviour-influencing illness	Questionnaires, tests
Reduction of anxiety, depression	Rating scales. Questionnaires: STAI, Poms, BDI, BSI, HADS-D, PAF
Coping with illness	Questionnaires FKV, FKV-LIS, BEFO, TSK, FIBECK
Clarification and improvement of vocational fitness	Resumption of vocation, length of time of inability to work
Reduction of necessity of nursing care	Questionnaires: Barthel index, FIM, ADL
Relief of physical and psychological symptoms	Questionnaire: POS

Abbreviations of questionnaire

ADL = Activities of Daily Life; CCM = Cancer Care Monitor; DDC = Daily Diary Card; EORTC-QLQ = European Organization for Research and Treatment of Cancer Quality of Life Questionnaire; ECOG = European Cooperative Oncology Group; Fact-An = Functional Assessment of Cancer Therapy Anemia; Fact-Ct = Functional Assessment of Anorexia and Cachexia; FIBECK = Freiburger Inventar zur Bewältigung einer chronischen Erkrankung; FIM = Funktional Independence Measure; FLI-C = Functional Living Index-Cancer; HADS-D = Hospital Anxiety and Depression Scale; KPS = Karnofsky Performance Scale; LCSS = Lung Cancer Symptom Scale; PDI = Pain Disability Index; POMS = Profile of Mood Status; POS = Palliative Care Outcome Scale; RSCL = Rotterdam-Symptom Checklist; SF-36 = SF-36 Health Survey; SIP = Sickness Impact Profile; SIRO = Stress Index Radio Oncology; STAI = Spiegelberger Trait Anxiety Inventory

Measurements of quality of life

Basically, improvement in quality of life is attained when less nursing care is necessary ("rehabilitation to combat the need of care"), when the patient can be vocationally reintegrated ("rehabilitation to combat early retirement"), when he/she feels secure and knows that his/her fate is in somebody's hands, in a positive sense ("rehabilitation to combat resignation and depression") and when the patient's physical handicaps and functional limitations are at a minimum ("rehabilitation to combat disability").

Quality of life questionnaires of the European Organization for Research and Treatment of Cancer such as EORTC QLQ C-30) and the functional assessment of cancer therapy (Fact) (Barat and Franchignoni, 2004) are internationally validated questionnaires and have been used on multiple studies. They are composed of multi-item scales and yes/no questions assessing physical, role functionning, cognitive, emotional, and social effects. The EORTC QLQ C-30 also includes symptom measures and a global health and QL scale.

Bibliography

- Alguacil J, Pollan M, Gustavsson P (2003) Occupations with increased risk of pancreatic cancer in the Swedish population. Occup Environ Med 60, 8: 570-6
- Aspinal F, Hughes R, Higginson I *et al.* (2002) A user's guide to the palliative care outcome scale. Palliative care & policy publications. Kings College, London
- Barat M, Franchignoni F (2004) Assessment in physical medicine and rehabilitation. Maugeri Foundation Books, PI-ME Press Pavia
- Bergasa NV (2006) Medical palliation of the jaundiced patient with pruritus. Gastroenterol Clin North Am 35, 1: 113
- Bausewein C, Fegg M, Radbruch L *et al.* (2005) Validation and clinical application of the German version of the palliative care outcome. J Pain Symptom Manage 30: 51-62
- Bundesarbeitsgemeinschaft für Rehabilitation (BAR) (2003) Rahmenempfehlungen zur ambulanten onkologischen Rehabilitation. Schriftenreihe der Bundesarbeitsgemeinschaft für Rehabilitation. Frankfurt
- Cella D (1997) The (Fact-An) scale: A new tool for the assessment of outcomes in cancer anemia and fatigue. Semin Hematol 34 (suppl 2): 13-9
- Delbrück H (2002) Bauchspeicheldrüsenkrebs. Rat und Hilfe für Betroffene und Angehörige. Kohlhammer, Stuttgart
- Delbrück H, Haupt E (edit.) (1998) Rehabilitationsmedizin. Ambulant – Teilstationär – Stationär. Urban & Schwarzenberg, München
- Delbrück H (2004) Krebsschmerz. Rat und Hilfe für Betroffene und Angehörige. Verlag W Kohlhammer, Stuttgart
- Dunn GP (2002) Surgical palliation in advanced disease: Recent developments. Current science 4: 233-41
- EAPC Expert Working Group (2001) Morphine and alternative opioids in cancer pain. The EAPC recommendation BJC 84: 587

- Epelbaum R, Rosenblatt E, Nasrallah S *et al.* (2002) Phase II study of gemcitabine combined with radiation therapy in patients with localized, unresectable pancreatic cancer. J Surg Oncol 81: 138-43
- Glimelius B *et al.* (1996) Chemotherapy improves survival and quality of life in advanced pancreatic and biliary cancer. Ann oncol 7: 593
- Gordon JN, Trebble T, Ellis RD *et al.* (2005) Thalidomide in the treatment of cancer cachexia: a randomized placebo controlled trial. GUT, 54: 540-5
- Hocht S, Wiegel T, Siegmann A *et al.* (2004) Radiochemotherapy in unresectable pancreatic cancer. Front Radiat Ther Oncol 38: 87-93
- Holt A, Patel M, Ahmed MM (2004) Palliation of patients with malignant gastroduodenal obstruction with self-expanding metallic stents: The treatment of choice.
- Jatoi A, Windschitl HE, Loprinzi CL *et al.* (2002) Dronabinol versus megestrol acetate versus combination therapy for cancer-associated anorexia. J Clin Oncol 20: 567-73
- Koski S, Venner P (2000) Chemotherapy-induced nausea and vomiting. In: Nabholtz JM Tonkin K, Aaapro MS *et al.* (edit) Breast cancer Management. Application of evidence to patient care. M Dunitz London 317-29
- Levy MH, Cohen SD (2005) Sedation for the relief of refractory symptoms in the imminently dying: A fine intentional line. Semin Oncol 32: 237-46
- Maguire P, Pitceathly C (2002) Key communication skills and how to acquire them. BMJ 325: 697-700
- McLeod RS (1999) Quality of life, nutritional status and gastrointestinal hormone profile following Whipple procedure. Ann Oncol 4 (suppl): 281-5
- Monti D, Yang J (2005) Complementary medicine in chronic cancer care. Semin Oncol 32: 225-31
- Moore M, Goldstein D, Hamm J *et al.* (2007) Erlotinib plus Gemcitabine compared with Gemcitabine alone in patients with advanced pancreatic cancer. J clin Oncol 25, 15: 1960-6
- Neoptolemos J, Cunningham D *et al.* (2003) Adjuvant therapy in pancreatic cancer: Historical and current perspectives. Annals of Oncology 14: 675-92
- Oyan N (2004) Chemoradiotherapy for pancreatic cancer: Current status and perspectives. Int J Clin Oncol 9, 6: 451-7
- Ogata Y, Hishinuma S (2002) The impact of pylorus-preserving pancreatoduodenectomy on surgical treatment for cancer of the pancreatic head. J Hepatobiliary Pancreat Surg 9, 2: 223-32
- Patel L, Lindley C (2003) Aprepitant – a novel NK-1receptor antagonist. Expert Opin Pharmacother 4: 2279-96
- Rosemeyer D (1996) After-care rehabilitation after pancreas operations. Z Gastroenterol 34, 2: 37-40
- Sanders M, Papachristou G, McGrath K *et al.* (2007) Endoscopic palliation of pancreatic cancer. Gastroenterol Clin North Am 36,2: 455-76
- Sehlen S, Fahrmüller H, Herschbach P *et al.* (2003) Psychometrische Eigenschaft des Stress Index Radio Onkologie (SIRO). Strahlenther Onkol 179, 4: 261-9
- Sharfman WH, Walsh TD (1990) Has the analgesic efficacy of neurolytic celiac plexus block been demonstrated in pancreatic cancer pain. Pain 41: 267-71
- Sindelar WF, Kinsella TJ (1999) Studies of intraoperative radiotherapy in carcinoma of the pancreas. Ann Oncol 10 (suppl. 4): 226-30

- Shah J, Muthusamg VR (2005) Endoscopic palliation of pancreaticobiliary malignancies. Gastrointest Endosc Clin N Am 15, 3: 513-31
- Shore S, Vimalachandran D, Raraty MG et al. (2004) Cancer in the elderly. Pancreatic cancer. Surg Oncol 4: 201-10
- Silverman D, Stewart PA, Blair A et al. (2001) Occupational exposure to pesticides and pancreatic cancer. Am J Ind Med 39, 1: 92-9
- Smeenk HG, Tran TC, Erdmann J et al. (2004) Survival after surgical management of pancreatic adenocarcinomas: Does curative and radical surgery truly exist? Langenbecks Arch Surg 14
- Tisdale M (2003) Pathogenesis of cancer cachexia. J Support Oncol 1: 159-68
- World Health Organization (1990) Cancer pain relief and palliative care. Technical report, series 804. Geneva
- World Health Organization (2001) International classification of functioning, disabilities and health. www. who.int/classification/icf

Rehabilitation and palliation of patients with colon cancer

Aims of rehabilitation and palliation: Their special features, value and limitations in curative follow-up care

The primary objective of all **potentially curative follow-up measures** (prevention of recurrence, early recognition of recurrence and treatment of recurrence) is to prolong survival time (fig. 1.3). To stop the progression of the cancer disease is clearly the prime concern in curative aftercare. In colon cancer, these measures are just as important as rehabilitation and palliation because, in contrast to many other tumours, these measures can significantly prolong life (fig. 1.1).

The objective of all **rehabilitation and palliation measures** is not to prolong life but to treat the problems caused by the tumour and the treatment (fig. 1.2). The negative physical, mental, social and occupational effects of the cancer disease and treatment are to be eliminated or at least alleviated. Numerous measures are used to achieve these objectives. Because of the holistic objective, they are provided not only by the physician but also by a team comprising a large range of professional groups. Their efforts are directed primarily at the severity of the consequences of the tumour and treatment and not at the severity or prognosis of the disease as is the case with potentially curative aftercare.

In rehabilitation, it is the ICF (International Classification of Functional Capacity, Disability and Health) and not the ICD (International Classification of Diseases), usually applied in curative oncology, that forms the basis for assessments, therapy and quality assurance (Barat and Franchignoni, 2004). It also covers psychosocial aspects.

In theory, the differences between the objectives of aftercare and those of rehabilitation and palliation are easily differentiated. In practice, however, there are many overlaps in the case of colon cancer. This relates in particular to treatment of recurrences which can both prolong life and alleviate symptoms in colon cancer patients.

Rehabilitation measures in follow-up care

The rehabilitation objectives listed in the tables 1.4 and 10.2, apply both to potentially cured patients and to patients with progressive tumours. The secondary diseases frequently present in elderly patients must also be treated during rehabilitation (Yancik et al., 2000).

A certain minimum amount of information on the disease status (table 10.1) is prerequisite before initiating rehabilitation measures. Without this information, it is difficult to carry out rehabilitation; valuable time is wasted in performing additional research, thus threatening the success of rehabilitation.

Table 10.1 - Minimum information before initiating rehabilitation measures.

– Extent of tumour (e.g., pTNM)
– Curative or palliative therapy approach (e.g., R0, R1 or R2-resection of the tumour)
– Localisation of the tumour (e.g., ascending, transverse, descending colon)
– In the case of progression information on the location, and any therapy performed so far (what were the results?)
– Which chemotherapy or radiotherapies have been performed? (Which cytostatics and what dosages were prescribed and what were the results?)
– Psychosocial information (e.g., the level of understanding, possible coping and compliance problems, family structure, amount of support given by relatives, social and occupational problems, etc.)

Before carrying out rehabilitative measures, a rehabilitative assessment is to take place, with rehabilitation planning and documentation of the goals to be achieved (tables 1.6, 1.7, 1.8). Here, the consequences of surgery constitute the main focus.

Rehabilitation measures aiming at reducing physical problems ("rehabilitation to prevent disability")

After a hemicolectomy, physical problems (table 10.2) are usually if not always only minor.

Table 10.2 - Somatic rehabilitation requirements after hemicolectomy.

– Hernias
– Diarrhea/Constipation
– Adhesions
– Anemia
– Diet/Obesity
– Neuropathies
– Hand-foot syndrome
– Sexual disorders

Prevention of an abdominal wall hernia

Aftercare is occasionally complicated by the formation of a scar hernia.

Overweight patients and patients with delayed wound healing are particularly at risk of hernia.

In the first six months after the operation, the scar tissue is particularly weak and precautionary measures are therefore advised (table 10.3).

Table 10.3 - Precautionary measures to prevent abdominal wall hernia.

– Caution in lifting and carrying heavy loads.
– Loads should never be lifted suddenly.
– Excess weight should be avoided.
– Straining should be avoided as far as possible.
– In the case of threatened or existing hernias, a fitted abdominal bandage should be worn.

Diarrhea

In general, a third of the large intestine is sufficient to bulk up stools. If diarrhea occurs, this is often caused by hyperperistalsis of the small and/or large intestine. Anti-motility drugs (e.g., loperamide) are then indicated.

If the whole large intestine has been removed, stools are inevitably liquid. This occurs in **ileostomy** patients. Ileostomies are mainly performed after intestinal resections within the context of inflammatory intestinal diseases and to a lesser extent in tumour patients. Exceptions include temporary or permanent ileostomies after colectomy because of a family history of adenomatosis and cancer.

After a total colectomy there is always diarrhea which leads to appreciable loss in quality of life irrespective of primary diagnosis (Lim and Ho, 2001).

There is a risk of diarrhea if the Bauhin's valve and large parts of the terminal ileum have been removed at the same time as the ascending colon. This can lead to uninhibited flow of bile acids and the liquid content of the small intestine into the large intestine, resulting in diarrhea (chologenic diarrhea). Chologenic diarrhea is treated with bile acid-binding (cholestyramine) and anti-motility (loperamide) drugs; there are few effective dietary measures.

Irinotecan, a cytostatic frequently used to treat colon cancer, can cause severe diarrhea. In elderly and weakened patients, the dose of this preparation should be reduced by 25%.

As with a cholinergic syndrome, the early occurrence of diarrhea on the first day of irinotecan administration is prevented by atropine (0.4mg s.c. or i.v.). Late onset diarrhea is more dangerous; it develops after several days and may persist for days (tables 10.4, 10.5).

Table 10.4 - Increased risk of irinotecan-induced diarrhea.

– After irradiation of the abdomen or the pelvis,
– In hyperleukocytosis,
– In the case of WHO Performance Status superior 2
– In patients with Gilbert Meulengracht's syndrome

Table 10.5 - Measures to prevent or alleviate irinotecan-induced complications.

– Administration only if strictly indicated in high risk patients.
– The 5-FU/folinic acid combination should not be administered as a bolus but in a long-term infusion.
– Nausea, vomiting and abdominal cramps are warning signs and the patient should be closely monitored if these occur.
– Even at the start of diarrhea and abdominal cramps, loperamide 2mg should be administered after each evacuation. As with diarrhea, cramps should be monitored.
– Due to the risk of paralytic ileus, loperamide should not be administered for longer than 48 hours.
– Loperamide should not be given as a prophylactic treatment.
– If diarrhea persists, treatment should be switched to octreotide 100 micrograms s.c. 3 times daily and parenteral fluid replacement given until it stops.
– In the case of neutropenia and diarrhea concurrently or in the case of fever, prophylactic antibiotic therapy with a broad spectrum antibiotic and vancomycin or metronidazole is required.
– Parenteral fluid replacement is important.
– If diarrhea persists and in the case of particularly severe diarrhea (grade 3-4), inpatient treatment should be initiated.

For the "diarrhea" frequently mentioned by patients after rectum resection, see the chapter on rectal cancer.

Constipation

If there was already a tendency for constipation before the operation, it usually returns shortly after the operation. However, if paradoxical constipation occurs, the possibility of adhesions and renewed tumour growth should be considered (tables 10.6, 10.7).

Table 10.6 - Main causes of constipation.

– Medication (e.g., opioid medication, sedatives, diuretics, medicaments containing iron, aluminium, calcium)
– Dehydration
– Insufficient intake of dietary fiber
– Hypokalemia
– Medications, such as opioids (e.g., codeine and morphine) and certain antidepressants
– Paralytic ileus due to some cytostatics (e.g., vinca alkaloids)
– Radiotherapy
– Functional constipation (e.g., psychosomatic-based on anxiety or unfamiliarity with surroundings)

Table 10.7 - Constrictions which do not allow feces to pass

– Tumour stenosis (e.g., intraluminal or extraluminal tumour growth, intestinal linitis plastica)
– Adhesions (e.g., benign oder malignant)
– Strictures
– Diverticula

Anemia

Anemia is the reason for many objective and subjective functional incapacities (table 12.24). It causes energy imbalance and emotional distress. Anemia has a negative impact on the majority of organs; in an elderly cancer population the consequences of anemia can be even more invalidating due to its contribution to the " fragility syndrome" (Mancuso *et al.*, 2006).

Operation-induced hypochromic anemia does not usually need iron substitution unless transferrin is reduced (empty iron reserve). However, hyperchromic anemia does require treatment. It is one of the possible late complications following an operation on a tumour in the ascending colon with loss of the terminal ileum. In this case prophylactic vitamin B12 must then be administered intramuscularly at three to six-monthly intervals.

Treatment with erythropoietin needs to be compared with the transfusion of red blood cells which also leads to a hemoglobin increase. Packed red blood cell transfusions are indicated for patients with severe or life-threatening anemia or with acute anemia associated with hemorrhage. Erythropoietin is almost devoid of side effects, but it is slow and ineffective in a substantial proportion of patients. Red blood cell transfusion is associated with a small risk of infectious, allergic or toxic complications, but it reliably induces a rapid hemoglobin increase in virtually all patients.

Adhesions

Adhesions in the abdominal cavity generally occur due to inflammatory processes following an operation or radiotherapy. Most adhesions cause no problems, but they can obstruct the intestine in about 2% of all patients. An ileus may develop and an operation is required to cut the fibrous tissue and free the intestinal loops. Obstructions can occur several years after operation and/or radiation therapy.

In the case of adhesions care should be taken to avoid excessive intake of cabbage, onions, vegetables, whole wheat bread, carbonated drinks, etc., because abnormal formation of intestinal gas should be avoided. Stools should be kept "soft". Laxatives containing lactose (lactulose) should be avoided because of gas formation. If there is a tendency for constipation, the administration of *plantaginis ovatae semen* (psyillium seeds) is recommended.

Artificial sweeteners can also cause increased gas formation. They are only partially absorbed in the intestine and reach deep-lying sections of the intestine in undigested form where their degradation by bacteria causes gas formation.

When there is no positive effect of dietary restrictions surgical removal of adhesions is indicated.

Nutrition deficiencies and general dietary recommendations

Special dietary recommendations are not necessary unless extensive intestinal resections have been performed (Lin, 2001) (table 10.8) or short bowel syndrome is present (table 10.9). Short bowel syndrome occurs in the event of extensive resection in the small intestine but no resections in the large intestine.

Table 10.8 - Dietary recommendations after extensive intestinal resections.

– Foods that stimulate intestinal motility and irritate the mucosa should be avoided.
– Milk is often poorly tolerated; in this case lactose-free basic diets are advised. In the case of milk intolerance, the diet can be supplemented with lactase.
– The diet should be low in fat, lactose and oxalate.
– Care should be taken to balance out any electrolyte losses (potassium). Many patients regularly take three to six magnesium-gelatin capsules prophylactically.
– Drug therapy can include bile acid inhibitors and pancreatic enzyme or secretion inhibitors (octreotide).
– Synthetic opioids such as loperamide, opium tincture and codeine sulfate frequently help to combat diarrhea. They reduce intestinal motility.
– Supplements should be iso-osmolar. Hyperosmolar drinks cause osmotic diarrhea.

Table 10.9 - Dietary restrictions with shortened small intestine.

– Due to the reduced utilization of nutrients, energy intake must be 25% to 75% higher than the theoretical level for healthy persons. Patients must therefore eat considerably more than their healthy counterparts.
– Food should be easily digestible and well chewed, making it easier and quicker for the remaining small intestine to function.
– For oral feeding, easily digested diets with special protein and fat components are suitable. Carbohydrates are tolerated best and fats are tolerated least well.
– It is important to use the remaining intestine throughout the day and not just at main meals. This means eight to ten small meals instead of three main meals.
– With large volumes, intestinal motility is excessively stimulated, resulting in poor utilization of the food and diarrhea.
– During the relatively short time spent in the remaining intestine, the best possible mixing of digestive enzymes should take place. This can be achieved by thorough chewing because this results in the release of digestive enzymes from salivary gland secretions in the mouth. Digestion is then aided by pancreatic enzymes.
– The diet should be high-protein, low-carbohydrate and low-fat.
– The fat portion should be about 30%, half of which should ideally be taken in the form of MCT fats. This will enable utilization of the fats even with impaired gall bladder and pancreatic function.
– If the end section of the small intestine is removed, vitamin B12 deficiency may occur, resulting in macrocytic anemia. Prophylactic vitamin B12 must therefore be administered at three-six monthly intervals.
– Since bile acids are absorbed in the end section of the small intestine, they may pass into the large intestine and damage the mucosa. Cholestyramine should therefore be taken in the case of diarrheal disorders.

Colon cancer patients should follow general dietary guidelines. These are necessary not only for "colon cancer prophylaxis" but also for protection against other modern diseases (table 10.10) (Bromer, 2005)

Table 10.10 - Nutritional advices to prevent colorectal cancer.

– The nutrition should be low-caloric.
– The nutrition should be low-fat and high-fiber.
– Excess weight should be avoided.
– Less meat and more fruit and vegetable.
– Alcohol only in small quantities (men less than 20gr./daily and women less than 10gr./daily).
– Daily physical activity.

Changing eating habits is more successful than low-calorie diets in the long term. Excess weight is not only a risk factor for cardiocirculatory diseases and orthopedic problems but also increases the risk of breast, prostate and large intestine cancer (table 10.11).

Table 10.11 - Reasons to avoid excess weight.

– Excess weight puts additional strain on the abdominal muscles and therefore increases the risk of abdominal wall hernia and suture dehiscence.
– Excess weight increases lethargy; physical activity may reduce the risk of disease recurrence.
– Association between body mass index and elevated risk for colon cancer in men.
– Excess weight makes radiotherapy planning and metabolism of cytostatics more difficult and complications therefore more frequent.

The diet should be low in animal fats because animal fats themselves (omega-6 fatty acids) are regarded as risk factors. Epidemiological studies showed a reduced tumour risk in people who eat poultry, olive oil and fish because of the omega-3 fatty acid contents of these foods.

High fiber foods are appropriate. They bring about an early feeling of fullness and accelerate intestinal transit, thereby shortening the exposure time of the intestinal mucosa to any carcinogenic substances. Plenty of fresh vegetable and fruit should be recommended. The intake of foods with a high folate and complex carbohydrate content reduces the risk of adenoma. High alcohol consumption, especially beer, is regarded as harmful. There is no objection to moderate alcohol intake. Highly concentrated alcoholic drinks should be avoided.

Calcium in the diet is helpful. Milk products contain a lot of calcium and vitamin D. The lactic acid bacteria found in yogurt, kefir or sour milk act on disturbed intestinal flora. Whether they actually improve immune defense, as repeatedly claimed by some representatives of "biological medicine", is not proven.

As colorectal cancers arise from adenomatous polyps, prevention of polyps growth has been a focus of considerable clinical research. To date, trials have failed to show benefits from taking antioxidant vitamins, fiber supplements or modest dietary changes with respect to preventing new polyps growth. The potential value of non-steroidal anti-inflammatory drugs (NSAIDs), including aspirin, for prevention of colorectal recurrence is being studied.

Physical activity

Most studies have shown an inverse relationship between physical activity and colon cancer incidence. The average relative risk reduction provided by regular physical activity is 40%. In men, physical activity for two hours or more a week is more associated with a reduction in risk of advanced adenomas than in a reduction in risk of non advanced adenomas. The mechanism of protection by physical activity is unknown but may be linked to effects on colonic mucosal prostaglandins (Wannamethee et al., 2001).

Neuropathy

See also chapter on ovarian cancer.

Adjuvant or additional chemotherapy for potentially curative or palliative purposes is not without side effects.

The sensory neuropathy that occasionally occurs during and directly after oxaliplatin administration (Junker et al., 2004) can be largely prevented by avoiding exposure to cold on the day of administration. More problems arise with the delayed onset of sensory neuropathy that occurs in many patients after a cumulative total dose of $510mg/m^2$ oxaliplatin. Nearly all patients treated with oxaliplatin develop a sensory-motor neuropathy after six to nine months of treatment. Oxaliplatin-induced neurological disorders usually recede after stopping the chemotherapy. Gabapentin (Neurontin® 600-1200mg/day and carbamazepine (Tegretal® 600-1200mg/day) and a magnesium supplement are most frequently used to treat the symptoms.

Hand-foot syndrome

The efficacy and tolerance of orally administered capecitabine (Xeloda®) and tegafur/uracil (UFT®) are relatively good. Tegafur/uracil is regarded as less effective but does not carry the risk of a hand-foot syndrome.

The range of side effects occurring with capecatibine includes hand-foot syndrome (approximatively 50%), diarrhea (approximatively 40%), vomiting and nausea (20%), mucositis/stomatitis (approximatively 20%) and hemorrhage (approximatively 5%) (Heo, 2004). Dose interruption and reduction of capecitabine usually lead to a rapid reversal of signs and symptoms without any long-term consequences (Lassere, 2004).

At the first sign of a hand-foot syndrome (Grade I = redness of the hand), the capecatibine dose should be reduced by about 20%. Unlike other chemotherapies, dose reduction (only in the case of a grade I side effect) does not cause any loss of effect. With grade II (pain in the hand or foot), in some people the therapy must be discontinued. With grade III (peeling of the skin), capecitabine must be stopped completely. Capecitabine administration is contraindicated in patients with impaired renal function (creatinine clearance inferior to 30mL/min.).

Biological therapy (immunotherapy) can cause flu-like symptoms such as chills, fever, weakness and nausea. Side effects of bevacizumab, which is highly effective in medical treatment of colon cancer include allergic reactions, stomach problems, bleeding problems, high blood pressure.

Sexual disorders

No organic sexual disorders are expected after colon cancer resections. If they do occur, there is more likely to be a psychological than an organic cause. (Andersen, 1985). Unlike erectile dysfunction after rectum amputation, drugs after colon resection combatting erectile dysfunction (e.g., sildanefil and vardenafil) may help.

Inherited cancer syndrome and counselling

Gene carriers and their relatives should be given the addresses of genetic advisory boards. About 5-10 % of colorectal cancers have a genetic background. Genetic counselling is necessary in patients with inherited cancer syndromes (table 10.12).

Table 10.12 - Clinical features of some inherited colorectal cancer syndromes (FAP = Familial Adenomatosis Polyposis, HNPCC = Hereditary Non-polyposis Colon Cancer, FAS = Flat Adenoma Syndrome).

Feature	FAP	HNPCC	FAS
Age of onset	Early	Early	Late
No. of adenomas	<100	<10	0-100
Adenoma distribution	Left of total	Mainly right side	Mainly right side
Cancer distribution	Random	Mainly right side	Mainly right side
Other cancers	Peri-ampullary	Endometrial, ovary, stomach	Peri-ampullary

Persons with **familial adenomatosis polyposis (FAP)** are born with normal-appearing colonic mucosa; polyps develop during the second and third decades of life. If surgical treatment is not performed, colorectal cancer is almost certain to develop by 40 years of age (Katz *et al.*, 2006).

Genetic testing is now the standard of care for FAP. Despite the detailed genetic knowledge of FAP that is now available, genetic testing is often poorly interpreted. Genetic counselling is an integral part of management and should precede genetic testing. Testing for FAP in a family is most informative when it begins with the affected family member, to identify the mutation responsible for FAP within that family. Once a causal mutation has been identified in an affected person, predictive testing can be done to identify other family members at risk. DNA testing for APC gene mutations has a sensitivity of 70% to 90% and a specificity of 100%.

If the test result is positive or the test is not available, flexible sigmoidoscopy is performed at 10 to 12 years of age. During the procedure, mucosal biopsy specimens are taken to identify subtle adenomatous changes. Colonoscopy with mucosal biopsies is advisable at 18 to 20 years of age. If adenomas are detected, surgical prophylaxis should be considered. Routine gastroduodenoscopic surveillance is also recommended for patients with FAP, because these patients are at high risk for potentially precancerous gastric and duodenal adenomas.

Surgical prophylaxis in FAP consists of resection of the entire large bowel, to prevent malignant transformation. In the past, surgical alternatives included total colectomy with a permanent ileostomy and subtotal colectomy with an ileorectal anastomosis; the latter procedure is complicated by the frequent appearance of rectal polyps, which often necessitates a subsequent proctectomy. Currently, total proctocolectomy with J-pouch ileo-anal anastomosis is advocated as surgical prophylaxis.

Celecoxib was shown to reduce the number of colorectal adenomas by an average of 28%, compared to a 5% reduction with placebo. On the basis of this study, the Food and Drug Administration approved celecoxib as oral adjunctive therapy for adults with FAP. Nevertheless, endoscopic surveillance and colectomy as indicated remain the standard of care.

HNPCC (Hereditary Non-Polyposis Colorectal Cancer), like FAP, is an autosomal dominant disorder (Katz et al., 2006). The median age at which adenocarcinomas appear in HNPCC is less than 50 years, which is ten to fifteen years younger than the median age at which they appear in the general population. In contrast to FAP, HNPCC is associated with an unusually high frequency of cancers in the proximal large bowel. Families with HNPCC often include persons with multiple primary cancers; in women, an association between colorectal cancer and either endometrial or ovarian carcinoma is especially prominent.

Several sets of selection criteria have been developed for identifying patients with this syndrome. The Amsterdam-2 criteria comprise the following: Histologically documented colorectal cancer (or other HNPCC-related tumour) in at least three relatives, one of whom is a first-degree relative of the other two, a family history of one or more cases of colorectal cancer diagnosed before 50 years of age, and cases of colorectal cancer in at least two successive generations of the family. Affected relatives should be on the same side of the family (maternal or paternal), FAP must be excluded in colorectal cancer cases, and tumours must be pathologically verified. Another selection set, the Bethesda criteria, is more sensitive than the Amsterdam criteria but is less specific.

If HNPCC is confirmed, affected family members should undergo colonoscopy between the ages of 20 and 25 or at the age of 10 years younger than the youngest age at diagnosis in the family, whichever is earlier. This procedure should be repeated every one to two years. Recommended screening for women includes an annual transvaginal ultrasound or endometrial aspiration, beginning at age 25 to 35 years.

If an adenocarcinoma of the colon is identified, total abdominal colectomy with an ileorectal anastomosis is recommended. In women, total abdominal hysterectomy and bilateral salpingo-oophorectomy are often considered, particularly if the patient has no intention of having children in the future, because of the increased risk of ovarian and endometrial carcinoma.

Necessity of information and patient education (discussion groups and health training)

Information and training are important in helping to cope with the disease (table 10.13). They can help the patient to understand what is happening in his/her body and why a certain therapy is proposed. The majority of patients do not want to decide themselves about the tumour therapy but like to know the reasons for pursuing a certain treatment strategy.

Table 10.13 - Subjects of health training and education in patients with colon cancer.

– Information on colon cancer and its causes
– Possible hereditary factors
– Available treatments and their side effects, including complementary, alternative medicine and paramedicine
– The possibilities and also the limitations of traditional medicine
– Recurrence prevention and therapies in the case of recurrences
– Adverse effects of various tumour therapies
– Aftercare examinations, content and timetable of follow-up examinations
– Diet, dietary recommendations, what to do in the case of constipation/diarrhea
– Coping with anxiety
– Ways of dealing with pain
– Recommendations how to deal with family members
– Information on social rights and assistance and occupational consequences
– General health-related topics

The negative effects of an unhealthy diet and certain lifestyle habits should be mentioned. Physical exercise, preferably a sporting activity, should be advised because an inverse association between physical activity and risk for colon cancer has been seen in studies of occupational activity and of job-related and recreational activity (Wannamethee *et al.*, 2001). In young patients in particular, any genetic-related causes for the disease should be mentioned (Matloff *et al.*, 2004).

The psychologist, nutritionist, physician and social worker should take turns to lead the discussion. Relatives should also be given the opportunity to participate in group discussions. Participation by relatives is particularly desirable with regard to dietary advice.

It is helpful if the information and advice included in the health training are also made available to the patients and their relatives in writing (e.g., in the form of a range of guidebooks giving independent advice). These guides can never of course replace medical consultation but should form the basis of useful discussions with the treating physician.

The Internet represents a growing source of information for those involved, such as relatives, but it is often difficult for the layperson to recognize whether the information available is serious. It is useful if the physician can recommend certain Internet sites that he/she considers to be serious, informative and helpful.

Stoma patients need special training (see chapter on rectal cancer).

Rehabilitation measures aiming at reducing psychological problems ("rehabilitation to combat withdrawal and depression")

See also chapter: "Psychological support and self-help groups in cancer rehabilitation and palliation".

Necessity of psychological support

Psychological problems are sometimes linked to pain, dietary problems, incontinence, impotence or other physical problems. Fears of progress and the uncertain future are frequent. Somatization of psychological disorders is not uncommon. The assessment of psychological symptoms, interpersonal or social consequences of the disease is sometimes more important than physical complaints and should be considered.

Some patients believe that psychotherapy could influence their cancer. As yet, however, it has only been proved that the effects and consequences of the tumour and the therapy can be influenced by accompanying psychological treatment. Professional psychotherapy may be necessary.

Fatigue syndrome

The term **"fatigue"** is defined as a syndrome of extreme (pathological) tiredness and exhaustion (table 2.8). Multiple factors are involved in its causes. Sometimes, fatigue symptoms are linked to the antidepressant medications themselves. Psychotropic drugs have, however, also been used successfully to treat fatigue.

The positive influence of erythropoetin on fatigue symptoms with low Hb has been proved in a series of international studies. For other, mostly unexplained causes, before initiating such high cost cytokine therapy, other non-medication measures should be used first (e.g., physiotherapy, ergometric training, conversation therapy, behavioural therapy, diet, change of environment) (Watson, 2004) (tables 2.9, 2.10).

Rehabilitation measures aiming at reducing social problems ("rehabilitation aiming at preserving social life and autonomy")

See also chapter: "Social support in rehabilitation and palliation".

The aim of these measures is to strengthen the patient's own resources and prevent the risk of a need for care, or at least reduce such a need. It is not uncommon for the additional burdens of the disease and therapy to cause a deterioration in domestic care, already at risk before surgery.

One of the purposes of rehabilitation is to plan measures for further care at home. These plans should be made jointly with the relatives: Care assistance such as "meals on wheels", nursing care, household help, home medical care and, in some circumstances, care in a nursing home or hospice must be organized if necessary. It is useful to pass on contact addresses (self-help groups, advisory bodies, etc.).

Rehabilitation measures aiming at reducing problems at work ("rehabilitation aiming at preventing unnecessary early retirement")

See also chapter: "Vocational integration in cancer rehabilitation".

Harmful occupational substances

There are no known links between harmful occupational substances and colon cancers.

Capaccity to work

Assessment of the capacity to work depends on the pain symptoms, the location of the tumour, whether an R0 or R1 resection has been performed, the extent and location of intestinal resection and any chemotherapy carried out. Accompanying diseases unrelated to the tumour and therapy must also be taken into consideration.

After a total colectomy irrespective of ileorectal anastomosis or stoma, activities involving physical exertion are considerably restricted (Lim and Ho, 2001). After operations on tumours in the ascending colon, there is a tendency for diarrhea if the Bauhin's valve and large parts of the terminal ileum have also been removed and bile acid loss syndrome has occurred. This tendency for diarrhea may be an occupational handicap and cause at least occasional incapacity to work.

Otherwise, after a hemicolectomy because of colon cancer, no occupational restrictions or long-term reduction of capacity to work are to be expected. Initial stool irregularities normalize within a few weeks and provided there is no secondary wound healing, no unfavorable incision with particular risk of hernia and no special psychological problems, it can be expected that work will be fully resumed a few months after completion of therapy. If there was no adjuvant chemotherapy, unrestricted capacity to work can usually be expected no more than three months after the operation.

During the phase of **adjuvant chemotherapy** it is unreasonable to expect the person concerned to perform physically difficult and moderately difficult tasks. Employability for light physical activities must be decided on an individual basis because not only the choice of cytostatics and their dose but also their tolerance may vary considerably between individuals. Basically, there is nothing against returning to a previous job one to two months after completing chemotherapy and gradually resuming work, depending on the physical and psychological burdens involved.

Tumour activity generally rules out going to work but even with ultrasound-confirmed liver metastases and minimal CEA increase over many months, in individual cases even over years, there may be freedom from pain and unrestricted capacity to work. If a patient expresses a wish to work, for psychological reasons, this should not be refused.

Palliative measures within the context of aftercare

Informing the patient about disease progression; breaking bad news

The physician must explain the situation and propose further therapeutic procedures to the patient in person. The risk ratio and consequences of the intended treatment must be explained in detail.

If patients ask questions, this should not be regarded as annoying but as a sign of positive compliance. The treating physician is highly dependent on the patient's cooperation.

Choice of treatment modalities

The decision for tumour therapy should be discussed jointly with the patient. The pros and cons must be discussed. Even palliative tumour therapies have subjective and objective side effects of varying severity, which must be taken into consideration, especially in elderly patients. In the elderly and in the case of secondary diseases (Yancik *et al.*, 2000), the potential benefits of chemotherapy may be reduced (tables 10.14, 10.15).

It is possible that surgical procedures may cure in case of anastomosis recurrence, solitary liver and pulmonary metastases. For all other recurrences, there is no possible curative therapy. In the latter case maintaining the quality of life (palliation) is the prime objective.

Table 10.14 - Causes for the frequent reduced tolerance of cytostatics in the elderly.

– Altered absorption of cytostatics because of slower intestinal motility
– Altered absorption of cytostatics because of achlorhydria
– Altered biliary and renal elimination of cytostatics
– Altered distribution and storage of lipophilic cytostatics in fat and muscle tissue
– Altered hepatic metabolism of cytostatics
– Reduced hematopoetic reserve
– Altered nutritional status
– Anemia
– Altered cardiac and pulmonary functional capacity
– Frequent comorbidity
– Varying levels of compliance

Table 10.15 - Contraindications to adjuvant chemotherapy.

– General status below level 2 (WHO Performance Status) or Karnofsky status below 70
– Uncontrolled infection
– Liver cirrhosis Child classification B and C
– Severe coronary heart disease; cardiac insufficiency (NYHA III and IV)
– Preterminal and terminal renal insufficiency
– Impaired bone marrow function
– Inability to attend regular check-up examinations

Localization of recurrences

The tumour may continue to spread to the peritoneum/omentum and other sections of the intestine.

Recurrences most frequently occur in the liver (30%), lungs (15%) and in locoregional lymph nodes (5% to 20%).

Local and regional problems and palliative therapies

Liver metastases

Solitary liver metastases should be resected surgically with potential cure. Today, the operative mortality rate for liver resections is less than 5%. Extrahepatic metastasis should have been excluded by FDG-PET. Radiologic evaluation is needed not only to identify extrahepatic disease but also to assess the adequacy of liver parenchyma after surgery. Some patients with a history of liver cirrhosis or liver steatosis may not tolerate liver resection.

In the case of unresectable multiple liver metastases or synchronous extrahepatic involvement, systemic chemotherapy should be considered. Temporary alleviation of symptoms may be possible from systemic therapy and, in individual cases, a R0 resection of liver metastases may be possible after "down-sizing" by chemotherapy.

Intra-arterial chemotherapy has a predominantly local and, to a lesser extent, systemic action. The substances used are administered via a pump over 24 hours. Comparatively high response and remission rates are then achieved but these do not necessarily prolong survival time. The disadvantages of this treatment are the uninhibited growth of extrahepatic metastases, problems caused by catheter complications, frequent problems with the pump and port system and, not least, also the toxicity that occurs with regional application.

Other therapeutic alternatives include radiofrequency ablation (RFA), laser-induced thermotherapy (LITT), local alcohol injection, cryo-ablation, chemo-embolization.

Radiofrequency ablation is safe and feasible but is less effective than surgical resection in prolonging survival. Complications include symptomatic pleural effusions, fever, pain, subcapsular and subcutaneous hematomas, biliary tree injuries, hepatic abscess, diaphragmatic necrosis, hepatic artery injury, renal failure, liver failure, coagulopathy, and ventricular fibrillation.

Cryotherapy can be used in conjunction with surgical resection, especially if the surgical margins are close. Cryotherapy is a good adjunct for local control but has little impact on overall survival. Complications include hemorrhage from a cracked and frozen liver, bile leak or fistula, right pleural effusion, thrombocytopenia, myoglobinuria, arrhythmias, acute renal failure, cryoshock from disseminated intravascular coagulation (DIC) and multi-organ shock. The overall mortality rate is 1.6% (Ruers *et al.*, 2001).

Low doses of cortisone have pain-relieving and anabolic effects and may have a positive effect on the patient's psychological state.

Pulmonary metastases

In the case of several pulmonary metastases in different pulmonary lobes, systemic therapy is indicated. For solitary metastases, resection is indicated if further metastases can be excluded.

Stenoses

The choice of surgical treatment procedure (table 10.16), with the aim of removing or bypassing the stenosis, depends on the number and location of the stenoses, the patient's general status or the severity of the ileus disease, the tumour stage and the extent of congestion-related damage to the colon sections lying in the proximal area of the tumour stenosis.

Surgery can effectively palliate symptoms in patients with advanced malignancy and thereby maintain quality of life. However, the goal of surgical palliation should be balanced with the associated risks, and the decision to operate can be challenging for even the most experienced surgeon.

A colorectal stent can be used in the palliative treatment of terminal patients before colostomy is considered. Experiences with the use of stents before elective surgery are also positive (Bosker *et al.*, 2005).

Table 10.16 - Surgical principles in colorectal stenoses.

– Oncological resection with primary anastomosis (curative approach)
– Oncological resection, with attachment of the part of the intestine closest to the mouth to an opening and closure of the part of the intestine closest to the anus (curative or palliative approach)
– Primary placement of a double artificial anus in front of the stenosis and secondary oncological tumour resection (curative approach)
– Bypass of the stenosis with a stent (palliative approach)
– Placement of a bypass anastomosis between the small intestine and the part of the colon on the anus side of the stenosis (palliative approach)

Systemic palliative therapies

Chemotherapies

In inoperable cases, systemic chemotherapy, anti-angiogenic agent bevacizumab and epidermal growth factor-receptor antibodies as well can be considered (Korfee *et al.*, 2004). Their objective is to improve survival time and quality of life. Both are possible thanks to the introduction of new cytostatics, chemotherapy combinations and the introduction of biological target therapies.

Monoclonal antibodies against vascular endothelial growth factor (e.g., bevacizumab) or against epidermal growth factor receptor (e.g., cetuximab or Panitumumab) provide clinically significant patient benefit, including statistically significant improvement in progression-free survival (Kabbinavar *et al.*, 2005). Bevacizumab has relatively few systemic toxicities. If added to standard chemotherapy biological target therapies may be even more effective. Bevacizumab may cause hypertension that requires medication in 10% to 20% of patients, bevacizumab should be discontinued permanently if nephrotic syndrome occurs; if gastrointestinal perforation has occurred during treatment and if arterial thrombotic complications or life-threatening hemorrhages have occurred. The most common grade 3 to 4 toxicities observed in patients treated with cetuximab are skin problems, allergic reactions, diarrhea, neurotoxicity, and leukopenia. The most serious panitumumab-related adverse events include pulmonary fibrosis, severe skin rash complicated by infections, infusion reactions, abdominal pain, nausea, vomiting, and constipation.

Palliative chemotherapy at an early stage, even before onset of symptoms, seems to prolong the symptom-free phase and also survival (Simmonds, 2000).

Pain therapies

See also chapter: "Pain treatment in rehabilitation and palliation".

In the case of metastases-induced pain, centrally acting analgesics should be initiated without too much delay. Long-lasting forms of morphine should be given preference in this case (tables 5.21, 5.22, 5.23). Transdermal forms such as fentanyl or buprenorphin have the added advantage that they cause few adverse effects. Supplementary measures that influence pain symptoms and the pain threshold include: Physiotherapy procedures, psychiatric pain control, psychosocial support and relaxation techniques. In the case of liver capsule pain, additional low-dose administration of corticosteroids may relieve pain and at the same time have a positive effect on the psyche and loss of appetite. The additional administration of psychotropic drugs raises the pain threshold. Percutaneous pain irradiation may be indicated in some cases.

Ensuring the quality of rehabilitation and palliative measures (structural quality, process quality and evaluation)

Quality of structural features, quality of medical and therapeutic processes

As with acute therapy, structural guidelines should also apply to follow-up care, including rehabilitation and palliation. The progress and results of rehabilitation and palliation must be recorded and evaluated (Delbrück, 1998, Barat and Franchignoni, 2004). There are unfortunately few guidelines on this subject.

In Germany, there are structural guidelines for rehabilitation institutions that provide rehabilitation treatment for ambulant or hospitalized patients with colorectal cancers (Bundesarbeitsgemeinschaft für Rehabilitation, 2003).

Regardless of whether the patient is ambulant or hospitalized, a senior physician who can demonstrate his/her experience of rehabilitation and oncological palliation is indispensable. The team (fig. 1.4) must include a nutritionist. Psycho-oncologists can be helpful. Social workers are essential for the necessary psychosocial rehabilitation objectives.

Outcome assessment and evaluation

There are objective and subjective measurement parameters for evaluating the rehabilitation procedures performed in colon cancer patients and assessing the success of the therapies carried out. Patient satisfaction (evaluation of the result by the person concerned) is also important and can be assessed through questionnaires.

Basically, therapy is regarded as successful if the need for care is reduced (rehabilitation to combat the need for care), if the person concerned can return to work (rehabilitation to combat early retirement), if he/she is not resigned (rehabilitation to combat resignation and depression), if the physical pain and physical handicaps are slight and if the patient can lead a satisfactory life with his/her disabilities (rehabilitation to combat disability).

Different outcome scales in palliative care of cancer patients have been developed (Aspinal *et al.*, 2002, Bausewein *et al.*, 2005). The scales cover physical and psychological symptoms, spiritual considerations, practical concerns, emotional concerns of the patient and family, and psychosocial needs of the patient and family. The Palliative Care Outcome Scale (POS) is a multidimensional instrument covering these physical, psychosocial, spiritual, organizational, and practical concerns.

Bibliography

- Andersen BL (1985) Sexual function morbidity among cancer survivors. Cancer (1985) 15, 55, 8: 1835-42
- Aspinal F, Hughes R, Higginson I *et al.* (2002) A user's guide to the palliative care outcome scale. Palliative care & policy publications. Kings College, London
- Balducci L (2000) The assessment of the older cancer patient. Euro J Ger, 2, 4: 168
- Barat M, Franchignoni F (2004) Assessment in physical medicine and rehabilitation. Maugeri Foundation books, PI-ME Press Pavia
- Bausewein C, Fegg M, Radbruch L *et al.* (2005) Validation and clinical application of the German version of the palliative care outcome. J Pain Symptom Manage 30: 51-62
- Bosker RJ, Eddes EH, ter Borg F *et al.* (2005) The use of self-expanding stent as palliation or before elective surgery in patients with obstructive colorectal carcinoma. Ned Tijdschr Geneeskd 149, 21: 1159-63
- Bromer M, Weinberg DS (2005) Screening for colorectal cancer-now and the near future. Semin Oncol 32: 3-10

- Bundesarbeitsgemeinschaft für Rehabilitation (2003) Rahmempfehlungen zur ambulanten onkologischen Rehabilitation. Publication series of the Federal Study Group on Rehabilitation, Frankfurt, Eyssenekstr
- Delbrück H, Haupt E (eds.) (1998) Rehabilitationsmedizin. Ambulant – Teilstationär – Stationär. Urban & Schwarzenberg, Munich
- Desch C, Benson ALB III et al. (1999) Recommended colorectal cancer surveillance guidelines by the American Society of Clinical Oncology. J Clin Oncol 17: 1312
- ESMO (2001) Minimum clinical recommendations for diagnosis, adjuvant treatment and follow-up of colon cancer. Ann of Oncology 12: 1053
- Heo YS, Chang HM, Kim TW et al. (2004) Hand-foot syndrome in patients treated with capecitabine-containing combination chemotherapy J Clin Pharmacol 44, 10: 1166-72
- Junker A, Kretschmar A, Bohm U et al. (2004) Treatment of patients with intestinal cancer. Increased neurotoxicity after oxaliplatin and related liver metastasis. Med Monatsschr Pharm 27, 10: 349-52
- Kabbinavar F, Schulz J, McCleod M et al. (2005) Addition of Bevacizumab to Bolus Fluorouracil and Leucovorin in First-Line Metastatic Colorectal Cancer. J Clin Oncol 23, 16: 1-9
- Katz A, Brentnell T (2006) Genetic testing for colon cancer. Nat Clin Pract Gastro-enterol Hepatol 3, 12: 670-9
- Korfee S, Gauler T, Hepp R et al. (2004) New targeted treatments in lung cancer – overview of clinical trials. Lung Cancer 45, 2: 199-208
- Lim JF, Ho YH (2001) Total colectomy with ileorectal anastomosis leads to appreciable loss in quality of life. Techniques in coloproctology 5, 2: 79-83
- Lassere Y, Hoff P (2004) Management of hand-foot syndrome in patients treated with capecitabine (Xeloda). Eur J Oncol Nurs 8: 31-40
- Mancuso A, Migliorino M, de Santis S et al. (2006) Correlation between anemia and functional/cognitive capacity in elderly lung cancer patients treated with chemotherapy. Annals of oncoloy 17: 146-50
- Matloff ET, Brierley KL, Chimera CM (2004) A clinician's guide to hereditary colon cancer. Cancer J 10, 5: 280-7
- Putnam JB Secondary tumours of the lung. In: Shields W (2000) General thoracic surgery. Lippincott Williams & Wilkins Philadelphia 1555
- Robinson BJ et al. (1999) Is resection of pulmonary and hepatic metastases warranted in patients with colorectal cancer? Thorac Cardiovasc Surg 117
- Ruers TJ, Joosten J, Jager G (2001) Long-term results after hepatectomy for colorectal cancer metastases. Br J Surg 88: 844-9
- Schlag P, Liebeskind U, Gütz H (2000) Postoperative follow-up for colorectal cancer. What is left? Onkologie 23: 202
- Schmid L, Delbrück H, Bartsch H et al. (2000) Zur Strukturqualität in der onkologischen Rehabilitation. Rehabilitation, 39: 350-4
- Simmonds PC (2000) Palliative chemotherapy for advanced colorectal cancer: Systematic review and meta analysis. Colorectal cancer collaboration group. BMJ 321: 531-5
- Yancik R, Wesley M, Ries L et al. (2000) Comorbidity and age predictors of risk for early mortality of male and female colon carcinoma patients. Cancer 82, 11: 2123-34
- Wannamethee SC, Shaper AG, Walker M (2001) Physical activity and risk of cancer in middle-aged men. Br J Cancer 85: 1311-6

– Ward W, Hahn EA, Mo F *et al.* (1999) Reliability and validity of the functional assessment of cancer therapy-colorectal (FACT C) quality of life instrument. Qual Life Res 8: 181
– Watson T, Mock V (2004) Exercise as an intervention for cancer related fatigue. Phys Ther 84: 736-43

Rehabilitation and palliation
of patients with rectal carcinoma

Goals of rehabilitation and palliation: Significance and definition as distinct from curative tumour aftercare

Some complaints differ from those that occur in colon cancer patients. This applies to rectal cancer patients having had a sphincter preserving procedure and to patients having had an abdomino-perineal resection with permanent colostomy as well. The value of **rehabilitation measures** (fig. 1.2) in these patients is undisputed. Disabilities and handicaps in these patients can be reduced by rehabilitation measures not only in the physical but also in the psychological, social and vocational area.

The value of **curative tumour aftercare** is uncertain (fig. 1.3). Whether potentially curative aftercare measures (prevention of recurrence, early diagnosis of recurrence and treatment of recurrence) are life-prolonging after anterior resection is doubtful. Sure is on the other hand, that there is often a loss of quality of life with curative therapy of recurrence.

The fact that disease recurrence may not be eliminated even when it has, by means of routine diagnostics, been detected at an asymptomatic stage, or very "early", calls the value of routine follow-up diagnostics into question. Therapy of disease recurrence brings about only – if any at all – marginal gains in survival time. As long as potentially curative measures (early detection and therapy of recurrence) (fig. 1.3) have failed to show a significant survival benefit, rehabilitative and palliative measures in the follow-up care of rectal cancer patients will remain the main focus.

The impairments requiring rehabilitation can be due both to the tumour itself and to the therapy. The nature and extent of the therapeutic measures necessary in rehabilitation (table 1.5) are determined primarily by the severity of the impairments. This is very different of curative care which is dependent on the extent and prognosis of the cancer.

Theoretically, the objectives of curative aftercare may be easily distinguished from those of rehabilitation and palliation. However, in practice there is significant a overlap. This applies particularly to the **therapy of recurrence**. Its primary goal is relief of symptoms (rehabilitative indication); however, it should also produce prolongation of life (curative indication).

The patient with persistent or recurrent colorectal cancer merits the entire range of medical skills of the family physician. He will have to keep in mind, that not all findings are attributed to the cancer; unrelated other treatable diseases should also be considered.

Rehabilitation measures

Rehabilitation of rectal carcinoma involves an extremely varied patient population with a wide range of different functional impairments and disabilities. The rehabilitation goals listed in the tables 1.4 and 11.2 apply both for potentially cured patients and for those with progressive rectal carcinoma. Palliative rehabilitation applies equally to patients with advanced cancer. Its primary goal is reduction of dependence in mobility and self-care activities in association with the provision of comfort and emotional support. Enabling patients to remain independent with bowel and bladder management is a prime goal. Faecal and urinary incontinence, in particular, engender psychological distress. Through provision of supportive devices and supportive instructions, patients maintain personal hygiene until the extremely advanced stages of the disease.

To avoid redundancy, please refer to the chapter on colon carcinoma regarding the disorders that are also possible after colon carcinoma resection and chemotherapy.

Comorbidities must also be treated during rehabilitation.

Before the start of rehabilitation an assessment with rehabilitation planning and definition of goals should take place. Many questions have to be answered. Without this preparation, there is a risk of failure of the rehabilitation measures. Certain minimum information about disease status (table 11.1) is a precondition before the start of rehabilitation and palliation measures.

Table 11.1 - Minimum information that should be available before the start of the rehabilitation measures.

– Extent of tumour (e.g., pTNM)
– Curative or palliative therapy approach (e.g., R0, R1 or R2 resection of the tumour?)
– In the case of tumour progression information about the site and extent of the tumour foci (metastases)
– Operative procedure (e.g., sphincter sparing surgery or permanent colostomy, colonic pouch?)
– Radiotherapy (location, dose, fractionation, what were the results?)
– Chemotherapy (which cytostatics, dosage, what were the results?)
– Psychosocial information (for example, about family structure, about statements given pertaining to degree of patient information, about any problems with coping or compliance, about amount of support given by family members, about social and occupational problems, etc.)

Rehabilitation measures aiming at reducing physical problems ("rehabilitation to combat disability")

Organ dysfunction is a crucial factor in determining quality of life after rectal cancer surgery.

There are different problems after an anterior resection and adjuvant radio-chemotherapy than after an abdomino-perineal rectal resection with permanent colostomy with or without adjuvant chemo or radiotherapy. Other rehabilitation measures are necessary. This is the reason why in the following the effects after:
– sphincter- (continence-) preserving operations;
–abdomino-perineal rectal amputation (colostomy) will be commented on separately.

For more details to physical problems in patients with ileostomy and/or short gut syndrome also refer to chapter: "Rehabilitation of patients with ovary cancer".

Rehabilitation measures aiming at reducing physical problems after sphincter preserving operation for rectal cancer

Although patients without a stoma generally fare better than do those with a colostomy, the former may suffer from physical impairments of bowel and genito-urinary function after sphincter-saving procedures. These impairments may become more prevalent as very deep resections are used more frequently.

Prospective evaluation of quality of life turns out sometimes better in patients receiving abdomino-perineal resection than sphincter-preserving procedures (Schmidt *et al.*, 2005). Sphincter preservation without good function is of questionable benefit. The functional result after low anterior resection may be disappointing because of an increased frequency of defecation, urgency and faecal leakage.

Table 11.2 - Physical rehabilitation needs after anterior resection (sphincter-preserving operation).

– Urinary and faecal incontinence
– Urogenital infections
– Sexual disorders
– Diarrhea
– Constipation
– General dietary recommendations
– Impaired mobility
– Chronic radiation side effects
– Chronic chemotherapy sequelae

Faecal incontinence and management

Faecal incontinence is a debilitating problem with significant medical, social and economic implications.

Postoperative defaecatory disorders are caused by many factors in addition to denervation of the neorectum. This is different from apparent sphincter weakness. In this functional disorder, the sphincter muscle itself is intact but because of the damaged innervation its function is impaired.

With a low rectal anastomosis, alterations of bowel movements are usual for weeks or even months after the operation. Irregularity appears to result from disrupted peristalsis and poor compliance in the remaining rectal ampulla but can also be related to a narrowed anastomosis. Loss of the rectal ampulla causes constant onward pushing contractions of the bowel, the feeling of defaecatory urgency, and the occasional faecal incontinence.

Sometimes there is defaecatory urgency as a result of the impaired reservoir function and holding capacity of the residual rectum. Some patients cannot distinguish wind from stool. Patients complain about this particularly often after radiotherapy.

An "anterior resection syndrome" is not rare after low anterior resection with formation of a neorectum (table 11.3).

Table 11.3 - Symptoms of anterior resection syndrome.

– Faecal incontinence
– Pain
– Irregular bowel movements (rectal tenesmus)
– Defaecatory urgency

Treatment options include conservative, non-operative interventions (e.g., pelvic floor muscle training, biofeedback, drugs) and surgical procedures. Surgery is used in selected groups of patients when the structural and functional defects in the pelvic floor muscles or the anal sphincter complex can be corrected mechanically.

In all of the mentioned forms training of the pelvic floor muscles is required. Electrostimulation with biofeedback can be employed as a supplement to pelvic floor exercises. There is no doubt that feedback and/or sphincter exercises help to reduce faecal incontinence (Norton *et al.*, 2003).

Foods that cause flatulence and promote motility should be avoided. No improvement can be anticipated from pelvic floor exercises when the sphincter is infiltrated by a tumour.

The therapy of incontinence is one of the main emphases in rehabilitation, so nursing staff with special training (incontinence counsellors) should be involved in the rehabilitation team (fig. 1.4, table 1.18b).

Urinary incontinence and management

The rate of reported urinary dysfunction after surgery for rectal cancer ranges from 30-70% presenting as various complaints. The most common symptoms are stress incontinence, urgency, elevated frequency of voiding, difficulty emptying the bladder, loss of sensation of fullness of the bladder and overflow incontinence.

Bowel and urinary dysfunction and impotence have a major adverse impact on the quality of life after rectal cancer surgery. These adverse effects need to be discussed with the patient and preoperative function needs to be taken into account when choosing between treatment options.

Information about frequency of micturition (PAD tests) and ultrasound measurements of residual urine volume are necessary at the start of rehabilitation. Additional urodynamic investigations can be useful.

Mesorectal excision can result in bladder dysfunction (Nesbakken et al., 2000). Stress incontinence is often present. The bladder sphincter itself is rarely involved. Sometimes injury of sacral nerve fibers is responsible for the loss of bladder function. Injury of the sympathetic nervous system (hypogastric nerve) can lead to increased urinary urgency or stress incontinence. Involuntary passage of urine occurs particularly together with physical complaints about the absence of the sensation of bladder filling.

In the case of compression of sacral nerves by a haematoma continence will improve spontaneously. Otherwise pelvic floor physiotherapy can be employed successfully. In the case of tumour infiltration, radiation injury or atony of the bladder muscle there is no effect.

If there is no improvement in the complaints despite intensive pelvic floor physiotherapy and electrotherapy, organic insufficiency must be considered. It can only be alleviated surgically. Cholinergic drugs can be indicated in disorders of bladder voiding.

With modern operation techniques permanent major urinary dysfunction is rare.

Urogenital infections and treatment

Bladder and urinary tract infections are common and must be treated with antibiotics. One cause among others is residual urine after inadequate bladder voiding. Nocturia and stress incontinence are frequent in women. This urogenital dysfunction is most marked in those women who had previously undergone a hysterectomy (Daniels et al., 2006).

Sexual dysfunction and recommendations

The effect of sexual dysfunction on quality of life is not very well known, as a high percentage of rectal cancer patients are elderly and often either not sexually active or choose not to answer the questions concerning sexuality (Rauch et al., 2004).

Mesorectal excision can result in erectile dysfunction and even impotence. Some men report retrograde ejaculation (Nesbakken et al., 2000). Radiation therapy to the pelvis may induce a more gradual process of fibrosis that eventually damages both the nerves and blood vessels involved in erection. Impaired sexual ability may occur after laparoscopic resection.

PDE-5-inhibitors (sildenafil, vardenafil, tadalafil) will help only in partial, but not in total denervation. PDE-5-inhibitors are contraindicated in patients with cardiovascular problems.

Table 11.4 - Therapeutic options in erectile dysfunction.

– Oral intake of PDE-5-inhibitors
– Intra-urethral application of Alprostadil (MUSE)
– Corpus cavernosum auto-injection of vaso-active substances (SKAT)
– External vacuum therapy (Osborne Erecaid System)
– Penile prostheses

In contrast to men, women after radical cystectomy or rectal cancer surgery have similar sexual function *versus* healthy controls (Schover, 2005). After radiation therapy, oestrogen-containing suppositories may prevent dryness and pruritus of vagina. Vaginal dilatation is widely accepted as a treatment to prevent vaginal fibrosis in women who have had pelvic radiation therapy.

Diarrhea and its management

Table 11.5 - Possible causes of diarrhea.

– Extended colorectal resection
– Chemotherapy
– Treatment with antibiotics
– Lactose intolerance
– Radiation therapy

In general one third of the colon is sufficient for thickening the stool. If diarrhea occurs nevertheless, this is often the result of hyperperistalsis of the small bowel and/or colon. Drugs that slow motility (e.g., loperamide) are then required.

If the entire colon has been removed, the stool is inevitably liquid. This is the case in **ileostomy patients**. Ileostomies are constructed predominantly after bowel resections for inflammatory bowel disease and rare in tumour patients. For the treatment of large-volume secretory diarrhea, octreotide may have beneficial effects.

The peri-anal skin may become excoriated as a result of severe diarrhea; creams containing zinc oxide promote healing.

Treatment with antibiotics may result in infections with clostridium difficile causing diarrhea.

Rectal carcinoma patients who have had continence-preserving surgery often suffer in the first postoperative months from **"imperative defaecatory urgency"**, which is incorrectly referred to diarrhea by the patients. The cause is that the rectal ampulla, which serves as a stool reservoir and for thickening the stool, was removed along with removal of the rectum. If this reservoir is lost, there are constant onward pushing contractions of the bowel and the sensation of urgency. This sometimes very troublesome defaecatory urgency (imperative defaecatory urgency) usually settles within a few months. The recovery process can be hastened by pelvic floor exercise.

Constipation and its management

Constipation may be a drug side effect (e.g., centrally-acting analgesics) or due to a functional tendency that was present preoperatively. Constipation is often due to inadequate intake of fluids or dietary fiber but may be successfully managed by increasing dietary fiber and fluid intake. Constipation is rarely a side effect of radiation.

It can be influenced by conservative treatment and behavioural changes (table 11.6). Severe constipation may occur in patients with advanced cancer because of their reduced activity, reduced fluid and fiber intake or use of opioid analgesics.

Table 11.6 - Recommendations for treatment of functional constipation.

– Correction of erroneous ideas about defaecation

– Change in living and eating habits

– Physical exercise to increase bowel activity

– Gastrocolic reflex (drinking a glass of cold water)

– No high-calorie large-volume evening meals

– No high-calorie low-fibre foods such as white bread, pasta, cakes, custard, chocolate and ice-cream

– Physical measures (colon massage)

– High-fibre diet (bran)

– Plentiful fluid intake

Strategies to prevent and to reduce late radiation side effects

Following postoperative radiotherapy, symptoms can occur for a long time (Reis, 2002; Burdeos et al., 2004). Postoperative combined chemo- and radiotherapy can have a major detrimental effect on bowel function, with softer stools, increased number of daily bowel movements (daytime and at night), incontinence, soiling and peri-anal irritation. There is also a possibility of chronic tendency to constipation, slimy and sometimes bloody diarrhea, abdominal cramps and defaecatory urgency along with disorders of stool control (Reis et al., 2002; Burdeos et al., 2004). Sometimes they necessitate operative intervention.

Radiation induced proctitis is rare. Sucralfate suppositories may relief symptoms. Pelvic radiation therapy and temporary faecal diversion may contribute to a narrowed anastomosis, especially if the anastomosis is stapled. If pencil-thin stools persist, bowel stricture due to radiotherapy should be considered. A narrowed anastomosis may require dilatation. The differential diagnosis to be considered is a recurrent tumour invading the bowel lumen.

The dietary recommendations in the case of radiation damage are a low-fat and low-fibre diet avoiding highly spiced foods. This can reduce the harmful surge of bile acids. Cholestyramine can be given in addition. "Softeners" (psyllium, lactulose) are indicated for constipation. Whether non-steroidal anti-inflammatories are effective is controversial. Routine local or even systemic use of steroids is unadvisable. The protective effect of amifostin remains unconfirmed. Topical use of sucralfate several times a day (twice daily enemas) occasionally leads to symptom relief and regression of the radiogenic ulcerative proctitis

Improvements in the radiogenic sequelae in the rectum are sometimes achieved with **hyperbaric oxygen therapy** (HBO). Rectal bleeding, diarrhea, faecal incontinence and pain decrease after HBO (Anderson, 2003).

If all these conservative measures do not help a **protective colostomy** should be considered. The colostomy must only be created in non-affected segments of bowel, otherwise there is a risk of dehiscence.

Nutritional problems and dietary counselling

Recovery also requires physical activity to rebuild muscle strength. Cancer survivors with treatment-related complications or any other disabilities that interfere with diet and physical activity should be referred as needed to the appropriate health care provider to establish nutritional and activity goals.

Gas-producing foods should be avoided if there is imperative defaecatory urgency (see chapter on "colon carcinoma"). (See below for diet after abdomino-perineal resection of the rectum).

Closure of a temporary stoma

A temporary stoma is often created for relief. Until it is closed, the patient should practise **pelvic floor exercises** so that faecal incontinence does not occur later.

Rehabilitation after abdomino-perineal resection with colostomy

Numerous problems can occur at the ostomy itself (table 11.6b). Better colostomy care and management can be achieved by thoughtful selection of the colostomy site on the abdomen, by the use of specially trained personnel to help people understand the nature of the stoma with its special care problems, and by an appreciation of a person's attitude about oneself in his own environment.

Ostomy education begins before surgery. The healthcare providers may use diagrams, photographs, and examples of equipment to explain what the person can expect after surgery. Concerns related to changes in body image and sexuality can be discussed.

Table 11.6b - The most common specific types of ostomies.

Colostomy	The surgically-created opening of the colon (large intestine) results in a stoma. A colostomy is created when a portion of the colon or the rectum is removed and the remaining colon is brought to the abdominal wall. It may further be defined by the portion of the colon involved and/or its permanence.
Temporary colostomy	Allows the lower portion of the colon to rest or heal. It may have one or two openings (if two, one will discharge only mucus).
Sigmoid or descending colostomy	The most common type of ostomy surgery, in which the end of the descending or sigmoid colon is brought to the surface of the abdomen. It is usually located on the lower left side of the abdomen.
Transverse	The surgical opening created in the transverse colon results in one or two **colostomy** openings. It is located in the upper abdomen, middle or right side.
Loop colostomy	Usually created in the transverse colon. This is one stoma with two openings; one discharges stool, the second mucus.
Ascending colostomy	A relatively rare opening in the ascending portion of the colon. It is located on the right side of the abdomen.
Ileostomy	A surgically created opening in the small intestine, usually at the end of the ileum. The intestine is brought through the abdominal wall to form a stoma. Ileostomies may be temporary or permanent, and may involve removal of all or part of the colon.
Ileo-anal anastomosis	The most common alternative to the conventional ileostomy. Technically, it is not an ostomy since there is no stoma. In this procedure, the colon and most of the rectum are surgically removed and an internal pouch is formed out of the terminal portion of the ileum. An opening at the bottom of this pouch is attached to the anus such that the existing anal sphincter muscles can be used for continence. This procedure should only be performed on patients with ulcerative colitis or familial polyposis, and who have not previously lost their rectum or anus. It is also called J-pouch, pull-through, endorectal pullthrough, pelvic pouch, or a combination of these terms.
Continent ileostomy	This surgical variation of the ileostomy is also called a Kock pouch. A reservoir pouch is created inside the abdomen with a portion of the terminal ileum. A valve is constructed in the pouch and a stoma is brought through the abdominal wall. A catheter or tube is inserted into the pouch several times a day to drain faeces from the reservoir. This procedure has generally been replaced in popularity by the ileo-anal pouch. A modified version of this procedure called the Barnett Continent Ileal Reservoir is performed at a limited number of facilities.
Urostomy	This is a general term for a surgical procedure which diverts urine away from a diseased or defective bladder. The ileal or cecal conduit procedures are the most common urostomies. Either a section at the end of the small bowel (ileum) or at the beginning of the large intestine (cecum) is surgically removed and relocated as a passageway (conduit) for urine to pass from the kidneys to the outside of the body through a stoma. It may include removal of the diseased bladder.
Continent urostomy	There are two main continent procedure alternatives to the ileal or cecal conduit (others exist). In both the Indiana and Kock Pouch versions, a reservoir or pouch is created inside the abdomen with a portion of either the small or large bowel. A valve is constructed in the pouch and a stoma is brought through the abdominal wall. A catheter or tube is inserted several times daily to drain urine from the reservoir.

A frequent reason for problems at the ostomy is an error in constructing it (e.g., failure to mark the site of the stoma preoperatively, bringing out the stoma in the region of scars or abdominal creases, etc.). If a few precautions are taken, many disorders can be prevented or at least alleviated (Doughty, 2005).

For those who do require a stoma, enterostomal therapists provide preoperative support, postoperative education, and state-of-the-art supplies (table 1.18b). The enterostomal therapist (ET nurse) plays a major role in helping the cancer patient with an ostomy (i.e., colostomy, ileostomy, or urostomy) to understand the principles of ostomy care, to learn the different aspects of ostomy management, and to adjust to the altered self-image. Their assistance should be maintained during home care and recovery.

A new patient who attends a local ostomy support group can gain valuable advice about techniques for stomal management.

Stomal prolapse: Strategies to prevent and to reduce problems

Stomal prolapse may be caused by inadequate intra-abdominal fixation of the bowel and by conditions resulting in increased abdominal pressure. There is a high incidence in transverse and ascending colostomy. Prolapse is frequently very upsetting to the patient, but it represents a surgical emergency only when it is associated with stomal ischemia.

Normally the bowel end should project only slightly above the abdominal wall in the case of a colostomy and about 2-3cm in the case of an ileostomy.

Conservative management of stomal prolapse includes application of a hypertonic substance (e.g., sugar or salt) to reduce bowel wall edema, followed by attempts to manually reduce the prolapsed bowel. Reduction may be sometimes maintained by applying a truss or hernia binder with prolapse overbelt. If a bowel prolapse of more than 5cm develops, operative correction should be considered. Persistent or recurrent prolapse typically requires surgical repair.

Stomal retraction: Strategies to prevent and to reduce problems

Stomal retraction to skin level or even below is common and is a frequent contributor to difficult pouching situations. Retraction may occur early after surgery due to difficulty in mobilizing the bowel, presence of a thick abdominal wall, or breakdown of the mucocutaneous suture line. Late retraction may be caused by postoperative weight gain, ascites, tension on the mesentery produced by intraperitoneal tumour growth, or chronic infections and irritation.

The management of stomal retraction can be particularly difficult because it is almost inevitable that the abdominal skin will come in contact with the intestinal contents. There are special stoma care products to protect against skin irritation. Operative correction is essential when there is pain on defecation or even stool retention.

Sometimes the fault is a pouch opening that is too big. Shrinkage of the stoma (1-2 ring sizes) in the first six months after the operation can be regarded as normal. If a finger can no longer be inserted into the stoma, it should be dilated with bougies.

Peristomal complications: Strategies to prevent and to reduce problems

Postoperatively, protecting the skin and collecting the drainage should be the primary goals. This is accomplished by a properly fitted appliance. Modern appliances with protective skin barriers cut to fit the exact size of the stoma will avoid postoperative peristomal skin excoriation and keep the patient dry and odour-free.

Common peristomal complications include epithelial denudation, yeast dermatitis and allergic dermatitis (table 11.7). There are a number of causes of sore skin and different ways to deal with it (table 11.6c).

Table 11.6c - Causes of sore skin.

— Too frequent pouch changes
— Allergy to pouch adhesive
— Leakage of faeces onto the skin
— Stoma may have changed size
— Uneven skin around stoma, e.g., scarring or creases
— Infection due to body hair growth under the adhesive
— Pre-existing skin allergies or food and drink allergies

Table 11.7 - Causes of chronic inflammation in the region of the stoma.

— Retracted stoma
— Incorrect removal of the adhesive surface
— Pouch opening too large
— Poor hygiene
— Aggressive adhesive materials
— Skin unevenness
— Folliculitis
— Allergic skin reactions
— Diet

Epithelial denudation occurs when enzymatic damage pools on the skin; it is typically caused by a poorly fitting or incorrectly sized pouch that permits contact between the skin and the drainage. The enzymes within the drained material literally digest the epithelial layer, producing an area that is red, wet and painful.

Management of epithelial denudation primarily focuses on modification of the pouching system to eliminate contact between the drainage and the skin. The damaged skin is treated with "crusting" before application of the pouch.

Allergic dermatitis is characterized by an area of erythema, pruritus and/or blistering that "matches" the area of skin in contact with the allergen.

The management of allergic dermatitis depends primarily on eliminating the offending substance. Secondary management includes minimizing product use until the dermatitis resolves and topical treatment with antihistamines or low-dose steroids. In selecting topical products, it is important to choose gels or vanishing creams instead of ointments, which may prevent pouch adherence. A change of pouch system may be useful.

Lack of stoma hygiene, incorrect cleaning or cleaning the skin with infected washcloths or sponges promotes colonization of the skin with yeasts and bacteria. **Yeast dermatitis** occurs when yeast penetrates the peristomal skin; this is most commonly seen among patients experiencing yeast overgrowth as a complication of antibiotic therapy, but it can also occur in areas exposed to moisture. Yeast dermatitis typically presents as a circumferential rash that appears solid in the centre and that features distinct "satellite" lesions at the edges; most patients describe the rash as "itchy and tender". Along with careful **hygiene** aqueous antifungal agents should be used exclusively as ointments and powders prevent adhesion of the pouch. Systemic therapy with fluconazole may be indicated if the patient also suffers from oral thrush and/or candidiasis in multiple body folds.

Acid-containing **foodstuffs** often cause inflammation in the stomal area in sensitive skin.

Pseudopolyps, which are harmless but subjectively troublesome for the patient, often develop due to mechanical irritation, particularly if there is a prolapse.

Stoma care products adapted to individual needs are important. Inflammation, eczema and allergies are often due to inadequate stoma care. In cases of doubt, a change in pouch type often helps. There is a large choice of different stoma care systems. The special experience of a stoma therapist is very useful here.

Peristomal hernias: Strategies to prevent and to reduce problems

Bringing the stoma out through the abdominal wall creates an artifical gap in the muscle layer. The intra-abdominal pressure increases considerably when straining and lifting or during heavy physical work, and playing an active sport. These activities can lead to an increase in the size of this muscle gap and to a peri- or parastomal hernia.

A few precautions should be observed in order to diminish strain on the abdominal wall and the risk of developing a hernia (table 11.8). These include risk patients wearing a truss when under strain. The truss should be custom-made and fitted. The greater the risk of hernia, the more often the truss should be worn even with the slightest strain. Excessively narrow trusses should be avoided. They can increase the risk of hernia.

Hernias are typically managed conservatively. The "usual" problems associated with hernias are difficulty in maintaining a pouch seal or difficulty with colostomy irrigation. Surgical repair is usually limited to hernias complicated by incarceration.

Table 11.8 - Precautions to prevent a parastomal hernia.

– Avoid activities that increase strain on the abdominal wall (lifting and carrying heavy loads, straining at stool)
– Avoid abrupt strains on the abdominal muscles
– Avoid overweight
– Wearing of a truss by those particularly at risk

Irrigation (bowel washout): Indications and contraindications

Patients who have a left-sided or sigmoid colostomy should learn to perform habitual stomal irrigation. The purpose of the irrigation is to establish a bowel routine, with the goal of evacuating only after the irrigation, rather than spontaneously or at inopportune moments (table 11.9). However, this is not always possible (table 11.10). Patients with a right-sided colostomy do not have as much remaining colon as those with a left-sided colostomy (fig. 11.1). There is usually too little colon left. This type cannot be controlled by irrigation, but instead behaves very much like an ileostomy with a fairly continuous discharge.

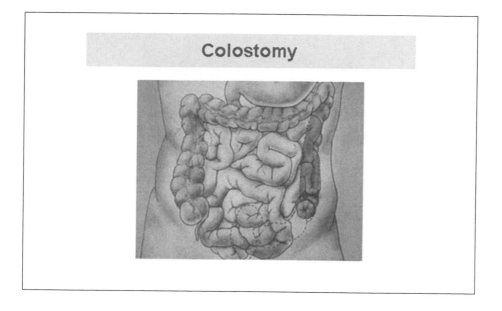

Fig. 11.1 - Colostomy.

The left-sided colostomy is often described as a dry colostomy because it discharges well formed stool. One has the choice of attempting to manage this type by either trained control or irrigation.

The irrigation should be done in private, preferably with the patient sitting by the toilet on a comfortable soft chair. A lubricated cone (fig. 11.2) is gently inserted into the stoma and one liter of lukewarm tap water is instilled over a period of approximately ten minutes from an enema bag placed no higher than a shoulder level, similar to administering an enema. The stretching stimulus of the bowel wall provoked by irrigation with water and the resulting mass peristalsis of the remaining colon leads to complete and targeted evacuation of the large bowel contents. This manoeuvre which lasts 30-50 minutes typically provides a "stool-free" period of 24-48 hours (fig. 11.3). Irrigation of the colostomy may be done daily, every other day, or even every third day, at the time of the patient's preference. Small security pads or pouches are available for use between irrigations.

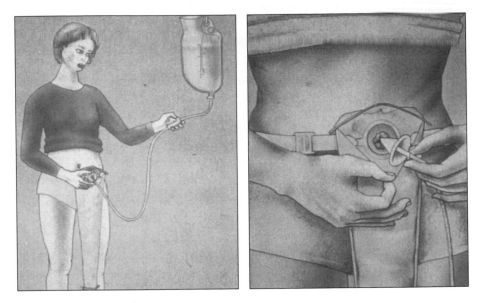

Fig. 11.2 et 11.3 - Irrigation

Those who practise self-irrigation have many physical and psychosocial advantages (table 11.9). Quality of life is far better in these patients than in patients wearing a pouch (stoma bag).

Table 11.9 - Advantages of irrigation for stoma patients.

– Irrigating stoma patients are largely independent of pouching. Pouch disposal problems do not arise.
– There is a stool-free period of 24 to 48 hours during which a stoma cap or plug must be worn. Mobility is largely problem-free.
– Irrigation shortens the time the stool is in the colon and so slows down the production of bacteria in the bowel. As a result gas does not develop as fast and there is less odour and borborygmi.
– Leisure activities, work and social life are often problem-free.
– Constipation occurs less frequently.
– Patients wearing a pouch are at a disadvantage in hot weather because eczema often occurs at the stoma as a result of sweat secretion or allergic skin reactions.
– Sex life is less affected.

Learning self-irrigation is one of the most important functions of rehabilitation. Unfortunately not all stoma patients can practise irrigation; there are a few absolute and relative contraindications (table 11.10). Stomal irrigation is avoided if ponderous obesity, poor vision, inanition, or another factor limits or precludes stomal management

Table 11.10 - Contraindications to performing irrigation.

– Ileostomy, caecostomy, transverse colostomy
– Liquid stool
– Frequent diarrhea
– Not during chemotherapy and not during radiotherapy
– Siphon effect of the terminal segment of bowel
– Very high or very low stoma
– Extensive diverticula
– Extensive abdominal adhesions
– Major prolapse
– Irritable bowel
– Limited when major retraction
– Limited when too little toilet space
– Limited when shortage of time
– Limited when poor compliance

Prior to irrigation an X-ray contrast enema should ideally be performed to rule out a siphoning effect or extensive diverticula.

Irrigation techniques cannot always be taught in the hospital setting, given the current pressure for early discharge. To teach irrigation techniques may be one of the missions in a rehabilitation clinic. A lot of experience is needed to assess which stoma care system is best and whether learning irrigation is useful. **Enterostomal therapists** (ET nurses) have great specialist and psychological competence in the area of stoma care (table 1.18b). Outpatient ET services and/or visiting nurses often teach or continue to teach irrigation in the home after discharge.

Posterior wound problems: Strategies to prevent and to reduce problems

The posterior wound over the coccyx usually heals after three months at the latest and apart from occasional discomfort does not cause any problems. However, if the wound becomes contaminated or inflamed, the healing process can take much longer. Often the wound is deliberately not closed at operation so that wound secretions can drain freely. In this case, hip-baths and dry dressings or pads are very useful. Camomile sitz baths are soothing for weeping wounds. If a secretion collection forms, the outflow channel must be opened.

Fistulas can be unpleasant. If they lead into the former wound cavity, they will heal faster with irrigation and regular camomile sitz baths. The direction and length of a fistula can be shown very well radiologically (with fistulography).

In the initial period after the operation, many patients complain of **pain** at the posterior wound and difficulties when sitting and walking. Experience has shown complaints subside after a time. Infection, abscess or tumour in the previous wound cavity should be considered if they persist or even occur after a prolonged asymptomatic period.

Patients often complain of problems when sitting. The problems are reduced by taking the pressure off the sensitive areas and distributing the pressure onto the pelvic bones and thighs. So-called postoperative pillows provide great relief and the use of swimming rings are very effective. The posterior scar can be kept more supple by regular sitz baths resulting in less problems while walking or sitting. Cycling is not recommended in principle until the posterior wound has healed. A wide saddle is recommended subsequently.

Sexuality/fertility problems: Strategies to prevent and to reduce problems

Sexual counselling is important. Disorders of sexual experience and behaviour often occur. They usually mean a considerable loss of quality of life for the patients and their partners. In many cases the development of severe neurotic behaviour disorders can be avoided with prompt and adequate counselling. After abdomino-perineal resection the risk for permanent impotence seems to be 35%-45% whereas low anterior resection carries about half the risk of impotence.

Experience has shown that only a small number of those affected raise the subject of sexuality themselves. The vast majority wait to be asked by the doctor or nurse (Black, 2004). There are considerable inhibitions associated with the subject of sexuality and particularly with "sexual failure". Fears and feelings of guilt play a central part. These can be reduced in discussion.

In the first weeks after construction of a stoma, pain can occur during sexual intercourse, particularly when the wound sutures after closure of the rectum extend to the region of the vaginal introitus. This also applies for the wound cavity within the abdomen, which can give rise to pain until final healing has occurred.

Many women experience dyspareunia, pain interfering with sexual pleasure, and fear of stool leakage, all of which limit sexual activity. Displacement of the vaginal walls is possible. Pain can occur in patients in whom a tuck had to be made in the vagina during the operation. A dilator hurts initially but makes problem-free intercourse possible later. After radiation therapy in fields that include the genital area, oestrogen-containing suppositories may prevent dryness and pruritus of the vagina.

Experience has shown that the sex life of irrigating women is impaired less than that of women using classical pouching.

Male patients may experience increased strain because of impaired sexual function (Schmidt *et al.*, 2005). Many patients find it difficult to discuss their sexual feelings; the nurse, e.g., rehabilitating professional, should be able to help patients to identify and adapt to alterations in sexual self-concept (Black, 2004). Disorders of erectile and ejaculatory function are due to the fact that the sympathetic and parasympathetic nerve paths responsible for potency run in the area of the rectal surgery. Libido is usually maintained.

Medical, psychological, mechanical and operative aids are available for erectile dysfunction. Intact pelvic nerves in the pelvis, which are required for perfusion of the penis, are a requirement for the action of chemically-defined agents to treat erectile dysfunction (e.g., sildenafil, vardenafil). However, this is often not the case with erectile impotence after rectal amputation.

The mechanical aids include external vacuum therapy (Osborne Erecaid System), the most well-known method. The costs of this are lower than the medical aids (corpus cavernosum autoinjection therapy, MUSE therapy, sildenafil).

(For more details on the medical and mechanical aids in erectile dysfunction, see chapter on "prostate carcinoma".)

Women with an ileostomy should be aware that the pill is not a reliable contraceptive for them because it is often excreted undigested. There are no such fears with a colostomy.

Pregnancy is possible; however, delivery should be by cesarian section because of the strain on the abdominal muscle during natural birth.

Dietary problems and counselling

Stoma patients have a need for precise dietary advice, although neither the cancer nor the stoma are reasons for restrictive dietary recommendations. However, if a few recommendations are followed, existing or imminent stoma problems can be prevented or at least alleviated (Fulham, 2004).

The avoidable disorders include overweight, flatulence and borborygmi, odour, tendency to diarrhea, stoma inflammation and stoma blockages.

Major weight gain is deleterious and often leads to complications such as parastomal hernia, stomal retraction, etc. Stoma will work best if patients eat regularly.

A high-fibre diet is regarded on the one hand as protective for the patient at risk from bowel cancer but on the other hand it is detrimental for stoma patients. Because of it, the irrigation intervals are shortened in the irrigating patient as it stimulates peristalsis and produces greater stool volumes. It also promotes flatulence and borborygmi. However, lactase deficiency or use of laxatives containing lactulose can occasionally also be the cause for flatulence.

The best thing is for the stoma patient to try out what agrees with him/her. This can be very different from one patient to another. It is beneficial to keep a food diary in which the patient writes down what and how much he/she has eaten. The diary should include time of the main evacuation, the consistency of the output, and whether anything particular (e.g., flatulence, odour, diarrhea, etc.) has occurred. That way, the stoma patient and his dietary counsellor gain the best overview of individual intolerances.

Flatulence: Strategies to minimize gas and odourous discharge

Because the small bowel has low bacterial levels, the individual with an ileostomy typically experiences less gas and less odour than does the patient with a colostomy.

Strategies to minimize gas and odour are to reduce intake of gas-forming foods, such as beans, broccoli and cabbage. Patients with colostomy should learn to limit activities that increase the volume of swallowed air (e.g., smoking, drinking through straws and chewing gum). Different foods cause more odour than others. Noxious odour may be increased by various foods and liquids (cabbage, eggs, onions, garlic, beer, coffee). What may adversely affect one person may not affect another. Deodourant tablets placed in the disposable colostomy pouch may help to diminish odours. Charcoal and other products to reduce the release of malodourous gas are widely available. Risk patients should use pouching systems with charcoal filters to vent and deodourants to minimize stool odour with pouch emptying. Routine use of oral deodourants, such as bismuth subgallate and chlorophyllin copper complex, also may reduce faecal odour significantly.

Irrigation slows down the production of bacteria in the bowel. As a result gas does not develop as fast and there is less odour and borborygmi.

Stoma (food) blockage: Strategies to prevent and to reduce this complication

"Food blockage" occurs when a mass of insoluble fibre becomes lodged near the stoma at the point where the bowel is brought through the fascia-muscle layer, a point of potential narrowing. There is a risk of stoma blockage in ileostomy patients and those with a very tight colostomy, so these patients should avoid foods that are difficult to digest or are very fibrous such as mushrooms, asparagus, nuts, etc. The risk of stoma blockage in patients with uncomplicated colostomy is low.

Patients must recognize and promptly report the signs of food blockage, which include no output or high-volume liquid malodourous output, cramping pain, distention, and, possibly, nausea and vomiting. Food blockage is managed by ileal lavage.

Non-specific postproctectomy complaints: Strategies to prevent and to reduce problems

After radical amputation of the rectum with removal of the surrounding lymphatic tissue and simultaneous construction of a stoma, non-specific complaints can occur that are known collectively as the postproctectomy syndrome. They are due particularly to the wound cavity which fills up slowly over time with connective tissue, small bowel and neighbouring organs.

If an abscess is suspected, MRI is a better choice than a CT scan.

In women, displacement of the internal genital organs into the wound cavity may cause prolonged complaints of varying intensity. Pain can occur as a result of division of the nerves supplying the rectum and anal region which is inevitable with organ removal. If adhesions are responsible for the pain, sitz baths, electrostimulation treatment, relaxation exercises and other "gentle pain therapies" can have an alleviating effect.

Retroperitoneal scar fibrosis can result in hydronephrosis, which is usually asymptomatic clinically. Loss of erection and ejaculation can occur in addition to disorders of bladder voiding including autonomic bladder and the infectious sequelae resulting from residual urine.

Sometimes pain is associated with the division of the nerves supplying the rectum and anal region. Besides the phantom feeling pain like that of a sphincter spasm can occur. Some patients complain of tenesmus-like urgency and paresthaesias including tingling, shooting or burning pains.

Perineal hernia and also tumour growth should always be considered in the differential diagnosis of pain in the low back and perineal region, especially as the former wound cavity and the tissue surrounding it are a frequent site of recurrence.

Sitz baths and warm baths have a calming and relaxing effect. A few authors report good experiences with infiltration treatments, low dose X-ray treatment, alcohol injections, acupuncture, electrostimulation treatment, and percutaneous laser therapy.

Late radiation side effects: Strategies to prevent and to reduce late side effects

See also the section on "rehabilitation measures after anterior resection".

The small bowel mucosa is much more radiosensitive than that of the large bowel. There is an increased risk if the small bowel is in the radiation field. This is the case when loops of small bowel become displaced into the pelvis postoperatively. Displacements of the small bowel into the pelvis must therefore be prevented during the operation.

When the stoma is in the radiation field, treatment must be modified to minimize the risk of peristomal skin damage. Stomatitis is a common complication of both radiation therapy and chemotherapy and is manifested by stomal edema and friability.

Necessity of information and patient education (discussion groups and health training)

Information promotes self-help. Self-help (empowerment) is an important goal of training (tables 2.12, 11.11).

Education and information are important aids in overcoming illness. Important topics include the patient's understanding of what is happening inside his/her body and why a certain therapy option has been chosen. Health training is a source of general information on rectal carcinoma, but mainly provide advice related to impairment and disabilities (tables 1.5, 11.12).

Table 11.11 - Key features of modern training.

– Communication of disease-specific knowledge and skills
– Assistance in formulating and achieving personal treatment goals
– Encouragement of training and experimentation
– Presentation of the advantages and disadvantages of various care recommendations
– Special emphasis on the difficulties in implementing therapy in daily life
– Active involvement of trainees
– Promotion of exchange among patients
– Involvement of relatives
– Evaluation of the results of training
– Appropriate dealing with fears and worries

Table 11.12 - Frequent questions which come up in group discussions.

– What are the various therapeutic possibilities?
– What can I do to prevent recurrence?
– Is there a genetic background of my cancer and is it necessary to counsel my relatives?
– What do I need to do for content regarding follow-up investigations?
– What are the dietary issues?
– What are the ways of coping with fear?
– What behavioural changes will occur in the event of pain?
– What information is available on topics regarding social legislation?
– What are my vocational consequences?
– What do I have to do for stoma care?

Training and discussion groups are particularly important for **stoma patients**. They make an important contribution to coping with the impairments. Colostomy and ileostomy patients are often dissatisfied with their opportunities to participate in the decision-making process (Persson *et al.*, 2005).

One-to-one and group counselling sessions are effective for this purpose; in the latter patients' family members may also participate (Fulham, 2004).

Since the questions raised about stoma care are sometimes highly specialized, the participation of a stoma therapist is advisable. A psychologist, dietary counsellor, psycho-oncologist, oncologist, social worker or representative of a self-help group should take turns in moderating the discussion groups.

It has proven to be beneficial if patients who have recently had surgery are introduced to other patients who had surgery and stoma construction a few years previously. The "more experienced" patients function as positive models encouraging the recently diagnosed patients.

The information and advice provided in health training and discussion groups should be made available to the patients and their relatives in written form (e.g., various guides or colostomy publications produced by support groups). Naturally, these written materials must never replace medical discussion. Rather, they should be the basis for useful discussions with the treating doctor.

Today, every layperson has access via the Internet to specialist literature/information including the sobering data on the life expectancy of patients with recurrence of rectal carcinoma. It is regrettable that the Internet passages often give rise to misunderstandings. This kind of information is as damaging as leaving the patient alone without an explanation.

Rehabilitation measures aiming at avoiding psychological problems ("rehabilitation to combat withdrawal and depression")

See also chapter: "Psychological support in cancer rehabilitation and palliation".

Necessity of psychological support

Psychological difficulties often occur because the patient has to cope with the fear of disease progressing, stoma acceptance and care issues. If stoma care problems (such as fear of odour, pain, and incontinence) are the sources of depression then good stoma counselling can make psychotherapeutic care unnecessary. In younger patients, sexual problems are often the cause of depression, while fatigue problems (table 2.8) may predominate in older patients (Black, 2004; Schmidt, 2005).

Psychological helps

It may be necessary to seek counselling in how to, accept and deal with disease and ostomy. This will reduce the fear and depression, increases compliance and improve quality of life (tables 2.4, 2.5). The help of a professional psycho-oncologist can be necessary (tables 1.19, 2.3). Stoma patients must feel that they still have a place in the family and in society. They can handle responsibility and make others happy.

It is important patients learn to talk openly with others who are affected about their problems. Discussion groups (e.g. during "health training") and/or self-help groups are very effective in aiding this process.

Support for family members

Cancer not only places strain on the patient but also has direct effects on the partner and entire family.

Distress affects the families of older tumour patients as well as the families of children suffering from cancer; the focus is merely shifted.

Cancer can cause considerable distress for the healthy partners of older patients, due to experiencing and supporting their partners coping with impairments. Ultimately the distress is magnified because they are also experiencing age related changes. They lose the security provided by continuity in their relationship prior to the cancer. Plans for a "peaceful retirement" are shattered, prospects for their life in old age must be reconsidered and redeveloped. The physical exertion involved in caring for the patient as well as the financial costs of old and new burdens pose substantial problems for the family. The transition in role allocation from "being provided for" to "being the provider" places high demands on the family's ability to adapt to the new situation. In addition to conflicts between the family members' own needs, the desire for autonomy, and obligations to the ill parent, conflicts also often arise between caring for the patient and fulfilling responsibilities in the adult child's own family or professional career. The partners of older cancer patients particularly experience emotional distress, while the adult children of cancer patients more frequently describe their stress as the result of a confusion in roles. This particularly applies to middle-aged daughters, who fulfill the responsibilities of several roles simultaneously, who more commonly experience stress and fear, and who are less able to fall back on support from their social environment.

It is helpful if carers can be seen alone from time to time, perhaps by the family doctor, asked how they are coping and invited to talk over any emotional distress.

Support options for families are internationally very limited with regard to financing by insurance companies or other cost carriers.

It may be desirable for the patient's partner to participate in educational cancer training. Informing patients and their families that physical inactivity can hinder the treatment of fatigue should be one of the problems focused upon in group therapy sessions. A number of German cancer rehabilitation clinics for gastro-intestinal cancer patients that have a basis on therapy close to the patient's residence explicitly integrate psychosocial care into both their inpatient and their outpatient/semi-outpatient treatment concepts. Self-help groups for family members have also been established. In some regions of Germany there are special centres and organizations (Alpha) that promote the support of family members of the terminally ill.

Rehabilitation measures aiming at reducing social problems ("rehab to prevent care")

See also chapter: "Social support in cancer rehabilitation and palliation".

Need of social support

If independent care is no longer possible, then corresponding outside care must be ensured as necessary. This is often prevalent in patients with advanced malignant disease.

Organization of outside assistance: Securing adequate care at home

Professional social work is highly important particularly in rectal carcinoma patients with an ostomy. Outside help and support are often necessary. Further care at home must be discussed with the relatives who must be informed about the possible problems that can be expected and put in contact with social aid organizations and institutions. Care aids such as "meals on wheels", nursing aids, in-home assistants, home nursing, and sometimes accommodation in a care home or hospice must be organized. It is necessary to provide contact addresses (self-help groups, stoma therapists, counselling centres, etc.).

Rehabilitation hospitals

If domestic care is not available or not yet arranged, temporary admission to a convalescent hospital is possible. In Germany there are rehabilitation hospital geared specially to the needs of patients with gastro-intestinal tumours. There are even special rehabilitation clinics for gastro-intestinal cancer patients with an ostomy. Over half of all cancer patients with an ostomy in Germany make use of these indoor rehabilitation measures. Adjuvant and additive cancer therapies, supportive therapies, stoma care, psychological support, and individual social counselling are being performed in these cancer rehabilitation centres (Delbrück and Witte, 2006).

In England and in Sweden as well as in some locations in Italy, every stoma patient is assigned a stoma care nurse as a continuous contact. The stoma care nurse discusses the diagnostic findings with the patient and his/her relatives and ensures correct stoma care and training. If the stoma cancer nurse has the impression that the patient has a particular need for support in the psychological or social area, the nurse arranges further contacts with psychologists and social workers. Following hospitalisation contact is maintained with the local community nurse. Regular team sessions are obligatory.

Procuring information about questions concerning medical care, nursing care, socio-legal and practical issues: Legally defined privileges for cancer patients

Assistance in social care is available in most countries. Cancer patients in most European countries are subject to legal privileges, ranging from tax reductions, financial grants, free use of public transport and a vocational protection against wrongful dismissal (table 3.9) (see for more information chapter: "Social support in cancer rehabilitation and palliation"). In addition to psychological support, self-help groups often provide their members with specific knowledge about medications and resources as well as social laws.

Self-help groups

The exchange of information between patients in self-help groups is the best source of advice in many cases. Questions about stoma care along with social legislation rights and psychosocial problems are often clarified. Self-help groups (colostomy associations – *fédération des stomisés*) have particular importance especially in the rehabilitation of cancer patients with an ostomy. The first formal organized ostomy group in the world began in 1950 (Lyons, 2001).

Patients receive enormous reassurance and support by the interacting with individuals in the same conditions. The experience of ostomy patients are also enlightening to each other, notably on sex, pregnancy, occupation, social helps and leisure activities. Among the greatest benefits are visits by these support group members to patients before and/or after operations. The ILCO Organisation (Ileostomy and Colostomy Organization), which is represented in nearly every country in Europe, is the most well-known support group today. Ostomy support groups should be regarded by the treating doctors as partners and not as competitors.

Rehabilitation measures aiming at reducing vocational problems ("rehabilitation to prevent early retirement")

See also chapter: "Vocational integration in cancer rehabilitation".

Harmful occupational substances

Associations between certain occupational toxins and rectal cancer have not been conclusively demonstrated.

Restrictions of working capacity

After **anterior R0 tumour resection** patients can usually return to work after three months at the latest. If there are complications after the operation and/or chemo-radiotherapy, physical symptoms then a medical leave from work can last longer. There are restrictions in the case of faecal incontinence (table 11.13) with imperative defaecatory urgency and lack of reservoir capacity in the residual rectum

Table 11.13 - Factors for vocational fitness.

– Tumour location
– Whether a R0 or R1 resection (an anterior or posterior resection) was performed
– Whether there is acceptance of the disease and ostomy
– Whether there are further functional disorders (e.g., incontinence)
– Whether there are concomitant diseases
– Whether adjuvant therapies were given
– Whether the patient is physically fit or not
– Physical symptoms, primarily fatigue
– Whether an anterior or posterior resection was performed

If **adjuvant radio-chemotherapy** is given, the resumption of work is postponed by four months. During adjuvant radiotherapy, patients are usually unfit for work. In the case of adjuvant chemotherapy, the therapy regime employed and how the patient tolerated the treatment are crucial in the decision whether or not to return to work. After 5-FU therapy, avastin or tyrosine kinase inhibitors alone, patients are often fit for work whereas oxaliplatin can considerably reduce physical fitness.

After **R1 resections or with tumour activity** there is usually unfitness for work. However, for psychological reasons, the desire to resume vocational activity should not be opposed. Gradual resumption of work can be recommended in these cases. Usually the patients very soon become aware during this "trial time" that they are no longer able to cope with the demands of work in a normal way.

Workloads to be avoided

Continuation of vocational activity is possible **after abdomino-perineal resection of the rectum with a colostomy**. However, there are a few occupational restrictions (table 11.14). The restrictions refer especially to jobs that are associated with physical strain. Many manual activities are no longer possible because of the weakened abdominal wall and the risk of hernia. On the other hand, desk jobs are still entirely feasible. Stoma patients, contrary to commonly held ideas, can also work in jobs involving frequent contact with the public or in hygiene industries.

Irrigating patients have greater opportunities for vocational re-integration because bowel evacuation is consciously controllable. There is less odour and noise and they have greater mobility than patients using pouches.

Table 11.14 - Workloads that cured rectal carcinoma patients with colostomy should avoid after an abdominal rectal resection.

- Severe physical workloads (this includes lifting, working above head height, jobs connected with severe vibrations and in which more than 5kg have to be frequently lifted)
- Unfavourable working posture (e.g., squatting or lying)
- Extreme climatic situations (e.g., working in the heat)
- Unfavourable working hours (shift and night work)
- Unfavourable working breaks (in order to be able to eat meals regularly and in peace, regular breaks of adequate length are required)
- Irregular working hours (require the opportunity to take individual breaks in the case of irregular evacuation of the bowels without interfering with colleagues' work flow)

How to return to work

In many countries assistance is available for returning to work. Gradual resumption of work is particularly recommended. The particular advantage of this arrangement is that the work load can be matched to the fitness level of the patient without financial disadvantages. Unfortunately this sensible vocational rehab measure is not possible in all countries and often only in large companies and the civil service.

Whether and how many patients with rectal carcinoma with or without a colostomy actually return to work and remain there in the long term depends on many factors. A few of the factors are the severity of the disease, the extent of therapy sequelae, and the quality of the vocational rehabilitation work.

Palliative measures

Informing the patient about disease progression: Delivering bad news

Despite the poor prognosis, there are more reasons to inform the patient than withold information. However, this does not mean the full extent of a recurrence and disease progression should be virtually forced on the patient unsparingly.

The patient has many fears associated with the disease. He does not know how to assess the situation or what awaits him. In any case, it is better if the patient receives information from the treating physician rather than through the "pulp magazines", "faith healers", "profiteers" or uncommented reports on the Internet. How to provide the information to the patient is as important as the information itself. Providing information without in the same time offering perspectives and help should be rejected.

It is important to communicate emotional support in dealing with the news at the same time. Unfortunately, some doctors discuss the essential questions of life expectancy with the patients and their relatives only when they are asked.

It makes sense to give the patient advance notice of the discussion. Ask him/her if he/she would like to involve relatives or other persons who are close to him/her. If other persons are to be involved, the patient must agree to it beforehand.

In the discussion, the seriousness and also the extent of the findings should be communicated to the patient but a time scale regarding the prognosis should never be made because diseases frequently can follow an unpredictable course. When the prognosis is poor, positive aspects should always be mentioned also (e.g., references to progress in palliative therapy, better pain control today, provision of constant medical/psychological accompaniment, etc.).

It is important to signal willingness for additional discussions, as many times as the patient needs them. It is important to listen and to ascertain what the patient has understood and what significance he/she assigns to the information content. A desire to suppress the problem temporarily or long-term can often be read from his/her behaviour. His/her feelings in this matter should be respected.

Choice of treatment modalities

Chemotherapy, possibly in combination with radiotherapy, can lead to significant prolongation of life, but, frequently unwanted side effects can considerably influence the quality of life. About 40% of patients above 70 years take more than seven medicaments daily. Comorbidity is frequent. The pros and cons of possible tumour therapies and possible alternatives must be discussed with the patient. Psychosocial factors should be included in the therapeutic considerations (tables 11.15, 11.16).

Table 11.15 - Factors to consider when making therapy decisions.

– What is the estimated biological age?
– Comorbidity?
– In what way will the patient benefit from the therapy?
– To what extent will he/she suffer from therapy-related morbidity?
– What is the social care like?
– Activities of daily life?
– Cognition?
– To what extent will his/her nearest relative assist with psychosocial care?
– Could concomitant diseases influence the efficacy and tolerability (e.g., diabetes, renal failure, cardiovascular diseases, poor nutritional status)?
– What is the patient's understanding of the disease?
– How strong is the patient's will to live?
– How strong is the patient's coping behaviour?

Table 11.16 - Principles of radiotherapy in the palliative situation.

– No additional "adjuvant" radiation of adjacent endangered areas
– Small safe distance
– High individual dose with rapid onset of effect
– Short fractionation
– Lowest possible total dose
– Pauses if any complaints

Many of the recommended chemo- and radiotherapy standards were tested in therapeutic trials in patients below 70 years. The median age of patients with rectal cancer is however in the seventh decade of life. The patient requirements for inclusion in these trials were as follows: They must be in good general condition and absence of concomitant diseases. The results obtained in these therapeutic trials can be translated only conditionally to the palliative treatment of elderly patients. The individual features of each patient must be taken into account in the therapy of recurrence (table 3.10).

The question of whether or not to have tumour therapy and if so, which therapy, should be decided on the basis of the patient's wishes, his/her functional status, psychosocial aspects, etc.

Local and regional problems and palliative therapies

Malignant stenosis (intralumina/extraluminal)

See also chapter: "Colon carcinoma".

Suture line recurrence in the rectum is usually the result of inward extension of persistent cancer in the pelvic side wall.

If surgical intervention is no longer possible in the case of intraluminal obstruction, there are alternatives to creation of a stoma for restoring stool passage (laser therapy, electro coagulation, cryosurgery, regional radiofrequency hyperthermia with and without insertion of a stent) (Hildebrand, 2004). Laser photo-ablation or stenting of obstructing rectosigmoid of rectal cancers should be considered if surgical decompression is not possible or advisable because of extensive metastatic disease or comorbidity.

Radiotherapy is the most proven palliative therapy in extraluminal involvement. Radiation therapy should be administered to patients with symptomatic metastases in the bone, brain, or presacral space. Its value is measured by its effect on tumour growth, prompt pain-relieving effect, restoration of stool passage, and arrest of bleeding and mucus discharge. Symptoms and the individual course are decisive for the dose, fractionation and radiation field. The risk of late radiation damage is of lesser importance than with primary therapy because of the limited survival time. The goal is to relieve symptoms and not to eliminate the tumour.

In individual cases, a second radiation treatment within a small space is possible. In addition, a prolonged 5-fluorouracil infusion, possibly combined with hyperthermia, can also be given simultaneously.

Table 11.17 - Symptoms indicating possible progression in the pelvis.

– Sciatica-like complaints
– Pressing and sometimes piercing and burning pain around the former anus
– Pain in the lumbar spine/sacrum
– Unilateral lymph edema

Pelvic floor recurrence

Pelvic floor recurrences are usually inoperable.

Apart from radiotherapy further chemotherapy or pelvis perfusion treatment through a percutaneous catheter can be considered. Regional chemotherapy through the internal iliac arteries can reduce the pain even if no arrest of tumour growth is demonstrable. If there is tumour occlusion of the rectum which can no longer be managed surgically, then there are other possibilities, besides cryotherapy. Construction of colostomy, brachytherapy and also insertion of a stent (Hünerbein, 2005; Hildebrandt *et al.*, 2004) should be considered.

Adequate pain therapy is important. Presacral and sacral invasion may be associated with severe and unrelenting pain. Although radiation therapy is the initial treatment of choice, management of persistent sacral pain is frustrating and difficult.

Bleeding

Patients with incurable distal rectal cancer often have persistent bleeding, and the risks and morbidity of a palliative abdomino-perineal resection may outweigh any benefits. Diathermy, cryotherapy of the rectal tumour and radiation therapy to the pelvis can control bleeding for an extended period and postpone or eliminate the need for a palliative colostomy.

Liver metastases

Icterus due to extrahepatic cholestasis or diffuse metastases must be differentiated by means of ultrasound.

In the first case, the obstruction can be bridged by ERCP using plastic or metal stents. In the case of diffuse intrahepatic metastases temporary alleviation may be possible from systemic therapy.

Solitary liver metastases should be resected surgically with potential cure. Systemic chemotherapy should be considered with **multiple non-resectable liver metastases**. Sometimes they become resectable after "down-sizing" by chemotherapy (Adam, 2001). Intra-arterial regional chemotherapy acts mainly locally but has also a systemic effect, however to a lesser extent. The response rates to regional chemotherapy are significantly higher than systemic therapy; however this is not identical to prolongation of life and certainly not with an improvement in quality of life.

Liver metastases which prove intra-operatively to be unresectable or do not respond to systemic chemotherapy can be an indication for placement of a hepatic artery port. Partial tumour remission can be achieved in a few patients with local alcohol injections or cryo-ablation. A less costly non-surgical treatment alternative that requires only very short hospitalization, if any, is high frequency-induced thermotherapy (HiTT®). It is given in combination with classical imaging techniques (ultrasound, CT or MRI).

Lung metastases

The cause of the relatively frequent lung metastases in rectal carcinoma is the special vascular supply of the tumour region. A resection of **solitary metastases** is indicated if the metastases occurred more than a year after the diagnosis of the primary tumour. The role of resection of synchronal or metachronal lung or liver metastases is currently controversial (Kobayashi *et al.*, 1999). Systemic therapy is indicated in the case of multiple non-resectable metastases in different lung lobes.

Brain metastases

Neurosurgical resection and the ablation by gamma knife or total brain radiation can be considered in the case of brain metastases depending on their number, size and location. Supportive therapies, such as corticosteroids, anticonvulsants, and anticoagulants are necessary for most patients to address the common medical complications that often accompany brain metastases.

Bone metastases

Low rectal carcinoma in particular leads to an increased incidence of bone metastases due to its vascular supply. Prophylactic orthopedic/surgical stabilization is indicated if there is an increased fracture risk. An increased fracture risk in the long bones can be anticipated with 50% destruction of the cortex and a defect size superior to 2.5 cm. There is a risk of vertebral fracture when there is destruction of the middle/central or anterior and posterior pillar of over 60% in the axial plane. Bisphosphonates are indicated if there are multiple bone metastases. They should be given parenterally if there are pain symptoms.

Systemic palliative therapies

Chemotherapy

The efficacy of chemotherapy for the relief of symptoms and improvement in quality of life makes these drugs a fundamental part of palliative care. If there is a late recurrence (later than one year after the conclusion of the previous adjuvant chemotherapy), the same therapy regime as in the adjuvant chemotherapy can be selected once more. However, 5-FU should not be given now as a bolus but as a 24-hour infusion and with the addition of leucovorin.

Other possible second line therapies include: Protracted infusion of 5-fluorouracil/folinic acid and treatment with irinotecan or oxaliplatin possibly combined with 5-fluorouracil/folinic acid over 24 hours. The length of remission is greater than after 5-FU/leucovorin alone but it also has more side effects.

Biologic therapies have become acceptable alternatives to traditional cytotoxic therapies with respect to disease control and quality of life. Clinical trials with newly introduced tyrosin kinase inhibitors (erlotinib) and antibodies involved in the epidermal growth factor receptor (EGFR) pathway and in anti-angiogenesis (cetuximab, bevacizumab) are showing promising results. They are even more effective when combined with standard chemotherapy. How long these therapies should be continued has not yet been clarified. While a few tumour centres recommend continuing chemotherapy until progression, others recommend a therapy pause when partial stable remission has been initiated.

Special features of pain therapy

See also chapter: "Pain management in cancer rehabilitation and palliation".

If the pain is associated with a presacral recurrence, primary radiotherapy can be considered. It can be combined with chemotherapy. Even low doses are adequate for pain relief. Fractionation is not indicated.

Orthopedic stabilization may be warranted for impending pathologic fractures. Anticholinergics are preferable for gastro-intestinal spasm and corticoids are useful for pain caused by nerve compression. Non-steroidal anti-inflammatory drugs are often more effective for bone pain than opioids.

There should not be hesitation to use centrally-acting analgesics when there are recurrences in the pelvis. Steroids and antidepressants have added benefits. Stepwise increments of opioids without an upper limit are given by the clock, not as needed, until pain is controlled. At the same time, a supplement of morphine is provided for breakthrough pain. Note non-steroidal analgesics will soon be ineffective and morphine preparations have fewer side effects in the long run. In several studies it has been shown that the physical and mental fitness of patients with tumour-related pain tends to increase with opioids. Note that opioids inhibit gastro-intestinal motility and cause constipation; such impaction can be more troublesome to the patients than cancer pain.

A requirement for successful therapy with morphine preparations is using a controlled-release formula. Long-acting morphines should be preferred. The advantages of using transdermal application are potential fewer side effects. Pain peaks can be covered with short-acting morphine preparations (e.g., Sevredol®, Temgesic sublingual® or Actiq®). The patches only have to be changed every 48 to 72 hours.

Complementary and alternative therapies

Numerous therapy forms are offered by various industries to which are ascribed the qualities of improving unspecific immune functions and activating the body's own immune defenses against the tumour (**immunostimulants or immune modulators**). Examples of such substances are mistletoe extract, enzyme and thymus preparations, snake venom, oxygen multistep therapy, phototherapy, symbiosis control, microbiological therapy, vitamins, among many others. All these therapy options are based on widely speculative assumptions, do not appear very plausible from a theoretical standpoint and are not recognized by standard medicine. Their therapeutic effects on tumours are at best only minimal.

So far there has been no scientific study that might have proven the tumour-inhibiting effects of mistletoe preparations. The assertion that the patient's quality of life can be improved through its use is very difficult to confirm. Yet these mistletoe preparations are not only used by those practicing alternative and nature-oriented forms of medicine, but also by some oncologists. The reason for this is less the belief in its effectiveness, than the possibility to offer the patient a further therapy option.

Experience has shown not only that "faith can move mountains", but that it can also improve the quality of life. One should not shatter these patients' faith in a particular therapy form with evidence-based arguments.

Quality assurance of rehabilitation and palliative measures
Quality of structural features

Therapies needed in rehabilitation and palliation should be provided by specialized rehabilitation services with a team of patient care specialists. Colorectal rehabilitation services include critical components of assessment, physical reconditioning, skill training, and psychosocial support. They may include vocational evaluation and counselling.

Special experience and a specialised infrastructure are essential.

Quality of medical and therapeutic processes

To study the quality of life of rectal cancer patients, most centres use the EORTC questionnaire (QLQ-C30 and its colorectal module QLQ-CR 38).

The therapies needed in rehabilitation and palliation are provided by the physician and an entire team of patient care specialists. They should be coordinated by a physician experienced in rehabilitation and palliation with demonstrable oncological knowledge. A stoma therapist and a nutritional adviser must be integrated in the team (fig. 1.4) if patients with a colostomy are to be rehabilitated. The collaboration of psycho-oncologists is useful particularly in the care of stoma patients. Social workers are essential because of the social aids that are often needed (Delbrück, 1998; Bundesarbeitsgemeinschaft für Rehabilitation, 2002). Cooperation and exchanging information with the previously and subsequently treating physicians are important.

Outcome assessment and evaluation

There are objective and subjective parameters for examining outcome quality of the rehabilitation measures. Some of them are listed in table 11.19. Patient satisfaction – as measured by the patient him-/herself – can be evaluated most readily by questionnaires.

Different outcome scales in palliative care of cancer patients have been developed (Aspinal et al., 2002; Bausewein et al., 2005). The scales cover physical and psychological symptoms, spiritual considerations, practical concerns, emotional concerns of the patient and family, and psychosocial needs of the patient and family. The Palliative Care Outcome Scale (POS) is a multidimensional instrument covering these physical, psychosocial, spiritual, organizational, and practical concerns.

Measurements of quality of life

Verifiability of the quality of rehabilitation and palliative therapies must be guaranteed.

Studies of quality of life in colorectal cancer patients have been performed mainly in therapeutic trials in order to assess the disease and treatment of specific symptoms. The studies mainly used performance status as a proxy regarding quality of life, even though there is only a weak association between the performance status such as the Karnofsky Performance Scale (table 3.4) and the quality of life as measured by the EORTC QLQ-C30. Palliation of symptoms, psychosocial interventions, and understanding patient's feelings and concerns all contribute to improving quality of life in cancer patients.

The most widely used tools to measure quality of life include the European Organization for Research and Treatment of Cancer Quality of Life. Questionnaire (EORTC QLQ –C30) (Aaronson *et al.*, 1993) and the US equivalent, the functional assessment of cancer therapy (FACT) questionnaire. These tools are self-reporting questionnaires designed for the patients.

Basically, improvement in quality of life is attained when there is less nursing care ("rehabilitation to combat the need of care"), when the patient can be vocationally reintegrated ("rehabilitation to combat early retirement"), when he/she feels secure ("rehabilitation to combat resignation and depression") and when the patient's physical handicaps and functional limitations are at a minimum ("rehabilitation to combat disability") (table 11.18).

Table 11.18 - Criteria for a successful rehabilitation.

– There is less need for nursing care (rehabilitation to prevent care).
– The patient can be reintegrated vocationally (rehabilitation to prevent early retirement).
– The patient is psychologically stabilised (rehabilitation to prevent withdrawal and depression).
– Physical complaints are slight (rehabilitation to prevent immobilisation).
– The patient masters stoma care.
– The patient leads a satisfactory life with his disabilities.

Table 11.19 - Possible goals of therapy and parameters of their effectiveness in the rehabilitation of rectal carcinoma patients.

Therapy goal	Parameters of effectiveness
Reduction of disorders resulting from surgery/chemotherapy/radiation therapy	WHO toxicity scale, CTC classification, EORTC-C30, EORTC-CR 38, FLIC, SIRO, assessment of organ function, neurological examination including sensory, motor and autonomous system
Optimization of stoma care, training in stoma use, prevention and hernia management	Number of pouches, learning irrigation objective and subjective criteria
Improvement of nutritional status	Weighing, determination of total protein and albumin concentration, biometric impedance analysis. Questionnaires: FACT-CT, MNA,

Reduction of faecal incontinence, compensation for incontinence	Stool frequency, patient diary, manometry, digital sphincter measurement
Reduction of urogenital symptoms	Number of pads, patient diary, length of micturition intervals, ultrasound measurements of residual urine, urine status, urodynamometry
Alleviation of diarrhea/constipation	Stool frequency, patient diary, questionnaires
Improvement of physical fitness, activities of daily living	Ergometry, Karnofsky index, WHO and EORTC performance status, walking distances, muscle force (hand-held dynamometry), exercise capacity (symptom-limited dynamometry), vigorimeter. Questionnaires: (EORTC) QLQ-C30, FACT-Ct, FACT-G, FACT-An, SIP, SF-36, Nottingham health profile
Family member counselling	Questionnaires
Information on illness, cancer therapies and follow-up, signs of recurrence, factors influencing prognosis, etc.	Questionnaires, tests
Reduction of anxiety, depression, fatigue	Rating scales. Questionnaires: DPS, POMS, STAI, BDI, BSI, HADS-D, PAF, MFI
Coping with illness	Questionnaires: FKV, FKV-LIS, BEFO, TSK, FIBECK
Clarification and improvement of vocational fitness, return to work	Resumption of work, length of time of inability to work
Reduction of necessity of nursing care	Questionnaires: Barthel Index, FIM, ADL, IADL, AADL
Sexuality/potency	Diary. Questionnaires: QLQ-PR2, IIEF
Pain relief	Pain diary, reduction of analgesic drugs, pain sensitivity scales. Questionnaires: PDI, EORTC QLQ- C30, SE36, SDS, RSCL
Improvement in feelings of self-worth	ISKN (self-concept scales). Questionnaires: HDS-D.
Relief of physical and psychological symptoms	Questionnaire: POS

Abbrévations meaning

ADL = Activities of Daily Life; DPS = Geriatric Depression Scale; ECOG = European Cooperative Oncology Group-Scale;; EORTC-QLQ = European Organization for Research and Treatment of Cancer: Quality of Life Questionnaire; PDI = Pain Disability Index; Fact-G = Functional assessment of cancer therapy: General; Fact-An = Functional assessment of cancer therapy: Anaemia; Fact-F = Functional assessment of cancer therapy: Fatigue; Fact-Ct = Functional assessment of anorexia and cachexia; Fact-P = Functional assessment of cancer therapy: Prostate; FIM = Functional Independence Measure; FLI-C = Functional Living Index-Cancer; IIEF = International Index of Erectile Function; MFI = Multidimensional Fatigue Inventory; POS = Palliative Care Oncology Outcome Scale; RSCL = Rotterdam Symptom Check List; STAI = Spiegelberger Trait Anxiety Inventory; SIRO = Stress Index Radio Oncology; FIM = Functional Independence Measure; FIBECK = Freiburger Inventar zur Bewältigung einer chronischen Erkrankung; HADS-D = Hospital anxiety and depression scale

Bibliography

- Adam R, Avisar E, Ariche A *et al.* (2001) Five-year survival following hepatic resection after neoadjuvant therapy for non-resectable colorectal hepatic metastases. Ann Surg Oncol 8: 347-53
- Anderson DW (2003) Using hyperbaric oxygen therapy to heal radiation wounds. Nursing. 33(9): 50-3
- Aspinal F, Hughes R, Higginson I *et al.* (2002) A user's guide to the palliative care outcome scale. Palliative care & policy publications. Kings College, London
- Bausewein C, Fegg M, Radbruch L *et al.* (2005) Validation and clinical application of the German version of the palliative care outcome. J Pain Symptom Manage 30: 51-62
- Black PK (2004) Psychological, sexual and cultural issues for patients with a stoma. Br J Nurs 7, 13: 692-7
- Bonthuis D, Landheer ML, Spillenaar B *et al.* (2004) Small but significant survival benefit in patients who undergo routine follow-up after colorectal cancer surgery. Eur J Surg Oncol 30, 10: 1093-7
- Bundesarbeitsgemeinschaft für Rehabilitation (2003) Rahmenempfehlungen zur ambulanten onkologischen Rehabilitation. Schriftenreihe der Bundesarbeitsgemeinschaft für Rehabilitation BAR, Frankfurt
- Burdeos MG, Botella MG, Pascual VV *et al.* (2004) Postoperative radiotherapy-induced morbidity in rectal cancer. Rev Esp Enferm Dig 96, 11: 765-72
- Daniels I, Woodward S, Taylor F *et al.* (2006) Female urogenital dysfunction following total mesorectal excision for rectal cancer. World J Surg Oncol 4: 6
- Delbrück H (1998) Rehabilitationsmedizin. Urban & Schwarzenberg München
- Delbrück H, Witte M (2005) Onkologische Nachsorge und Rehabilitation in Ländern der europäischen Gemeinschaft (in press)
- Doughty D (2005) Principles of ostomy management in the oncology patient. J Support Oncol 3: 59-69
- Fulham J (2004) Improving the nutritional status of colorectal surgical and stoma patients. Br J Nurs 7, 13 (12): 702-8
- Hildebrand B, Wust P, Gellermann J *et al.* (2004) 27, 5: 506-11
- Höfler H (1999) Beckenbodengymnastik für sie und ihn. BLV Verlagsgesellschaft mbH, München
- Hünerbein M, Krause M, Moesta KT *et al.* (2005) Palliation of malignant rectal obstruction with self-expanding metal stents. Surgery 137: 42-7
- Kobayashi K, Kawamura M, Ishiara T (1999) Surgical treatment for both pulmonary and hepatic metastases from colorectal cancer. J Thorac Cardiovasc Surg 118: 1090-6
- Lyons A (2001) Ileostomy and colostomy support groups. The Mount Sinai J Med 68, 2: 11-113
- Nesbakken A, Nygaard K, Bull-Nija T *et al.* (2000) Bladder and sexual dysfunction after mesorectal excision for rectal cancer. Br J Surg 87, 2: 206-10
- Norton C, Chelvanayagam S, Wilson J *et al.* (2003) Randomized controlled trial of biofeedback for faecal incontinence. Gastroenterology 125: 1320-9
- Persson E, Gustaffson B, Hellstrom AL *et al.* (2005) Ostomy patients' perceptions of quality of care. Adv Nurs 49, 1: 51-8

– Rauch P, Miny I, Connoy T *et al.* (2004) Quality of life among disease-free survivors of rectal cancer. J Clin Oncol 22: 354-60
– Reis E, Vine A, Heimann T (2002) Radiation damage to the rectum and anus: Pathophysiology, clinical features and surgical complications. Colorectal Dis 4: 2-12
– Schmidt CE, Bestmann B, Kuchler T *et al.* (2005) Impact of age on quality of life in patients with rectal cancer. World J Surg
– Schmidt C, Bestmann B, Küchler T *et al.* (2005) Prospective evaluation of quality of life of patients receiving either abdominoperineal resection or sphincter-preserving procedure for rectal cancer. 12: 117-23
– Schover L (2005) Sexuality and Fertility after Cancer. American society of haematology 523-6

Rehabilitation and palliation of patients with bronchial cancer

Aims of rehabilitation and palliation: Significance and definition as distinct from curative tumour follow-up care

The aims of after-care in the follow-up are to lengthen survival time and to improve quality of life as well (fig. 1.1). Recurrence prevention, early detection of recurrences and therapy of disease recurrence (potentially curative follow-up measures) serve to lengthen survival time (fig. 1.3). Supportive, rehabilitative and palliative measures serve to improve quality of life and activities of daily living (fig. 1.2).

The fact that disease recurrence may not be eliminated even when it has – by means of routine diagnostics – been detected at an asymptomatic stage or very early on, calls the value of routine follow-up diagnostics into question. The value of prophylactic forms of therapy (adjuvant chemotherapy and radiation therapy) is controversial, and therapy of disease recurrence has only –if any at all– marginal effects in survival time.

As long as potentially curative measures (recurrence prevention, early detection and therapy of recurrence) have failed to show a significant survival benefit, rehabilitative and palliative measures in the follow-up care of bronchial carcinoma patients will remain the main focus (table 1.4, 1.5). Since more than 80% of lung cancer patients with recurrences die within a year, the issue of quality of life in this group of patients is paramount. The need of palliation is the first priority.

With rehabilitation and palliation it is not the influencing of the illness, but rather the reduction of disabilities due to the tumour and therapy and improvement of quality of life which constitute the aims of therapeutic procedures (table 1.4). It is the intention to alleviate the negative effects of the cancer disease and therapy, not only physically but also psychologically, socially, and vocationally. It is not influencing the illness, but rather the improvement of activities in daily life for the rest of life which constitute the aims of rehabilitative and palliative procedures.

In theory, the aims of curative follow-up care can be differentiated simply and clearly from those of rehabilitation and palliation. In practice, however, there is much overlapping. This involves in particular tumour recurrence therapy and palliative measures. Here we find a lot of common ground for both rehabilitative/palliative steps along with potential curative treatments. Potentially curative recurrence therapy does not only serve to prolong survival time, but also to alleviate symptoms

Rehabilitative measures in follow-up care

Rehabilitative measures can be considered for patients undergoing potentially curative as well as palliative treatment (tables 1.12, 1.13).

A certain minimum amount of information (table 12.1) on disease status is required before initiating rehabilitative measures (tables 1.6, 1.7, 1.8). Without it is difficult to carry out rehabilitation. Before carrying out rehabilitative measures, a rehabilitative assessment has to be conducted, including rehabilitation planning and documentation of the goals to be achieved (Barat and Franchignoni, 2004).

Table 12.1 - Minimum information required before initiating rehabilitative measures.

– Extent of tumour (e.g., pTNM?)
– Curative or palliative therapy approach? (e.g., R0, R1 or R2 resection of the tumour?)
– Localisation of the tumour (e.g., mediastinal, peripheral, systemic metastases?)
– Which therapeutic procedure has been used? (e.g., surgery, radiotherapy, chemotherapy or no treatment at all, e.g., wait-and-see policy?)
– Which surgical procedure has been used? (e.g., pneumonectomy or resection?)
– Which chemo- or radiotherapies have been performed? What dosages were prescribed and what were the results?
– Psychosocial information about the family structure is essential and helpful, particularly with social and occupational problems (statements given pertaining to degree of patient information, about any problems with coping or compliance, amount of support given by family members, etc.)

Rehabilitative measures aimed at reducing physical problems ("rehabilitation to combat disability")

The physical disabilities associated with lung cancer and its treatment include respiratory insufficiency, shoulder pain and stiffness, scoliosis, the remote effects of certain lung cancers that cause a neuromuscular disorder that becomes manifest as weakness and incoordination.

Physical impairments are often present against a background of comorbidities and polypharmacy in older patients.

Comorbidity, side effects of chemo- and radiotherapy, the age and compliance of the patient, and the prognosis influence the nature and scope of rehabilitative measures (table 1.12). Complications of cytotoxic chemo- and radiotherapy are more common in older patients than in younger ones and the occurrence of myelosuppression, mucositis, cardiodepression, peripheral neuropathy, and the central neurotoxicity can influence and complicate the rehabilitation process. COPD, overweight, and chronic coronary artery disease are independent predictors of postpneumonectomy complications.

Nature and scope of rehabilitative measures depend, among other factors, on whether an exclusive operation, only radiotherapy with or without adjuvant therapy have been carried out. Depending on radiotherapy and/or chemotherapy, segmental resection, lobectomy or pneumonectomy with or without bronchoplastic interventions, rehabilitative measures differ from case to case.

Reduced respiratory capacity

Pulmonary function studies to assess the capacity of the remaining parenchyma (spirometry, arterial blood gases, diffusion/capacity and, if necessary, ventilation-perfusion scans) are necessary to estimate the proportions of functioning pulmonary tissue.

As a rule, 25%-30% of previously functioning pulmonary tissue get lost after lobectomy and bilobectomy; after pneumonectomy – depending on left – or right – between 40% and 60% get lost. Lobectomy is very well tolerated and is associated with only minor deterioration of lung function and exercise capacity. Pneumonectomy causes a decrease in pulmonary volumes to about 75% of the preoperative values, but this loss of volume is partly compensated by better oxygen uptake, which postoperatively was about 85% of the preoperative values.

Most patients had already a history of lung restrictions such as emphysema, chronic obstructive pulmonary disease or chronic bronchitis. A worsening of these restrictions has to be prevented, including assistance for cessation of smoking.

The best and most frequently used indicators for postoperative lung function are the FEV1 predicted, postoperative diffusion capacity of the lung for carbon monoxide, and maximal oxygen uptake during exercise.

Reduced respiratory capacity after pneumonectomy, especially when combined with pre-existing chronic obstructive pulmonary disease (COPD), may result in respiratory complications and insufficiency during both the postoperative period and the long-term follow-up.

Oxygen should be prescribed with as much care as any other drug. Its misuse is potentially harmful. The principal goal of long-term domiciliary oxygen therapy in obstructive airway disease is to prevent the development or progression of right heart failure as a consequence of pulmonary hypertension. Cognitive function and exercise tolerance may also be improved.

Respiratory physical therapies

Pulmonary rehabilitation is mainly based on exercise training and physical therapies. Respiratory physical therapy is one of the most important rehabilitative measures in the case of reduced respiratory capacity (Donner, 2006; Edel and Knauth, 1999). Physical therapy is directed towards relaxation, improving the breathing technique, drainage of secretions, and bodily conditioning. Correction of posture, mobilization of joints and strengthening of respiratory muscles may all be required. Exercises based on activities of daily living may be more meaningful to the patient than abstract gymnastics, and therefore more likely to encourage his co operation. Some exercises contribute to the patient's relaxation and others to a coordinated and effective breathing. Patients should be given written information about breathing exercises from the physiotherapist and should be encouraged to continue the exercises at home.

Respiratory therapies affect both breathing technique and the breathing process, in turn helping to relieve pain. Thoracotomised patients tend to fear pain and become tense, which increases resistance in the respiratory tract. Thanks to breathing exercises and relaxation techniques the breathing rate lowers, the respiratory volume increases, and a more natural, efficient and effective breathing pattern becomes possible. Anxiety, tension and pain decrease.

The effective use of abdominal muscles and diaphragm may need to be relearned.

Training in the techniques of chest percussion, postural drainage, assisted coughing, and proper use of nebulizers and ventilatory equipment is often needed. Without proper training, the medication delivered by hand-held nebulizers is too often deposited uselessly on the tongue.

Breathing exercises should be used with the goals of modifying the breathing pattern, strengthening respiratory muscles, improving the cough mechanism and coordinating the breathing pattern. The preferred breathing technique may vary, depending on whether the pulmonary problem is obstructive or restrictive. Slow, relaxed breathing, with use of diaphragm in preference to accessory muscles in the neck is usually most efficient.

An effective method for releasing sputum from bronchi involves an assistant, who places his hands on the chest of the patient with sputum retention and applies pressure toward the tracheal bifurcation along the direction of the movements of the ribs during expiration.

Pursed lip breathing is often recommended when the obstructive component dominates. Pursed lip and diaphragmatic breathing decrease the respiratory rate.

Glossopharyngeal breathing ("frog breathing") may be of value in the presence of restrictive ventilatory deficit when the problem is muscular weakness.

Air shifting techniques should be taught. The air, thus, shifts to less ventilated areas of the lung and may help to prevent microatelectasis.

Drainage of secretions may be enhanced by humidification, improving the cough by postural drainage and percusssion.

An effective method for stopping the vicious cycle of respiratory panic attacks is constituted by the extracorporal assisted ventilation. It is a method of supporting sufficient expiration using compression of the lower part of the chest in time of expiration.

Relaxation exercises such as Jacobson exercises and biofeedback may be used to decrease tension and anxiety.

Radiation pneumonitis

Moderate to severe radiation pneumonitis occurs in an estimated 2-9% of patients treated for lung cancer with combination chemotherapy and irradiation. Classically, radiation pneumonitis manifests from two weeks to six months after completion of radiation therapy (Robnett et al., 2000; Abid, 2001).

The treatment which includes the mediastinum or hilum and the adjoining lung carries the highest risk of radiation injury. Mediastinal displacement of the remaining lung towards the surgical side (with inclusion of lung parenchyma within the "mediastinal" radiation portals) often results in a radiation pneumonitis. Additional treatment with chemotherapy can enhance the incidence of pneumonitis. Underlying pulmonary disease has been shown to modify the radiation effect. Baseline impairment of pulmonary function will add to radiation damage and cause symptoms with smaller radiation doses than in patients with normal function. While radiation pneumonitis is often thought to affect only the lung within the zone of irradiation, pathologic changes outside the zone of irradiation, including the contralateral lung, may happen (Arbeiter, 1999).

There are various classifications from grade I to grade IV according to the gravity of pneumonitis, which are based on clinical symptoms and radiologic criteria (Seegenschmidt, 1998).

When symptoms occur, dyspnea is the most common complaint. Usually, the patient has a non-productive cough and fever, which can range from low grade to high and spiking. On physical examinations, signs of pulmonary involvement are minimal. Occasionally, moist rales, a pleural friction rub, or evidence of pleural fluid may be heard over the area of irradiation. The most common laboratory findings are a polymorphonuclear leukocytosis and an increased erythrocyte sedimentation rate (table 12.2).

Table 12.2 - Symptoms and biological signs of radiation pneumonitis.

- Dyspnea
- Non-productive cough or a cough productive of small amounts of pinkish sputum
- Tachypnea
- Slight cough
- Low grade fever
- Fullness in the chest
- Elevated erythrocyte sedimentation rate
- Polymorphonuclear leukocytosis

Radiological changes are often discovered in asymptomatic patients. In most cases, radiological findings are confined to the radiation field. Usually, the first radiological change is a diffuse haze in the treatment zone which progresses to patchy alveolar infiltrates and air bronchograms. Air bronchograms are commonly present and volume loss of the affected portion of the lung may be observed. There is usually a sharp boundary crossing the normal anatomic structures without segmental or lobar distribution. Rarely an entire lung or both lungs are involved.

Radiological findings and symptoms can be difficult to distinguish from a number of illnesses that commonly occur in patients with lung cancer on therapy. Differentiating radiation pneumonitis from recurrent cancer is important. False positives include recurrent disease, drug-associated pneumonitis, infection/pneumonia and other inflammatory diseases, cardiac disease, fluid overload, chronic obstructive pulmonary disease and lymphangitic carcinomatosis. CT is useful in detecting recurrent tumour in an irradiated area. Nuclear medicine ventilation/perfusion scans are frequently abnormal following radiation treatment of lung cancer. Perfusion defects are more common than ventilation defects.

In **asymptomatic pneumonitis** (grade I) treatment is not necessary. Corticosteroids given prophylactically fail to prevent symptomatic pneumonitis. In **symptomatic pneumonitis** (grade II) bronchodilators and corticoid therapy may provide symptomatic relief. In **severe pneumonitis** (grade III-IV) bed rest, oxygen therapy and even respirators assistance may be necessary.

Most authors report improvement of symptoms with corticosteroids; others have noted exacerbation of pneumonitis under abrupt steroid withdrawal (Petzner, 1984). Prednisone is used most frequently at doses of 60-100mg/day. The initial dosage of corticoids should be continued until fever, dyspnea and cyanosis are completely eliminated and the chest radiograph returns to normal. To avoid recurrence, corticosteroids should be gradually tapered at the rate of 5-10% of the initial dose every two-four weeks, depending on symptoms. Inhaled steroids may minimize systemic side effects of corticoids; however, relatively high doses of inhaled steroids are needed to maintain control of symptoms. Other agents that have been used for treatment of radiation pneumonitis include azathioprine and cyclosporin A. Azathioprine may be a well-tolerated option in patients with radiation pneumonitis and concomitant corticosteroid toxicity.

In severe pneumonitis there is a high risk of right heart failure.

Drug-associated pneumonitis and interstitial lung disease

With the concomitant use of irradiation and chemotherapy, distinguishing the effects of the irradiation versus the effects of the cytotoxic agents is difficult. The chemotherapy-induced lung damage is diffuse, rather than nodular. About 10% of patients receiving chemotherapy develop pulmonary toxicity. Non-specific interstitial pneumonitis and interstitial lung fibrosis are very frequent. Depending on the antineoplastic agent the damage can happen immediately, later in the course of the treatment and even several weeks after the end of the therapy. Non-specific interstitial pneumonia is one of the most common forms of drug-associated pneumonitis.

In cancer patients, drug-associated interstitial lung disease (ILD) is most commonly observed during mitomycin, paclitaxel, docetaxel or gemcitabine therapy. The diagnosis depends upon a history of drug exposure, and, most importantly, the exclusion of other causes leading to lung damage, including progression of the cancer, radiation-related lung injury, congestive heart failure, infections, fluid overload, pulmonary edema, pulmonary embolism. Infiltrative lung disease is the most common form of antineoplastic agent-induced respiratory disease. Entities include non-specific interstitial lung fibrosis, bronchiolitis, acute respiratory distress syndrome, also termed diffuse alveolar damage, and alveolar hemorrhage (Akira, 2002; Limper, 2004).

There are no firm guidelines for the treatment of drug-associated interstitial lung disease, and therapy tends to be on an empirical basis. Withdrawal of the drug suspected is the first step in treatment. For patients with respiratory failure, high-dose methylprednisolone (250mg four times a day i.v.) for several days is commonly used. Immunosuppressive agents such as azathioprine have been used as steroid-sparing agents in the treatment of drug-associated ILD, particularly in chronic cases of bleomycin-associated ILD.

Pulmonary fibrosis and recommendations for treatment

Radiation fibrosis is presumed to be the end result of radiation pneumonitis, occurring approximately one year after completion of radiation treatment. Usually, the fibrosis is mild and asymptomatic. Radiation pneumonitis is often reversible with corticosteroid therapy, whereas fibrosis is usually irreversible. Established fibrosis will not improve with corticosteroid therapy.

Pulmonary fibrosis may develop following successful chemotherapy for malignancy, even if such therapy is not combined with radiotherapy. Bleomycin, which is known to induce acute pneumonitis and lung fibrosis, is especially associated with chemotherapy-induced pulmonary fibrosis that can occur more than five years after such therapy (Sleijfer, 2001). Additionally, supplemented oxygen therapy can trigger the onset of pneumonitis and lethal pulmonary fibrosis in patients who have previously received bleomycin therapy. Careful assessment of lung function via spiro-ergometry and arterial blood gas analysis during exercise are required if the administration of supplemental oxygen is considered.

Cardiovascular complications and recommendations for prevention and therapy

The most common complications after **resectional surgery** are not technical failures of the operation but cardiopulmonary problems. Cardiovascular and/or pulmonary complications occur in almost half of all patients who underwent pneumonectomy (Licker *et al.*, 2002). Cardiac morbidity is higher in elderly patients. Cardiovascular complications of pneumonectomy seen in the rehabilitation phase include arrhytmias, myocardial infarctions, acute heart failure, pulmonary emboli, and strokes.

Improved preoperative assessment of cardiac risk and postoperative care to identify high-risk patients may decrease cardiovascular complications.

The presence of chronic respiratory symptoms and lung function abnormality in pneumectomised patients may be due to a variety of other factors, including the presence of comorbid diseases such as heart disease, in addition to underlying chronic lung disease.

As a rule there is a **relative tachycardia** which is a compensation for the lost gas exchange tissue that has been resected. Heart rates up to 120 per minute are still tolerable and do not need any treatment. Pneumectomised patients with a tachycardia above 110/min should be treated with beta blockers to slow down the heart rate.

Relative tachycardia must be distinguished from tachycardia due to pneumonitis after radio- and/or chemotherapy.

Arrhythmias after pneumonectomy are common complications. Right pneumonectomy versus left pneumonectomy is identified as a strong predisposing factor for the establishment of postpneumonectomy cardiac rhythm disturbances (Algar et al., 2003). Cardiac tachydysrhythmias occur in 20-25% of patients undergoing pneumonectomy. Atrial fibrillation is the most common dysrhythmia, followed by supraventricular tachycardia and atrial flutter. An increased incidence of tachydysrhythmia is noted in patients undergoing intrapericardial dissections and those who developed postoperative interstitial or perihilar pulmonary edema. Tachydysrhythmias after pneumonectomy are associated with significant mortality.

Adjuvant/additive radio- and/or chemotherapy are additional risk factors.

The extent of cardiac damage of **mediastinal irradiation** is related to the radiotherapy dose, volume and treatment technique. Patients with high blood pressure have a particular risk. Today, modern techniques (i.e., three-dimensional conformal tangential irradiation) have significantly reduced the incidence of radiation-induced heart disease. Pericarditis and pericardial effusion that were considered the most common side effects of cardiac irradiation are now infrequent. Radiation-induced coronary artery disease is the most concerning long-term cardiac side effect.

Accounts of radiation-associated pacemaker failure, regional heart perfusion changes, myocardial infarction, and coronary artery spasm with cardiac arrest have been reported (Ampil and Caldito, 2006).

The most frequent symptoms of acute pericarditis are fever, tachycardia, substernal pain and dyspnea. Pericarditis is accompanied by an asymptomatic effusion in 40% of cases. A fibrosis of the myocard with or without cardial insufficiency may happen. Pericarditis can occur up to two years, coronary artery disease up to fifteen years after radiotherapy.

Cardiotoxicity is a dose-limiting toxicity occurring with several **cytotoxic drugs** that may cause severe morbidity in long-term surviving cancer patients. Cardiotoxicity induced by anthracyclines has been extensively studied. Important risk factors associated with cardiotoxicity are cumulative doses, infusion schedule, and high blood pressure (Chanan et al., 2004).

Anthracyclines induce an acute/subacute toxicity and a chronic progressive cardiotoxicity. Acute cardiotoxicity occurs within a week of the administration, is usually transient and characterized by transient electrocardiographic abnormalities in 20-30% of patients and arrhythmias in 0.5-3% of patients. Subacute cardiotoxicity has resulted in acute left ventricular failure, pericarditis or a fatal pericarditis-myocarditis syndrome in some rare cases. Chronic progressive cardiomyopathy, clinically the most significant subtype of cardiotoxicity, can have an early onset within a year of treatment or progress slowly to become manifest only years to decades after chemotherapy completion. It is characterized by a decrease of left ventricular function, changes in exercise-stress capacity and overt signs of congestive heart failure.

The most important prognostic factor for chronic cardiotoxicity is cumulative dose of anthracyclines. The probability of doxorubicin-induced cardiotoxicity is estimated at 3% or less with a cumulative dose of 400mg/m^2, 7% with 550mg/m^2 and 18% with 700mg/m^2.

Many strategies have been adopted to counteract anthracycline-induced cardiotoxicity: Limiting the cumulative dose, using less cardiotoxic anthracycline analogs such as epirubicin and employing liposomal anthracyclines. Liposomal doxorubicin (Myocet®) or pegylated liposomal doxorubicin (Caelyx®) have shown similar efficacy and less cardiotoxicity than doxorubicin (table 12.3).

Table 12.3 - Measures to reduce cardiotoxic risks of chemotherapy.

– Respect the cumulative dose. (With epirubicin cardiotoxicity occurs at a higher cumulative dose; (more than 900mg/m^2, compared to 550mg/m^2 with conventional doxorubicin.)
– Prolong the time of administration. (A prolonged continuous intravenous infusion over more than 48-96 hours is less cardiotoxic.)
– Patients submitted to anthracyclines should be monitored.
– High-risk patients (e.g., high blood pressure, pre-existing cardiac disease, advanced age) should get liposomal anthracyclines such as liposomal doxorubicin (Myocet®) or pegylated liposomal doxorubicin (Caelyx®).

Patients treated with anthracyclines should be monitored to identify subclinical myocardial dysfunction that could be present for many months or years before its overt manifestation. Serial measurements of left ventricular ejection fraction (LVEF) evaluated by means of echocardiography or scan have been recommended by some consensus guidelines even if early cardiomyopathic changes may not be detected by echography and may not be specific in assessing left ventricular afterload.

Loss of weight which is not induced by tumour and advice for prevention

For a more in-depth description see chapter: "Rehabilitation and palliation of patients with pancreatic cancer".

Many bronchial cancer patients experience weight loss. Apart from cancer activity, non-tumour related weight loss has to be considered (table 12.4). Fatigue, anxiety, depression as well as resulting therapy problems can all contribute, in addition to tumour progression, to loss of appetite and weight.

While corticosteroids (e.g., prednisolone 10-30 mg/die or dexamethasone 2-4 mg a day) have a short-term appetite-stimulating effect of two to four weeks as well as a reconstituting effect, and after this time typical side effects become predominant, the weight-increasing effect of megestrol acetate (160 to 480mg a day) lasts significantly longer (Mateen and Jatoi, 2006).

Appetite can be influenced with psychopharmacological drugs, especially tricyclic antidepressants.

Table 12.4 - Most common causes of non-tumour related weight loss in patients with bronchial ꞏꞏꞏꞏꞏꞏ

– Decrased food intake due to pain (e.g., due to radio-chemotherapy-induced mucositis, esophagitis, gastritis), and to vomiting.
– Loss of energy-rich body substance through fistula secretion.
– Increased energy demand due to cytokine therapy (e.g., tumour necrosis factor).
– No synchronization of deglutition due to wrong coordination of different muscles and displacement of esophagus and stomach towards the operated side.
– Lack of appetite due to psychologic reasons (e.g., fatigue, anxiety, depression).

The food industry produces high-caloric, protein-enriched drinks in the form of flavoured liquid nutrition (astronaut food) which can either be taken between or in addition to meals. Drinks containing 1kcal/mL are tolerated best. These can lead to noticeable weight gain. Unfortunately, many patients report that they do not tolerate this "astronaut food". There are many reasons for this (for more details see chapter: "Pancreatic cancer" and table 9.8).

Oesophagitis, mucositis and recommendations for prevention and treatment

Radiotherapy and chemotherapy can be associated with oral mucositis which can impact severely on quality of life. Risk factors are bad mouth hygiene, plaques, paradontosis, diabetes. Combined radio-chemotherapy worsens the risks.

Treatment of established mucositis remains a challenge and focuses on a palliative management approach (table 12.5). Topical anesthetics, mixtures (also called cocktails), and mucosal coating agents have been used despite the lack of experimental evidence supporting their efficacy. Agents which are under study are targeting the specific mechanisms of mucosal injury. While chlorhexidine is commonly recommended and used, its effectiveness remains uncertain and has yet to be shown to be more effective than water. Sucralfate has been the subject of many studies, however its effectiveness has yet to be shown. There is no evidence to support the use of beta-carotene or vitamin E. Prostaglandin E may well exacerbate mucositis.

Table 12.5 - Advices to prevent radio- chemotherapy-induced mucositis and esophagitis.

– Clean teeth and gums after meals and before sleep with tooth brush or swab as tolerated.
– Rinse the mouth with water regularly.
– If dentures are worn, remove and clean them daily and leave out while at rest.
– Avoid painful stimuli such as hot food and drinks, spicy food, alcohol and smoking.
– Regular inspection of mouth by the patient and health professionals.
– Report any redness, tenderness or sores on the lips or in the mouth.
– Provide comfort measures such as lubrication of the lips, topical anaesthesia and analgesics.
– Prompt treatment of mucositis symptoms and oral infections.
– Stop smoking.

Nutrition deficiencies and general dietary recommendations

Cancer survivors often receive dietary advice from family, friends, and health care providers, as well as from the media, health food stores, and the nutritional supplement industry. Magazine articles, books, Internet, family, and friends present cancer survivors with a wide range of options and choices about what to eat and what types of supplements or herbal remedies might improve the outcome of standard cancer therapy. The value of this information is at best minimal.

For many recommendations of the most important nutrition questions faced by cancer survivors, the scientific evidence comes only from *in vitro* and laboratory animal data or anecdotal reports from poorly designed clinical studies. Moreover, the findings from these studies are often contradictory. Very few controlled clinical trials have been done to test the impact of diet, nutritional supplements, or nutritional complementary methods on cancer outcome among cancer survivors.

Special dietary recommendations are not necessary in rehabilitation of lung cancer patients unless there are symptoms of malnourishment, anorexia and cachexia. Nutrition recommendations focus mainly on the importance of obtaining micronutrients from healthy eating, rather than the use of supplements. The additional administering of vitamins is not necessary. Exceptions are heavy smokers in whom food should be supplemented by polyvitamins.

There is no objection to moderate alcohol consumption. Highly concentrated alcohol, however, should be avoided.

Lung cancer treatment often causes side effects such as esophagitis resulting in dysphagia, fatigue, nausea, and vomiting that can impinge on nutritional well-being. Some survivors exihibit low blood nutrient levels, even before diagnosis, due to inadequate diets and/or to the adverse effects of smoking on micronutrients. For these patients it is important to make special efforts at regaining nutritional health during treatment and recovery. In such situations, a multivitamin-multimineral supplement may be advisable. High doses of vitamins and minerals, however, should be used cautiously. During treatment and the immediate recovery period, these patients may benefit from eating foods that provide concentrated calories and are easy to swallow. Small, frequent meals may be easier to manage than three large meals per day.

Immunosuppression and how to take preventive measures to avoid infections

Most episodes of pneumonia in patients with lung cancer are due to bacteria. This is particularly the case when risk factors like neutropenia, endobronchial lesions, or COPD are present. Although opportunistic infections are not common, fungal infections should be considered if the patient has received a high dose of corticosteroids. Viral infections with herpes simplex, cytomegalovirus or respiratory syncytial virus may also result in pneumonia in patients who have received high-dose corticosteroids or very intensive chemotherapy. Infections have to be treated at an early stage. Influenza and pneumococcal vaccinations are recommended.

Table 12.6 - Reasons for fever in cancer patients.

– Tumour growth
– Treatment with growth factors
– Bacterial/fungal/viral infections
– Abscess formation
– Bronchial fistula
– Empyema

Tuberculosis may exacerbate in these often immunosuppressed patients. Be aware that classical Tine and Mendel Mantoux tests may be negative despite active tuberculosis due to immune insufficiency. Measurements of antibodies and bacteriological examinations of the bronchial lavage are more reliable. In the case of fever fluctuations an abscess or a bronchial fistula has to be considered. Diagnosis will be confirmed by computertomography and bronchoscopy. Letality of empyema with or without bronchial fistula is high even in the case of therapy (e.g., antibiotics, thoracentesis, drainage, operation) (Deschamps, 2001).

Purulent sputum may be the consequence of a bronchial stump which is too long or of bronchectasis.

Intercostal neuralgia and what to do in the case of intercostal neuralgia

Scars may cause pain for years, especially during a change of weather. This (usually) nagging pain may be referred to more remote regions. They are frequently mistaken for signs of disease progression.

If ultrasound treatment, anaesthetic treatment and conventional analgesics like carbamazepine- containing drugs have no effect, morphine-based painkillers may be necessary. Ultrasound therapy may be helpful in the case of scar pain.

Chemotherapy-induced peripheral neuropathy and advice for treatment

For more details see chapters: "Pain therapy in cancer rehabilitation and palliation" and: "Rehabilitation and palliation of patients with ovary carcinoma".

Specific drugs involved in the development of peripheral neuropathy are the plant alkaloids, antimitotics, taxanes, and platinum-based compounds. Drug-induced peripheral neuropathy is sensory and dose-related. Its effect is often delayed, appearing weeks after initiation of therapy (Paice, 2003).

Polyneuropathies induced by paclitaxel, docetaxel, platin, carboplatin and vinca-alkaloids are dose-related. Sometimes symptoms can further deteriorate even after stopping cisplatin. Also, after stopping taxol symptoms often improve only slowly. Cisplatin leads to a mainly sensory polyneuropathy when cumulative doses of 200mg/m^2 are reached. Almost all patients will develop polyneuropathies after oxaliplatinum above 540mg/m^2. In typical cases this progresses for a further three months after stopping therapy ("coasting").

There is no equivocal proof of efficacy for pyridoxine and vitamin B preparations, which are often prescribed. The use of alpha-liponic acid is controversial and views on efficacy of the topical agent capsaicin are divided. There are a few positive reports on prophylactic administration of vitamin E and glutamine; once symptoms have developed there are no positive reports.

Mild sensory neuropathies appear to be often reversible within a few months whereas more severe forms may persist significantly longer. Anticonvulsants (carbamazepine 600-2,400mg a day in slow release form and gabapentin 300-18,00mg a day) are widely used in the treatment of neuropathic pain. Additional administration of antidepressants (e.g., amitriptyline) may be useful. However, this leads to dry mouth, which can be disturbing. Possible side effects of carbamazepine are sedation and cardiac arrhytmias.

Pain relief is one of the main therapeutic indications for low frequency electrotherapy which includes Stanger bath treatment, diadynamic current therapy, and transcutaneous electrical nerve stimulation (TENS). Ice packs and contrast hydrotherapy may improve the patient's well-being. Temporary relief of pain symptoms in the hands and feet is achieved by manipulating structured sand, but the relief provided by these physical measures unfortunately does not last. Many patients say that autogenic training helps.

Emesis and nausea following radiation and chemotherapy

Cytostatic agents and, to a much lesser extent, radiation therapy, have different emetogenic potential.

The incidence and severity of chemotherapy-induced emesis are dependent on several factors, including the emetogenicity of the chemotherapeutic agent and the risk factors of the patient (tables 12.7, 12.8). For bronchial cancer therapy, highly emetogenic chemotherapeutic agents (causing severe vomiting in more than 90% of patients), moderately emetogenic agents (causing vomiting in 30-90% of patients) and mildly emetogenic agents (inducing vomiting in the minority of patients) are used. Some drugs cause emesis; others delayed emesis (Koski and Venner, 2000).

5-HT3 antagonists have nearly completely replaced the use of other antiemetics. Within the context of highly emetogenic chemotherapy, parenteral administration of ondensatrone and dexamethasone should take place; with moderately and mildly emetogenic chemotherapy, dexamethasone is administered orally (as an alternative, for example for diabetics, a 5-HT3 antagonist such as ondensatrone can be used). With some cytostatic agents (for example, cisplatin) vomiting already occurs during or shortly after application of chemotherapy; with other cytostatic agents (for example, cisplatin combined with cyclophosphamide, or after procarbazine or mitomycin), as well as with radiation therapy, onset of nausea and vomiting is delayed. NK1 antagonists (acrepitant) are helpful in the case of delayed-onset emesis. These too should be combined with dexamethasone.

Acrepitant is very effective in combating platinum- and radiation-induced emesis (Patel, 2003).

Table 12.7 - Risk factors associated with emesis.

– Emesis present in prior chemotherapy cycles
– Younger age (below 35 years)
– Female sex
– Low chronic ethanol intake
– Karnowsky index inferior to 80

Table 12.8 - Classification of emetogenicity.

Highly emetogenic emetogenic	Moderately emetogenic	Mildly emetogenic	Minimally
Cisplatin >50mg/m^2	Cisplatin 20-50mg/m^2	Mitoxantrone	5- Fluorouracil
Cyclophosphamide	Carboplatin	Etoposide	Bleomycin
>1,500mg/m^2	Oxaliplatin	Irinotecane	Busulphane
Dacarbazine	Doxorubicine	Docetaxel	Vinca-alkaloids
Nitrogen mustard	Epirubicine	Paclitaxel	Methotrexate
Carmustin	Idarubicine	Cyclophosphamide	>100mg/m^2
<250mg/m^2	Cyclophosphamide	<750mg/m^2	Hydroxyurea
	>750mg/m^2	Gemcitabine	Chlorambucil
	Ifosfamide	Cytarabine<1g/m^2	Fludarabine
	Cytarabine <1g/m^2	Topotecane	Cladibrine
	Procarbacine		

Anticipatory vomiting can cause major problems for patients and for patient compliance as well. Benzodiazepine preparations are most effective for anticipatory vomiting. With very anxious patients, antiemetic therapy should be supplemented with lorazepam (1-2mg i.v. or 0.5-3mg orally). Nonetheless, psychological intervention should always be tried first.

Gastro-intestinal complications and recommendations

Gastric pain and indigestions often occur. They may be explained by stress, by medication side effects (take care of NSAID analgesics!) and by the displacement of the esophagus and stomach towards the surgical side (table 12.9).

Table 12.9 - Possible organ displacements after a right-sided-pneumonectomy.

– Displacement of the trachea towards the resected lung
– Compression of the distal trachea and main bronchus
– Displacement of the esophagus
– Mediastinal displacement towards the empty pleural space
– Marked reduction of the venous blood flow to the heart
– Elevation of diaphragm and liver
– Deviation of the vertebral column

Gastritis and esophagitis are frequent complaints. This is the reason why antacids or H2 inhibitors should be given during the first months after pneumonectomy.

In extended operations there is the possibility of damaging nerves affecting the patient's swallowing. One cause can be the removal of or damage to the vagal nerve during surgery. As a result the digestion system can be adversely affected. Disturbances in motility or even gastric atonia occur. Stomach motility may be dramatically shortened or lengthened. The tendency, especially in the first months following surgery, for diarrhea to occur for this reason, generally disappears spontaneously. Codeine drops or Imodium® alleviate symptoms.

Many patients complain of flatulence. Flatulence is usually a result of incomplete breakdown of nutrients.

Peritoneal carcinosis should always be considered as a possible cause as well. This condition manifests itself through paradoxical diarrhea. Calmative intestinal medications (for example, imodium®), sometimes also spasmolytic agents, may alleviate symptoms.

Constipation is almost guaranteed in a cancer patient receiving opiates. Unfortunately, this potentially serious problem is often overlooked and undermanaged. Although constipation may seem like a minor complication when compared to a life-threatening disease such as cancer, it can become a major detriment to quality of life if it is not well managed. For more details see chapter "Pain therapy in cancer rehabilitation and palliation".

Abuse of nicotine and ways to quit smoking

Whether a lung cancer patient keeps on smoking or not, does not change the course of the malignant disease itself. Nevertheless, smokers should be motivated to give up smoking altogether. There is hardly a function which is not negatively affected by smoking.

Non-smoking courses and assistance for those who want to stop the habit should be offered. During training priority should be focused to the repercussion of smoking-related complaints (e.g., dyspnea, cough or being easily prone to infections, etc.). Smoking family members should also be motivated to break the habit, because the patient will then find it easier to stay away from nicotine. Primary care physicians should enlist and educate available family members to aid in the patient's smoking cessation efforts. There are many different ways how to stop (table 12.10). It is even more important patients to promote the willpower by talking to him/her face to face, in a group or with other family members to give up the habit for good.

Table 12.10 - Ways to quit smoking.

– **Suggestive methods:** Hypnosis, acupuncture, laying on if hands, etc. Smoking cessation is one of the most popular medical uses of hypnosis. Hypnosis helps a person learn to deeply relax, be open to suggestions that strengthen the resolve to quit, and increase negative feelings toward cigarettes.

– **Medicinal treatment:** Medicinal treatment is more or less another suggestive method, too. It is not the choice of the drug, but rather the suggestive way it is prescribed that iss crucial for success.

– **Aversion therapies:** They are supposed to create the unpleasant and adverse consequences of smoking. Smoking shall be deprived of its positive psychotropic effect with, for example, the help of electric shocks and drugs causing nausea.

– **Behaviour modification training:** Often a standard approach to a smoking cessation program. It is based on the smoker's idiosyncrasies, expecting the smoker to take part in an analysing process. Smoking does not stop at once, but step by step. Learning to change the automatic nature of habitual behaviours is often a standard approach to a smoking cessation program.

– **Nicotine replacement therapy:** Based on the hypothesis that the addiction rests on a constant substitution of nicotine. By means of plasters nicotine is administered through the skin thus achieving a well-balanced nicotine level 24 hours a day. The strength of plasters is being reduced stepwise. Nicotine replacement therapy involves "replacing" the nicotine in a cigarette with another form of administration and helps relieve some of the withdrawal symptoms people experience when they quit smoking.

Information and patient education (discussion groups and health training)

Patients with lung cancer who are surgical candidates are often diagnosed and treated very quickly. In most cases they do not have a chance to assimilate all the information they are given.

One of the tasks in rehabilitation is patient education and health education (tables 2.12 12.11). The main aim of health education is to optimise the patient's compliance with treatment, in order to ensure a long-term commitment to regular physical activity. Explanation and information are important aids in helping to cope with the disease and overcome illness. This involves the patient's understanding of what is happening in his/her body and why a certain form of therapy has been suggested. The majority of patients do not wish to make decisions about tumour therapy themselves, but they would like to know the reasons for pursuing a certain treatment strategy.

Patients can get all sorts of information about the prognosis of their disease on the Internet and other media. Explaining the information and the consequences to the patient, however, is a matter for professionals. They can help to get the grips with this information.

It is vital that those concerned can talk unbiased to friends and relatives about their illness and their problems.

Table 12.11 - Subjects of education and counselling programmes for patients with lung cancer.

– Information about the disease, about the various possibilities of treatment, about possibilities to prevent recurrence, about the various prognosis criteria
– Information on necessity of aftercare, content and timetable of follow-up examinations
– Information about symptoms of recurrences
– Information about therapies in the case of recurrences
– Information about alternative therapy forms and complementary therapies
– Information about pain, therapy induced neuropathies and possible therapeutic helps
– Information about postpneumonectomy complaints and possible therapies
– Information about reduction of lung capacity after surgery, radiotherapy and chemotherapy, possible therapies, etc.
– Information about the consequences of nicotine abuse, necessity to stop smoking, ways to quit smoking
– Information about dietary recommendations
– Information about adverse effects of radio-chemotherapy. Prevention and therapy of side effects
– Information about interpersonal and social consequences of the disease
– Information about questions concerning medical care, nursing care, socio-legal issues, and practical issues
– Information about rehabilitation clinics, further care at home
– Information about vocational consequences; workloads to be avoided, harmful occupational substances
– Recommendations about how to cope with fears, depression and fatigue symptoms
– Recommendations about how to deal with family members
– Information about the significance of physical activity

Health education takes place in discussion groups in which psychologists, dietary advisors, physicians and social workers all take turns moderating the groups. Their task is to inform on possibilities and limits of the standard medicine and to protect patients from useless and maybe harmful alternative therapies; interest and use of follow-up examinations will be explained. For that reason single and group discussions are organised where relatives are always welcome. Patients with accompanying COPD need additional training to improve lung function (Celli, 2004).

Besides questions concerning origin, diagnosis, treatment, follow-up examinations, symptoms of recurrences, prevention of recurrence of lung cancer, diets, complications of therapy, coping with fears and pain, information on social rights and assistance as well as occupational consequences of the illness should be discussed. Patients should be counselled to avoid atmospheric or vocational pollutants and other aggravating factors such as pollen, aerosols, excessive humidity, stress, large meals, people with respiratory infections, etc.

It has been proven to be helpful for those patients who have undergone treatment recently to meet with others who have had the same treatment several years earlier.

It is useful for patients and their family members also to have access to printed versions of the information and advice which they have received in health education sessions (for example, in the form of differentiated and industry-unaffiliated self-help literature). This printed material should of course never take the place of medical consultations, but it should rather provide the basis of productive discussions with the attending physician.

Patients more and more go on fact-finding missions themselves, using books or the ever-present Internet to quench their thirst for knowledge. It is often difficult for the lay patient to recognize whether the information available is serious. It is useful if the physician can recommend certain Internet sites that he/she considers to be serious, informative and helpful. Further, explanatory information and – in particular – assistance in dealing with this information are necessary. These may be given to patients in health education within the context of a one-on-one meeting or in a group discussion.

In Great Britain specialised nurses (specialist lung cancer nurses) fulfil rehabilitative and educative duties as well. They are both vital in providing information about the disease and its treatment, as well as advice and support for patients and their families. Their role is crucial in guiding the patient through the complexities of the multidiciplinary team and in accessing help from other services, such as social work, community follow-up and physiotherapy. Patients and carers feel reassured that the nurse is an approachable point of contact at any stage in their illness. Specialist nursing support at home can have a significant impact on a patient's experience of living with lung cancer (Stanley *et al.*, 2004).

Rehabilitative measures aimed at reducing psychological problems. ("rehabilitation to combat resignation and depression")

See also chapter: "Psychological support in cancer rehabilitation and palliation".

Need of psychological support

Lung cancer patients report more unmet psychological concerns than other cancer patients (Hill *et al.*, (2003). Fear of progress, reduced physical activities, dyspnea, pain, immobility, loss of weight and social and vocational uncertainty are some of the reasons for the need of psychological help (Hopwood, 2000). The assessment of psychological symptoms, interpersonal or social consequences of the disease seems to be similarly, if not more, important than physical complaints and should be considered. It is the task of all members of the rehabilitation team to alleviate these problems as well.

Depressions

Depressions and fears in the face of uncertain future are frequent. In contrast to patients with a different cancer disease, such as breast cancer, patients with lung cancer have the tendency to speak only little about their problems, to isolate themselves, to dissimulate and to avoid professional help.

It has been pointed out that the patients tend not to complain about depression, and this condition is often neglected and considered a natural reaction of cancer patients.

It is to note that depressions may simulate brain metastases or hypercalcemia. Depression can be both a consequence and an aggravator of chronic pain syndrome. An effective pain therapy may alleviate depressions; on the other hand antidepressants also have a firm place in analgetic treatment (for more details see chapter: "Pain therapy in cancer palliation and rehabilitation). The reduction of somatic causes is a prerequisite before starting psychotherapy.

If antidepressants become necessary, tricyclic antidepressants are the medicaments of choice. Their doses should be increased step by step from 75mg to 150mg to achieve an antidepressive effect (table 12.12). It is important to heed that in contrast to the sedative effect, the antidepressive effect may take up to two weeks to develop.

In the terminal stage tricyclic antidepressants are of little use. Side effects, e.g., sedation and xerostomia, may predominate.

Table 12.12 - Dosage of antidepressants given in cancer patients.

Drug	Dosage	Application
Amitriptylin	10-150mg	p.o., i.m., rectal
Imipramin	12,5-150mg	i. m.
Bupropion	200-450mg	p.o.
Mapropilin	50-75mg	p.o.
Lithium	600-1200mg	p.o.
Dextroamphetamin	5-40mg	p.o.

Fears

Fears of progress and the uncertain future are frequent (table 2.5). It is the task of the physician and the psycho-oncologist to deal with these fears (table 2.3).

Medicinal support may be considered, but it cannot replace cognitive therapy. Benzodiazepines should be preferred to other substances due to their tolerability. Neuroleptic drugs also have strong anxiolytic qualities. Tricyclic antidepressants are primarily considered when fear emerges in conjunction with depression. However, these drugs may not become effective for up to two weeks. Anxiolytic drugs (such as lorazepam 1-2mg/ per day) may be indicated in insomnia.

Even when the very popular hypothesis of extended survival in positive thinkers cannot be scientifically explained, a positive compliance of the patient should be strived for (Schofield, 2004). There is no standardised procedure to encompass positive compliance, since those who are concerned always react differently and need a very individual approach.

Those patients who are rooted in a religious faith often do not ask for professional help.

Basically the patient should have the feeling that he/she is never left alone and always has a partner to tell about his/her fears, sorrows and problems.

Fatigue syndrome

A fatigue syndrome may be caused by various factors (tables 2.8, 2.9). In the case of anemia, blood transfusions or erythropoetin may decrease fatigue, increase motivation, enhance appetite, elevate a patient's mood and counter the effects of opioids. If no somatic cause can be found and treated, non-medication measures should be used first (e.g., physiotherapy, ergometric training [table 2.7], conversation therapy [table 2.4], behavioural therapy, diet, change of environment) (Watson, 2004).

Sometimes, fatigue symptoms are linked to the antidepressant medications themselves. Psychotropic drugs have, however, also been used successfully to treat fatigue.

Physical activity may be recommended after a somatic cause had been excluded (Spruit et al., 2006). Particularly in Germany group activities such as „sport after cancer" are being supported by the health insurances. Apart from the positive effects on the lung function and physical health these activities are expected to have positive repercussions on the social integration and last not least on fatigue (table 2.10).

Support for family members

Cancer not only places strain on the patient but also has direct effects on the partner and entire family (Keller, 1995). Research surveys show that depression and anxiety are almost as common among patients' partners as among patients themselves. It is helpful if carers can be seen alone from time to time, perhaps by the family doctor, asked how they are coping and invited to talk over any emotional distress.

Distress affects the families of older tumour patients as well as the families of children suffering from cancer; the focus is merely shifted. Tremendous communication problems often arise. Previously existing tensions and conflicts can emerge in the form of aggressions or feelings of guilt. This can place great stress on the patient and can negatively affect the patient's ability to cope with the illness. Psychological support for both the patient and family members, provided by the physician, the spiritual counsellor, or a psycho-oncologist, can be helpful in these cases.

Cancer can cause considerable distress for the healthy partners of older cancer patients, which is experienced in addition to the impairments resulting from age-related changes in their own lives. They lose the security provided by continuity in their relationship prior to the cancer. Plans for a "peaceful retirement" are shattered, prospects for their life in old age must be reconsidered and redeveloped. The physical exertion involved in caring for the patient as well as the financial costs of old and new burdens pose substantial problems for the family. The transition in role allocation from "being provided for" to "being the provider" places high demands on the family's ability to adapt to the new situation. In addition to conflicts between the family members' own needs, the desire for autonomy, and obligations to the ill parent, conflicts also often arise between caring for the patient and fulfilling responsibilities in the adult child's own family or professional career. The partners of older cancer patients particularly experience emotional distress, while the adult children of cancer patients more frequently describe their stress as the result of a confusion in roles.

Support options for families are internationally very limited with regard to financing by insurance companies or other cost carriers. In Germany, these options are restricted to "family health care" within pediatric oncological rehabilitation clinics, in which children suffering from cancer are cared for together with their parents for a period of three to six weeks. Most German cancer rehabilitation clinics offer the spouse/partner the option of residing in the clinic with the patient for the cost of room and board.

It is desirable for the patient's partner to participate in educational cancer training. Informing patients and their families that physical inactivity can hinder the treatment of fatigue should be one of the problems focused upon in group therapy sessions. A number of German cancer rehabilitation clinics that have a basis on therapy close to the patient's residence explicitly integrate psychosocial care into both their inpatient and their outpatient/semi-outpatient treatment concepts. Spiritual guidance is given emphasis in such cases, especially since it provides the opportunity for further care by placing the patient in contact with the local religious congregations. Self-help groups for family members have also been established. In some regions of Germany there are special centres and organizations (Alpha) that promote the support of family members of the terminally ill.

Rehabilitative measures aimed at reducing social problems ("rehabilitation to combat the need of care")

See also chapter: "Social support in rehabilitation and palliation".

Need of social support

One of the aims in rehabilitation is to strengthen the patient's own resources and to prevent the risk of the need of care, or at least reduce such a need (tables 1.9, 3.2). If the patient is no longer able to care for himself/herself, support must be organized. In patients with bronchial cancer, this situation arises particularly frequently. Early organization of assistance and social support is crucial in patients with poor prognosis and a rapidly progressing disease.

Organization of outside assistance: Securing adequate care at home

The planning of further care must be arranged with both the patient's and the family's consent. The patients and his adherents are confronted with a complexity of problems. Services such as "meals on wheels" or household assistance, home nursing, care assistance and in some circumstances the arrangement of nursing care or a hospice have to be arranged.

Providing addresses (e.g., self-help groups, charity organizations, counselling centres, etc.) is helpful.

The first step for the patient is to get in touch with social workers. They work at primary care hospitals, rehabilitation clinics, cancer counselling centres, health insurance companies and charity organizations. The importance of self-help groups is often underestimated within the context of the aims of a follow-up treatment on the social level.

If home care cannot or cannot yet be arranged, the time spent in hospital can be followed by a temporary stay in an institution for follow-up care. In Germany "AHB clinics" are especially designed for the patient's social assistance, in addition to medical and psychological guidance. Some of the maisons de repos in France have a similar function.

Rehabilitation hospitals

Most European countries prefer the out-patient rehabilitation, which is carried out in most of the cancer centres. In Germany there are rehabilitation hospitals specialised to meet the different needs of patients with pulmonary diseases. They provide accompanying medical follow-up as well as further social assistance (AHB hospitals). The average stay is about three-four weeks. Here, experienced physicians, psychologists and representatives of self-help groups share their experiences, information and helpful advice. Adjuvant and additive cancer therapies, supportive therapies, psychological support, counselling of the patients and their families are some of the tasks of these AHB hospitals.

Apart from the physical recovery programs to improve respiratory function and exercise capacity and the psychological guidance the stay incorporates the preparation of future life activities including the social, financial and vocational situation. In Germany, every cancer patient has a legal claim to a three-five week stay in such an institution. About 50% of all German cancer patients being pneumectomized prefer staying at a rehabilitation hospital.

Procuring information about questions concerning medical care, nursing care, socio-legal issues, and practical issues: Legally defined privileges for cancer patients

Assistance in social care is available in most countries. Cancer patients in most European countries are subject to legal privileges, ranging from tax reductions, financial grants, free use of public transport and a vocational protection against wrongful dismissal (table 12.13) (see for more information in the chapter "Social support in cancer rehabilitation and palliation"). In addition to psychological support, **self-help groups** often provide their members with specific knowledge about medications and resources as well as social laws. The concept behind self-help groups is based on the idea that sharing of mutual experiences and situations offer a person more strength. Self-help groups for patients with cancer exist in most countries.

In some countries, like Germany, there are special compulsory insurances in the case when the patient is unable to take care of himself. Hospital and nursing charges are split between the employer and employee. Retired people pay a minimum amount, the rest is paid by the government.

Table 12.13 - Legally defined priviliges for cancer patients in Germany.

– Increased dismissal protection at the workplace.
– Assistance in keeping or acquiring a workplace appropriate for a disabled person, e.g., technical aids or wage subsidies.
– Acceleration of pension provision.
– Exception from overtime and exemption from night-shifts if so desired.
– Right to 5 days additional holiday per year with a five day working week.

Rehabilitative measures aimed at reducing vocational problems ("rehabilitation to combat early retirement")

See also chapter: "Vocational integration in cancer rehabilitation".

Restrictions of working capacity

Patients with inoperable lung cancer and with active tumour are not usually able to work. They should ask for early retirement on grounds of ill health as soon as possible. Exceptions apply for psychological reasons, if the patient is keen on continuing to work. More often than not, however, these patients soon realise that they are not up to their job once they try to phase back in.

For lung cancer patients who have been treated potentially curatively, there are professional limitations, which are mainly due to pneumonectomy and/or radio- and chemotherapy side effects.

Apart from disabilities due to the treatment accompanying illnesses, in particular the obstructive bronchitis, often hamper the vocational performance.

Physically demanding activities should not be performed by pneumectomised patients (table 4.9).

Approximately one-quarter of long-term lung cancer survivors are significantly restricted in their physical ability or report significant depressive symptoms (Sugimura and Yang, 2006).

Harmful occupational substances

All occupational groups exposed to asbestos and radon decay products are especially endangered. Activities including crystalline silicondioxide with established silica sand lung disease, with chromium, nickel and arsenic are dangerous (tables 12.14, 12.15) (Neuberger and Field, 2003). Workers producing accumulators find themselves exposed to nickel. Workers producing chromate will be exposed to chrome, farmers and foresters will be exposed to arsenic.

With mesothelioma you always have to think of the vocational aspect. Patients suffering from a mesothelioma have to be reported to the health authorities in some countries (e. g. in Germany), even if there is no known exposure to asbestos. In these countries it is not the patient, but the accident insurer who has to prove that there is no correlation with previous occupational asbestos exposure. Simultaneously, an expert judgement of the clinical symptoms is conducted.

Table 12.14 - Vocational activities with frequent exposition to asbestos.

– Activities in shipbuilding
– Activities in construction industry
– Activities in asbestos mines
– Activities in the fuel-trade, activities with oil, coal, gas

Table 12.15 - Professional groups exposed to repirable quartz dusts.

– Ore and uranium ore miners
– Tunnellers
– Casting fettlers
– Sandblasters
– Furnace bricklayers and moulders in the metalworking industry
– Personnel in fine-china companies
– Personnel in dental laboratories

Basically, job-related lung carcinoma cannot be differentiated from those with less vocational history. Every type of histology is possible, small-cell lung cancer and non-small-cell lung cancer as well. Also the localisation referring to the different lobs and the distribution of peripheral and central bronchial carcinoma do not differ.

Type of work to be avoided

Even if most of the carcinogenic substances concerned with problems listed in the tables 12.14, 12.15 above have a long induction period, cancer patients should discontinue any activities in which they are exposed to these carcinogenic substances. It is presumed that potentially carcinogenic substances have a stronger carcinogenic effect in the case of "cured" cancer patients than in the case of healthy people. A workplace transfer or even a vocational reorientation may be necessary.

Vocational restrictions for patients who have had a pneumonectomy (R0 resection) are first and foremost the consequences of the pneumonectomy. Accompanying illnesses, particularly the obstructive bronchitis, reduce the vocational performance even more. With physiotherapeutic measures and consistent (consequent) treatment of the frequently simultaneous chronic obstructive bronchitis one can achieve an amazing adaptation of cardiopulmonary parameter functions and an increased performance, which only in single cases can equal the preoperative situation and therefore regain the initial performance and ability to work. In contrast, office work and non-physical activities are quite feasible.

R0 pneumectomized patients under 55 who carried out heavy workloads before they developed cancer should be given a physically less strenuous activity or a complete change of activity as early as possible.

The bulk of potential curative pneumectomized lung cancer patients belong to a group which find it difficult to get a job, because they are unfit to correspond to the vocational burdens of the labour market. After a **potential curative lobectomy or bilobectomy** it is possible to adapt a satisfactory performance (Donner, 2006). These patients should be given the opportunity to use the possible period to get on the sick list and have a period of rest to stabilize their health before a final expert report. It also makes sense to return to work in a stepwise fashion.

Return to work

Whether or not the patient is capable of working depends on tumour spread, whether resection was done R0 or R1, or whether only chemotherapy or radiotherapy was performed. It also depends on the severity of concurring diseases and on whether additional chemotherapy was done. Last but not least, subjective ability to work plays a role.

When judging the chances of professional reintegration it should be kept in mind that the risk of cancer relapse is high during the first 12-24 months, and that side effects of therapy such as platinum or taxol-induced polyneuropathy may take months to resolve.

Since the adaptation mechanisms of the cardio-respiratory system after a pneumonectomy take a long time to restore, in particular after an adjuvant chemo- or radiotherapy, it is advisable that the earliest time to return to work is six months after pneumonectomy. The patient's long-term restriction performance is highly dependent on his or her individual recovery. Dependent on the type of treatment and on individual disposition the recovery phase can differ in duration. Average duration of working incapacity following potentially curative pneumonectomy is six months, and after lobectomy/bilobectomy three months.

Gradual resumption of work is recommended. The particular advantage of this arrangement is that the work load and the fitness level of the patient can be matched without financial disadvantages. Unfortunately, this sensible vocational rehabilitation approach is only possible in a few countries and even there often only in large companies and in the civil service.

Palliative measures in follow-up care

At least half of all bronchial cancer patients already have an extended disease at the time of diagnosis of lung cancer and cannot be operated (stage IV). Furthermore, most of those lucky patients having been "successfully" operated (situation R0) will metastasize in the following two years (Earle, 2001; Bunn, 2003).

In the case of recurrence it is very rare to apply curative treatments. The issue of quality of life in this group of patients is paramount. The need of palliation has first priority in the case of recurrences.

Informing the patient about disease progression: Delivering bad news

Despite the unfavourable prognosis in the case of tumour recurrence, there are more points in favour than against patient information. This does not mean, however, that the patient should be forced to confront the full implications of his or her illness. Information without the simultaneous offering of prospects and assistance is never constructive. Many fears associated with the illness originate from the fact that the affected person does not know how the situation should be assessed or what he/she should expect. It is better in any case for the patient to be informed by the attending physician than by prayer healers, moneymakers, or by random information found on the Internet. Patients without a good foundation of knowledge tend to look for alternative medicine and to consult quack-doctors.

Even when prognosis is desperate, positive aspects can be mentioned (e.g., references to progress in palliative therapy, better pain control, provision of constant medical/psychological service, better supportive care in the case of dyspnea, etc.).

The assessment of emotional and physical costs must be carefully considered with any patient before deciding further cancer therapies. The physician has to inform the patient about all therapies at disposition, no matter if curative, supportive or palliative.

In the discussion, the seriousness and also the extent of the findings should be communicated to the patient but a time scale regarding the prognosis should never be made, all the more because diseases can quite frequently follow an unpredictable course.

It is important to signal willingness for discussion again and again, to listen and to ascertain what the patient has understood and what significance he assigns to the information content. A desire to suppress the problem temporarily or long-term, which can often be read from his/her behaviour, should be respected. Often doctors ignore patients' perceptions of their physical, emotional and social impact of the problems. They pay little attention to checking how well patients have understood what they have been told. Statistics show that less than half of psychological morbidity in patients is recognized.

Table 12.16 - Paraneoplastic syndromes of bronchial cancer.

- Osteoarthropathies (e.g., clubbed fingers)
- Endocrinopathies (e.g., ACTH syndrome, Cushing's syndrome)
- Auto-immune hemolytic anemia
- Disorders of hemostasis
- Disorders of hematopoesis
- Hypoglycemia
- Myopathy, neuropathy, cerebellar dysfunction
- Eaton-Lambert syndrome
- Pruritus
- Fever
- Acanthosis nigricans, acroceratosis, erythema gyratum repens, hypertrichosis
- Torre-Muir syndrome, dermatomyositis
- Hypercalcemia
- Schwartz-Bartter syndrome
- Neurological symptoms such as polyneuropathies, myasthenia

Symptoms that may require palliation include those of the cancer itself (table 12.16), of regional metastases within the thorax, or of distant metastases (table 12.17).

Table 12.17 - Symptoms hinting towards possible tumour progression and localisation of recurrences.

– **In the lung** (endoluminal stenosis, peribronchial stenosis, esophageal fistulas, bulky lymphadenopathy, tumour masses, esophago-tracheal fistulas): dyspnea, hemoptysis, pain on inspiration

– **In the regional metastases within the thorax** (e.g., superior vena cava syndrome, tracheo-oesophageal fistula, pleural effusions, chest wall, pericardium, pericardial and pleural effusions, mediastinum): cough, tachyarythmias, pain, hoarseness, sudden hoarseness, Horner syndrome

– **In distant organs** (e.g., brain, spinal cord, bone): anorexia, fatigue, ascites, pain, upper abdominal pain, neurologic symptoms, night sweat

Accompanying illnesses, altered pharmacodynamics, coping, social care may influence therapeutic strategies; comorbidity, quality of life scores and toxicity have to be taken into account (Earle *et al.*, 2001). A decline in organ functions can alter the pharmacokinetics and pharmacodynamics of many commonly used chemotherapeutic agents in some elderly patients, making toxicity less predictable. Most lung cancer patients are older than 65 years (Bunn and Lilenbaum, 2003), but most cytostatics have been tested in younger patients being in good shape. As a consequence conditions and results of these trials are scarcely comparable with the real situations.

This does not mean that elderly patients should not be treated. However, elderly patients should be assessed and treated differently from younger patients, as age-related physical changes affect the biology of cancer. Treatment must be tailored to the individual patient.

Answering the question: "How much therapy, and which one?" not only requires oncological expertise. Ethical competence and communication skills are just as important. Under no circumstances should a therapeutical decision be made exclusively depending on response in terms of likelihood of remission; goals such as reduction of physical symptoms, emotional stabilisation, and maintenance of daily activities are pre-eminent.

Surgical procedures are limited primarily to palliation (table 12.18). In most cases they are supplemented by radio- and/or chemotherapy.

Table 12.18 - Palliative situations when surgical interventions may be justified.

– Hemoptysis
– Poststenotic complications
– Unbearable pain because of perforated thorax
– No response to other forms of treatment
– Imminent fractures
– Stabilization of the vertebral column
– Brain metastases

One of the advantages of **radiotherapy** as administered externally is immediate relief from the symptoms. Irradiation in itself should concern palliation of the tumour region only and not focus on prevention of the region around at risk (table 12.19).

Table 12.19 - Palliative situations when radiotherapeutic interventions may be justified.

– Local progression of cancer despite of chemotherapy
– Local recurrences of cancer
– Symptomatic bone metastases
– Symptoms like dyspnea, cough, chest pain, hemoptysis
– Brain metastases and spinal cord compression syndrome
– Singultus due to irritation of nervus phrenicus
– Superior vena cava obstruction
– Bronchus stenosis with retention pneumonia
– In the case of refusal of surgical intervention or of chemotherapy, pain relief (e.g., bone metastases, lung cancer causing chest pain, nerve root or plexus compressing/invasion, soft tissue infiltration)
– Control of hemoptysis
– Control of ulceration
– Relief of impending or actual obstruction (e.g., bronchus, esophagus)
– Shrinkage of tumour mass(es) causing distressing symptoms (e.g., brain metastases, hepatic capsule stretching, skin lesions)
– Prevention of significant morbidity (e.g., impending bone fractures, spinal cord compression, superior mediastinal obstruction, superior vena cava syndrome)

In contrast to a conventionally fractionated radiation over several weeks, short-term and hypofractionated radiation has the advantage of rapid response and symptom relief. Rapid palliation and not the risk of late effects should dominate the planning of palliative therapy. Survival time of patients with recurrences is too short to experience the late effects.

Local and regional problems and palliative therapies

Hemoptysis

Bleeding from central airway tumours can be stopped by coagulation preferably with the argon plasma coagulator. Patients with endobronchial stenoses are ideal candidates for Nd-Yag laser, electrocautery, argon plasma coagulation, cryotherapy or photodynamic therapy. Extrinsic compression or airway wall destruction requires the placement of an airway stent. An additional use for laser therapy is retention pneumonia.

Brachytherapy and afterloading can destroy submucosal and peribronchial cancer tissue. In contrast to laser therapy the effects of brachytherapy is delayed. Several sessions are necessary.

Liver metastases

Solitary liver metastases are extremely rare. Therefore, neither surgical resection of metastases nor isolated regional chemotherapy or embolization can be expected to bring about any significant benefit of survival time. Systemic chemotherapy, on the other hand, can have an alleviating effect. Low doses of cortisone have pain-relieving and anabolic effects and may have a positive effect on the patient's psychological state.

Pleuritis carcinomatosa

Pleuritis carcinomatosa with pleural effusion is the most frequent cause of dypnea, cough and chest pain.

Options include thoracocentesis, chesttube placement, video-assisted thoracoscopy and pleurodesis. For patients in the terminal stage, pleurodesis is evident only in cases in which the space between the visceral pleura and parietal pleura is eliminated by continuous drainage. Intermittent needle drainage at about 500-1,000 mL is preferred in many cases.

Most intrapleurally instilled chemical agents (bleomycin, tetracyclin, mitoxantrone, asbestosis-free talc) incite an inflammatory reaction, which ultimately causes the visceral pleura to adhere to the parietal pleura, thereby eliminating the potential space in which fluid can accumulate. Cancer growth is not being influenced by the agent if there is a large residual effusion at the time a sclerosing agent is administered; the likelihood of success is low, and the possibility of turning a simple effusion into a multi-loculated collection requiring further intervention is high. Disadvantages of local instillation therapy are possible pain on inspiration, and re-formation of encapsulated collections, that are more difficult to access.

Pericardial effusion

The presence of pericardial effusion in patients with non-small cell lung cancer indicates a grave prognosis. Surgical approaches to malignant effusion are applicable only for limited cases. Since radiation therapy and systematic chemotherapy are not helpful in controlling the pericardial effusion, treatment with an initial pericardiocentesis followed by indwelling pericardial catheters is currently appropriate.

Peritoneal carcinosis

For more details see chapter about ovary carcinoma.

Neither surgery nor radiation therapies extend life or improve the quality of life in these patients. Systemic chemotherapy may be attempted but experience has shown that it is less effective in the case of peritoneal carcinosis than in other metastases locations.

Peritoneal carcinosis is often accompanied by an ascites. Cholesterol levels above 60mg/dL, and CEA levels above 12ng/mL in the ascites are a strong indicator of malignancy.

In the case of a symptomatic ascites, good, although temporary, relief of symptoms related to the build up of fluid can be achieved by paracentesis. Rapid re accumulation can necessitate frequent procedures, thus subjecting the patient to the risks of bleeding, infections, visceral perforation, and hypotension associated with invasive drainage. Repeated large volume paracenteses without plasma volume expansion may be associated with significantly higher incidence of hypotension and renal impairment.

Hiccup

Singultus (hiccup) can be caused by irritation of the phrenic nerve or the diaphragm (tumour, distention of the ventricle, enlarged liver) or brain metastases. Non-pharmacological treatments (sitting up, breathing into a paper bag, drinking ice cold water, or swallowing two teaspoons of sugar) are often inefficient.

Table 12.20 - Pharmacological treatment of hiccup.

– Metoclopramide 10 to 20mg, 3 to 4 times daily p.o./p.r. or parenterally.
– Haloperidol 0.5 to 2mg, 1 to 3 times daily p.o., or 2.5 to 5mg i.m. 1 to 3 times, 5 to 10mg/day s.c./i.v. infusion.
– Chlorpromazine 25 to 50mg, 1 to 3 times daily p.o. (may cause sedation).
– Baclofen 5 to 20mg, 2 to 3 times daily p.o.
– If the cause is a brain tumour, anti-epileptic medication may be effective.
– In the case of tumour invasion of the diaphragm radiotherapy is most effective.

Brain metastases

The management of patients with brain metastases can be divided into symptomatic and definitive therapy. Symptomatic therapy includes the use of corticosteroids for the treatment of peritumoural edema, anticonvulsants for control of seizures, and anticoagulants (low molecular heparine) for the management of venous thrombo-embolic disease. Definitive therapy includes treatments directed at eradicating the tumour itself, such as surgery, radiotherapy, radio surgery and chemotherapy.

The optimal combination of therapies for each patient depends on a careful evaluation of numerous factors, including the histology, location, size, and number of brain metastases; the patient's age, general condition, and neurological status; and the extent of the systemic cancer, as well as its response to past therapy and its potential response to future treatments.

More than 50% of all patients with **small-cell lung cancer** (SCLC) will develop brain metastases. Most of them are diffuse. They are not always symptomatic (Seute *et al.*, 2004).

Whole-brain radiation, followed by chemotherapy, is indicated in **symptomatic metastases**. In most cases this treatment will alleviate symptoms and improve quality of life. The risk of late complications (leuko-encephalopathy, brain atrophy, neurocognitive deterioration and dementia, brain necrosis) from whole-brain radiation is related to total dose, fraction size, patient age, extent of disease, and neurological impairment at presentation. Most patients, however, will not live long enough to suffer from these complications.

Temporary relief of symptoms after chemotherapy without irradiation is more than 70%.

In **non-small-cell lung cancer** it is important to differentiate patients with a single or solitary metastasis from those with multiple brain metastases since their subsequent treatment differs. In contrast to small-cell lung cancer **"solitary brain metastasis"** dominates in non-small-cell lung cancer. Surgery and/or radio surgery play an important role in their treatment.

For patients who are candidates for surgery, the most important factor to consider is the extent of extracranial disease. Patients with extensive systemic disease generally have a very limited prognosis and only rarely benefit from surgery. Important factors influencing the decision concerning surgery include the presence of single or multiple metastases, the location of the tumour, the neurological status of the patient, and the interval between diagnosis of the primary neoplasm and the brain metastases.

Studies support the use of surgery and eventually whole-brain radiation, or radio surgery in patients with a **single brain metastasis** and stable extra cranial disease.

The role of surgery in patients with **multiple brain metastases** is usually limited to resection of large lesions or symptomatic lesions or life-threatening lesions. Whole-brain irradiation or chemotherapy should be performed. In asymptomatic multiple brain metastases many authors start with chemotherapy, followed by whole-brain radiation in the case of symptomatic progression (Kelly, 1998).

The main goal of radiation therapy is to improve neurological deficits caused by the tumour deposit. Symptoms such as headache, focal neurological dysfunction, cognitive dysfunction, and seizures will improve.

Symptomatic therapies such as corticosteroids, anticonvulsants and anticoagulants are often necessary (Mamon, 1999). Dexamethasone has relatively little mineral corticoid activity thus reducing the potential for fluid retention. In addition, dexamethasone may be associated with a lower risk of infection and cognitive impairment. Dexamethasone therapy is usually started with a 10mg loading dose followed by 4mg, four times a day.

In addition to the usual complications of anticonvulsants, brain tumour patients experience an increased incidence of side effects, especially drug rashes. Approximately 20% of brain tumour patients treated with phenytoin and undergoing cranial irradiation develop a morbilliform rash and a small percentage develop Stevens-Johnson syndrome. Patients receiving phenobarbital have an increased incidence of shoulder-hand syndrome. Because of the increased incidence of allergic reactions in patients with brain metastases receiving anticonvulsant therapy and the lack of clear evidence that anticonvulsant therapy reduces the incidence of seizures, routine anticonvulsant therapy is considered to be unnecessary in patients with brain metastases who have not experienced a seizure.

Venous thromboembolic disease occurs approximately in 20% of patients with brain metastases. Anticoagulation (low molecular heparine) is more effective than inferior vena cava filter placement.

Unfortunately, for most patients with brain metastases, overall survival is more likely to be determined by the activity and extent of the extracranial disease than by success or failure of radiation therapy or surgery in controlling brain metastases.

Spinal cord compression syndrome

About 95% of cases with spinal cord compression are caused by the epidural infiltration of vertebral metastases. Most patients having paralysis experienced pain coming from the spinal cord or spinal roots several weeks or several months before the onset of paralysis.

Acute spinal cord compression syndrome requires prompt treatment within a few hours. Even in the case of chronic compression, paralysis is inevitable unless radiotherapy is initiated within two or three days.

Patients with corresponding symptoms (progressive back pain, spinal cord compression syndrome) should be promptly referred to a centre which can offer complete diagnostic tests and has the appropriate departments (neurosurgery, radio-oncology, orthopedics, and hematology). Meanwhile the patient should get corticosteroids.

Magnetic resonance imaging is the gold standard for diagnosis and is needed in any patient having new back pain, whether or not plain films or bone scans show metastases. On principle, the further course of action (surgical intervention, if necessary followed by postoperative radiotherapy, or immediate radiotherapy alone) should be decided individually for each patient by the interdisciplinary team. Symptomatic therapy addresses pain, constipation, spinal instability, and the psychological and social consequences of the associated disability (Abrahm, 2004).

The neurological status of the patient at the time the therapy is started determines the outcome.

Superior vena cava obstruction (SVCO)

Superior vena cava syndrome is the clinical appearance of an obstruction of the superior vena cava, acutely or subacutely threatening mainly small-cell lung cancer patients. It usually presents insidiously. Most patients have dilated neck veins and facial edema, while 15% to 20% of patients have arm edema. Treatment is purely palliative.

Generally, radiotherapy in combination with corticosteroids is the first treatment of choice. Treatment brings a fast response that lasts, in many cases, for a long time.

Vascular stenting has been established in the last decades. It is a very fast and effective therapy for occlusion of the superior vena cava syndrome (De Gregoirio et al., 2003).

Pancoast tumour

The classic superior sulcus syndrome (Pancoast tumour) includes lower brachial plexopathy, Horner's syndrome and shoulder pain. It usually manifests with local chest pain due to local invasion of the ribs. The pain may later extend to the inner side of the arm, elbow, and the pinky and ring fingers. If the tumour extends to the sympathetic chain Horner syndrome may develop (ptosis, anhidrosis, enophtalmos, and miosis). In as many as 10-25% of persons with Pancoast tumour, compression of the spinal cord and paraplegia develop when the tumour extends into the intervertebral foramina.

The standard of care is radiation followed by removal of the tumour and chest wall, when possible. Most centres offer a combination of chemotherapy and radiation followed by surgery. All persons with Pancoast tumours that are directly invading the parietal pleura and chest wall should undergo surgery, provided that no preoperative evidence of extensive mediastinal adenopathy exists.

Steroids are also given to reduce swelling.

Osseous metastases

The management of bone metastases depends on a number of factors: The histology of the lung tumour, the location and extent of bone destruction, the severity of morbidity, the availability of effective systemic therapies, and the overall status of the patient. In most cases of small-cell lung cancer, osseous metastases are present at the same time in other organs as well.

If X-ray shows a metastatic lesion in a long bone with cortical destruction, particularly the femur or humerus, pathologic fracture must be prevented if possible. Generally this will require local irradiation and internal fixation with or without systemic therapy. If the patient has or develops a pathologic fracture, **internal fixation** followed by radiotherapy is a most effective approach, assuming the patient can undergo the operative procedure.

If bone metastases are not complicated by pathologic fracture or do not involve the spinal cord or nerve roots, treatment is dictated by symptoms, by the risk of pathologic fracture, and by the potential for effective systemic therapy.

In symptomatic bone metastases of non-small-cell lung cancer **percutaneous cement injection** and **thermal ablation** are alternative or additive treatment options to standard therapy. Thermal ablation could achieve spontaneous pain relief due to the destruction of sensitive nerves surrounding the tumour. Thermal ablation and percutaneous cement injection seem to be a reasonable combination as thermal ablation destroys sensitive nerve ends, whereas cement injection increases stability.

Prophylactic **orthopedic/surgical stabilization** is required if there is an increased risk of fracture. An increased risk of fracture of the long bones can be anticipated with 50% destruction of the cortex and a defect size superior to 2.5cm. There is a risk of vertebral fracture if there is destruction of the middle/central or anterior and posterior pillar of over 60% in the axial plane.

Bisphosphonates and **bone-seeking radiopharmaceuticals** have entered the therapeutic armamentarium for the treatment of multiple painful osseous lesions. **Radio-isotopes** such as strontium-89 and samarium-153 have been shown to decrease pain in patients with osteoblastic metastases in contrast to osteolytic metastases, which respond better to bisphosphonates.

Cough

Cough is a defense mechanism that prevents the entry of noxious materials into the respiratory system and clears foreign materials and excess secretions from the lungs and respiratory tract (table 12.21). Cough interferes with the patient's daily activity and quality of life (table 12.22).

Table 12.21 - Frequent reasons for cough in lung cancer patients.

- Infections
- Bulky lymph-adenopathy or tumour masses, lymph-angiosis, endobronchial tumour, extrinsic bronchial compression
- Foreign materials in the respiratory system
- Esophago-tracheal fistulas
- Irritation of other structures associated with the cough reflex: Pleura, pericardium, diaphragm
- Pericardial and pleural effusions
- Bronchiectasis
- Pneumonitis
- Chronic obstructive pulmonary disease
- Pulmonary edema: Congestive heart failure, vascular heart disease

Table 12.22 - Possible consequences of persistent cough.

- Sleep disorder
- Dyspnea
- General malaise
- Pain
- Anorexia
- Hemoptysis
- Pneumothorax

The optimum solution is to treat the causes of coughs, if such an approach is possible. This may apply to wet coughs from heart failure, pleuritis carcinomatosa and infection and interstitial pneumonia as a complication of radiotherapy and anticancer chemotherapy.

Sputum retention and wet coughs from a loss of ciliary movement caused by radiotherapy should be treated with expectorant and inhalation therapy, combined with respiratory physical therapy for sputum removal. Suppression of coughs should be attempted, if coughs are persistent and not contributing to the clearing of airways. Sufficient pain control should be practiced, because pain in the ribs and lumbar vertebrae prevents coughing and sputum removal, leading to a risk of complications such as pneumonia.

Infections are treated with antibiotics. Pericardial and pleural effusions may be managed by drainage or sclerotherapy. Radiotherapy has been shown to improve cough in bulky lymph-adenopathy or tumour masses. Stenting of esophagotracheal fistulas (esophageal, tracheal, or double stenting) may offer symptom relief and better quality of life. Stents can also be used to open obstructed airways that might cause cough (Estfan *et al.*, 2004).

Sedation may be useful, especially at night.

Two classes of antitussive drugs are available: Centrally-acting (opioids and non-opioids) and peripherally-acting (directly and indirectly). Many antitussives, such as benzonatate, codeine, hydrocodone, and dextromethorphan, were extensively studied in the acute and chronic cough settings and showed relatively high efficacy and safety profiles. Benzonatate, clobutinol, dihydrocodeine, hydrocodone, and levodropropizine are the only antitussives specifically studied in cancer and advanced cancer cough. They all have shown to be effective and safe in recommended daily doses for cough control. In advanced cancer the following have a role in the selection of antitussives for prescription: The patient's current medications, the previous antitussive use, the availability of routes of administration, any history of drug abuse, the presence of other symptoms and other factors. Excellent knowledge of the pharmacokinetics, dosage, efficacy, and side effects of the available antitussives has a major effect on the overall management.

Codeine has been used as a cough suppressant for over 150 years. Dextromethorphan has been shown to be as effective as codeine in suppressing cough. Hydrocodone has been found to be effective at a median dose of 10mg/d in divided doses. It is considered to be the drug of choice. Hydrocodone has the advantage of less gastro-intestinal and central nervous system toxicities compared with codeine. When the cough is resistant to this, second line of therapy would be the addition or substitution of a peripherally-acting antitussive, e.g., benzonatate. The recommended oral dose is 100-450mg/d in divided doses. Benzonatate is a synthetic drug that inhibits cough through anesthetizing the vagal stretch receptors in the bronchi, alveoli, and the pleura.

Opioids reduce the sensitivity of the respiratory centre, possibly decreasing the respiratory rate to the point of apnea. The antitussive effect is based on the suppression of the excitability of the cough centre and is not dependent on the respiratory depressant effect. Buprenorphine reaches a ceiling effect at fairly low doses and, as a result, virtually never causes clinically relevant respiratory depression.

Despite pulmonary function impairment, morphine derivatives have proved effective in lung cancer patients because of their concomitant antitussive effect. In pain patients the respiratory depressant effect of opioids is compensated by the stimulating effect of pain on respiration, with the result that the risk of respiratory depression is low in patients in pain.

Systemic palliative therapies

Chemotherapies and biological therapies/targeted therapies

Evaluation criteria of chemotherapy include amelioration of symptoms (table 12.23), making activities of daily life possible and giving the chance of survival advantage (Pawel et al., 1999, (Huisman et al., 2000; Stinnett et al., 2007).

Table 12.23 - Symptoms which have to be evaluated in palliative chemotherapy in bronchial cancer.

– Dyspnea
– Anorexia
– Hoarseness
– Fatigue
– Daily activities
– Pain

In small-cell lung cancer chemotherapy should start early at an asymptomatic stage. The risk of rapid progression with untreatable symptoms is high in small-cell lung cancer patients. While SCLC initially responds quite well to first-line chemotherapy, relapsed disease is exceedingly difficult to treat. There is no established role for maintenance therapy following the initial course of treatment

Therapy differs according to the recurrence free time. If the remission after a certain chemotherapy lasted more than 90 days the same cytostatics may be applied (rechallenge). If recurrences occur before 90 days, a different chemotherapy should be used. The advantages of poly-chemotherapy as opposed to monotherapy are not unequivocal. Few of the currently available drug combinations have a clear survival advantage. Polychemotherapies may have higher response rates but the rate of unwanted side effects is higher as well as demanding more supportive measures (Fryback, 2004; von Pawel, Gatzemeier, Pujol *et al.*, 2001). In the case of reduced physical state monotherapy is primordial. Elder patients should be given the option of receiving chemotherapy in addition to supportive care as well (Earle, 2001; Ramsey, 2004).

In non-small-cell lung cancer (NSCLC) chemotherapy should be applied only after symptoms have appeared and not at an asymptomatic stage. For patients with advanced **non-small-cell lung cancer,** there is no agreement upon standard for chemotherapy. Taxotere, Pemetrexed, carboplatinum and vinorelbine, given alone or in combination with other drugs, are often chosen.

Recent results from early clinical trials when **chemotherapy and radiotherapy** were administered concurrently yielded impressive improvements in overall response rates and median survival. Unfortunately, the grade III and IV toxicities of these treatment schedules were significantly greater than those with the sequential approach (Zatloukal *et al.*, 2004). These factors have to be discussed honestly with patients as some will accept a large degree of toxicity for just a small potential benefit whereas others may want a bigger survival gain before accepting a well-tolerated treatment schedule.

Several new targeted therapies have demonstrated encouraging response rates and have improved survival outlook for patients with advanced **non-small-cell lung cancer (NSCLC).** These therapies have become acceptable alternatives to traditional cytotoxic platinum-based therapies with respect to disease control and quality of life. The epidermal growth factor receptor (EGFR) has been identified as an important target in cancer therapy. In addition, the anti-angiogenic agent bevacizumab, a monoclonal antibody to vascular endothelial growth factor (VEGF), has been associated with a survival advantage when added to chemotherapy. Targeted therapies such as **tyrosinkinase inhibitors (erlotinib)** have been shown to be effective even in patients who have failed first- or second- line chemotherapy (Korfee *et al.*, 2004). Erlotinib has shown to prolong survival and to relieve symptoms such as dyspnea and cancer pain without some of the unpleasant side effects of chemotherapy, such as myelosuppression, neuropathy, nausea, of diarrhea and vomiting and alopecia (Shepherd *et al.*, 2005).

The trade-off of Erlotinib is a higher incidence of cutaneous adverse effects resulting in follicular eruptions, seborrhea and painful fissures in the palms of the hands and soles of the feet. Several months after administration of the EGFR inhibitor, abnormal hair growth could occur, appearing in some cases as abnormally long eyelash growth or a slowing of scalp hair growth.

Hypertension is the most common toxicity with Bevacizumab, Bevacizumab should be discontinued in nephrotic syndrome, in hemorrhagic events, in venous thrombotic events and in gastrointestinal perforation.

Anemia

Anemia is the reason for many objective and subjective functional incapacities (table 12.24) (Mancuso *et al.*, 2006). It causes energy imbalance and emotional distress. Anemia has a negative impact on the majority of organs; in an elderly cancer population the consequences of anemia can be even more invalidating due to its contribution to the "fragility syndrome".

Table 12.24 - Effects of anemia on functional capacities.

– Decline of physical capacities
– Decline of functional functioning
– Decline of emotional functioning
– Higher risk of therapeutic complications
– Cardiovascular and central nervous comorbidity
– Mental decline
– Depression
– Fatigue

Anemia can be tumour-associated, e.g., cytokine-induced. It can occur as a result of chemotherapy or radiation therapy, or in connection with bone marrow infiltration, hemolysis or it can be nutrition-dependent. Considerable improvement of physical condition and functional/cognitive capacities and quality of life can be achieved when the hemoglobin level is raised (Cella, 1997).

The beneficial effects of erythropoetin on quality of life and functional/cognitive capacities have been proven (Mancuso *et al.*, 2006). The treatment should be started at Hb levels inferior to 9/dL and continued as long as Hb level remains below 12g/dL (Rizzo *et al.*, 2002). When Hb level is superior to 13g/dL there is a greater risk for thrombo-embolism.

Erythropoetin is effective in the case of anemia due to bone marrow infiltration as well; however, in this case, cytostatic or radiation therapies would generally be the preferred treatment.

Dyspnea

The reason for having dyspnea during terminal stage is often multifactorial. (Thomas et al., 2003). Lung cancer more frequently causes dyspnea than other types of cancer (Bruera et al., 1998).

In contrast to respiratory insufficiency documented by arterial blood gas analysis, dyspnea is a subjective feeling described as the "sensation of respiratory effort" and "discomfort in breathing". Dyspnea cannot be defined by physical abnormalities alone.

It is essential to find out whether dyspnea is caused directly by the tumour or associated with the treatment, or whether its aetiology has nothing to do with the tumour (table 12.25).

Table 12.25 - Causes and nature of dyspnea in terminal lung cancer patients.

- Decrease in respiratory surface
- Airway obstruction
- Hypoxemia
- Psychogenic dyspnea
- Concomitant disease
- Cardiovascular failure
- Neurologic disorder
- Anemia
- Cerebral vascular accident

Many different causes may co-exist in a lung cancer patient. Patients with bronchial cancer often suffer from chronic obstructive pulmonary disease, congestive heart failure, non malignant pleural effusion, pneumonitis, air flow obstruction, or bronchospasm associated with asthma. The accumulation of fluid in the pleural space is often associated with dyspnea, cough, and chest pain (Covey, 2005). In the absence of lung or heart disease, dyspnea may be a clinical expression of the syndrome of overwhelming cachexia and asthenia or of severe asthenia.

Whenever possible, an attempt should be made to treat the underlying cause of dyspnea. Radiotherapy, chemotherapy and target therapies may relieve dyspnea in the case of tumour-related shortness of breath. Symptomatic medication and non pharmacologic intervention in addition to specific treatments for the underlying cancer and/or other pulmonary and cardiovascular diseases are indicated. Drainage of pericardial or pleural effusions, treatment of pulmonary infections, and successful therapy of cardiovascular complications such as pulmonary embolism or congestive heart failure will all improve shortness of breath and the patient's ability to withstand cancer therapy.

In the case of dyspnea due to a bronchial stenosis the bronchus has to be opened. Patients with endobronchial stenoses are ideal candidates for Nd-Yag laser, electrocautery, argon plasma coagulation, endobronchial brachytherapy, cryotherapy or photodynamic therapy. Extrinsic compression or airway wall destruction requires the placement of an airway stent and eventually external beam radiation therapy.

While the administration of oxygen is effective in patients with hypoxemia, there are large individual variations in hypoxic respiration response and the placebo effect may be considerable. Patients should be freed from oxygen supplementation when they are at rest and experience fewer symptoms.

The role of transfusion therapy to relieve anemia-related dyspnea in advanced and terminal cancer patients has been proven. Blood transfusions or erythropoetin may decrease dyspnea due to anemia induced by chemotherapy.

Opioids improve dyspnea via the mechanism of respiratory depression. They reduce the respiration rate and weaken the sensation of the need of respiration effort. Oral or subcutaneous morphine should be started from small doses. For dyspnea due to multiple metastases, lymphangitis carcinomatosis and pneumonitis, oral, subcutaneous opioids (2-2.5mg s.c. morphine) or nebulised morphine are all useful agents in the management of pain and dyspnea. Morphine inhalation exerts direct effects on the suppression of airway secretion smooth muscle, as well as a systemic effect after absorption.

Aids for expectoration may be useful (mucolytic agents, nebulised saline, expectorants and physiotherapy). Non pharmacologic interventions such as positioning and scheduling activity, pursued lip breathing, relaxation, music and other therapies may relief breathlessness.

In some patients, benzodiazepines may be used when dyspnea is considered to be a somatic manifestation of a panic disorder or when patients have a coexisting anxiety disorder. Tested drugs include diazepam, lorazepam, alprazolam, promethazine and chlorpromazine.

A strong association has been found between airflow obstruction and dyspnea in some patients. Studies have shown that untreated airflow obstruction is often present in patients with bronchial carcinoma and is strongly associated with breathlessness. Bronchodilator therapy combining nebulized adrenergic and anticholinergic agents given four times per day relieves symptoms of cancer dyspnea.

It is important to help patients and families recognize the types of activities associated with increased dyspnea and accordingly plan anticipatory relief measures and avoidance of undue activity. Anticipatory relief measures may include premedicating with opioids or initiating behavioural techniques such as relaxation or imagery before a dyspnea-inducing activity. Avoidance includes assisting the patient to the maximum during an activity to minimize muscle effort and consequent dyspnea such as using a wheelchair and portable oxygen during hygiene or toiletting or for an outing.

Most endoscopic procedures are possible on an outpatient basis. They improve quality of life in a significant way (table).

There are different types of endoprotheses. If the tumour penetrates the stent it can be removed by the bronchoscope. Palliative chemotherapy is indicated in dyspnea due to lymphangiosis. Corticoids (6-12mg dexamethason) alleviate symptoms.

Pulmonary embolism is particularly common in patients with lung cancer, with as many as 20% of patients estimated to develop a deep vein thrombosis or pulmonary embolism during the course of their disease.

Hypercalcemia

The frequency of hypercalcemia in lung cancer is reported to be 12-35%. Unless treated promptly, hypercalcemia is life-threatening. Care must be taken not to confuse clinical symptoms of hypercalcemia (table 12.26) with the terminal-stage symptoms of cancer.

The standard treatment of moderate and severe cases is the intravenous infusion of bisphosphonates.

Table 12.26 - Major clinical symptoms of hypercalcemia.

– Extreme muscle weakness
– Fatigue
– Loss of appetite
– Nausea, vomiting
– Polydipsia and polyuria
– Constipation
– Anorexia
– Weakness
– Changes in heart rate
– Sleepiness
– Confusion
– Coma

Characteristics of pain therapy

See also chapter: "Pain management in cancer rehabilitation and palliation".

It is important to differentiate malignant from non-malignant aetiology. It is important to evaluate how much of the patient's complaints are, in fact, fear of malignant pain.

Palliative percutaneous (external) radiation therapy is primarily used to control pain due to bone metastases (table 5.15). Patients with a short life expectation may be treated safely with a single fraction of 8Gy.

Two different mechanisms apply. The first mechanism is that of reducing tumour volume (curative radiotherapy), involving elevated cumulative therapeutic doses and fractionation (e.g., 5 x 4Gy or 10 x 3Gy). The analgesic effect of fractionated radiotherapy correlates with cancer cell kill and occurs after several days or weeks of treatment. The second mechanism is that of symptomatic radiotherapy, requiring lower doses and only one shot (e.g., 1 x 8Gy). Pain relief is rapid. The "only" effect is reduction of peritumoural inflammatory acidosis, i.e., reduction of tumour swelling but not of actual tumour size.

Both regimens are equivalent in terms of pain and narcotic relief at three months and are tolerated with few adverse effects.

Pharmaceutical therapy of bone pain includes **non-steroidal analgesics and opiates** (tables 5.6, 5.9, 5.20, 5.21). Periphery-acting pain medications frequently have only short-term effects, if any at all, for this reason they should be administered very early together with long-term morphine preparations.

Bisphosphonates are excellent painkillers in osteolytic metastases. They do not influence tumour cell growth but decrease the proliferation and functional activity of osteoclasts. They may also be beneficial in subjects with predominantly osteoblastic metastatic processes. Parenteral administration of biphosphonates is indicated in symptomatic and oral administration in asymptomatic bone metastases. They should be already given in an asymptomatic stage because of reducing the risk of pathologic fractures, the need of bone irradiation, hypercalcaemia., immobilisation, spinal cord compression and last not least need of care (Rosen *et al.*, 2004).

Radionuclide therapy with bone seeking radiopharmaceuticals is one of the oldest interventions in nuclear medicine. It is an effective method of palliating **painful bone metastases** (Maini *et al.*, 2003).

Chronic pain patients frequently suffer from insomnia, anxiety, hopelessness and despair. They are prone to depression. All these symptoms lower the pain threshold and result in more severe pain and a higher analgesic requirement (fig. 5.2). Psychosocial support should always be considered as an adjunct to pharmacotherapy (fig. 5.1). If relaxation techniques and other non-medical measures are unsuccessful, pharmacotherapy is necessary (e.g., in the form of benzodiazepines). Anxiety affects the severity of pain. Tricyclic antidepressants and/or benzodiazepines may be administered in addition to analgesics for pain relief based on anxiolysis. The mood-uplifting effect of antidepressants helps to reduce the quantity of analgesics required.

Tricyclic antidepressants are mainly indicated in neuropathic pain. Antidepressants and antiseizure medications are commonly administered for continuous burning pain and painful dysaesthesia. A treatment strategy combining opioids and antidepressants is particularly effective in subjects with plexus involvement. Antidepressants are also used with success in painful iatrogenic polyneuropathy. In addition to their antidepressant and analgesic effect, some antidepressants (amitriptyline and doxepine, for instance) also have sedative effects and may be indicated for patients with sleep disorders.

In the case of painful cough, dihydrocodein works best. Sedation may be useful, especially at night.

Corticosteroids are indicated in numerous areas of pain management. One important feature is their anti-oedematous and inflammatory effect, which provides rapid relief in the presence of peritumoural oedema, nerve compression, joint pain, etc. Low-dose corticosteroids may have positive effects on mental status and appetite.

Long-term opioid therapy may be appropriate for carefully selected patients who can be monitored by their physicians and who can appropriately manage their medication (table 5.21). Opioids should be prescribed by only one physician (case manager). Long-acting opioids should be given on a time-contingent dosing schedule rather than as needed. Regular timed dosing intervals for opioids minimize the risk of psychological dependence. Oral preparations and opioid patches reduce the risk of addiction (table 5.23). Slow influx and constant levels provided by oral sustained release formulations and opioid patches minimize the euphoriant effect.

In contrast to people who are in normally health the physical and mental capacity of patients with tumour pain will improve after taking opioids. The risk of addiction is low.

Sleeplessness influences the level of pain sensitivity. Sleep quantity and quality are important in people living with cancer. If relaxation techniques and other non-medical measures are unsuccessful, pharmacotherapy is necessary (e.g., in the form of benzodiazepines).

Despite pulmonary function impairment, morphine derivatives have proven effective in lung cancer patients because of their concomitant antitussive effect. In pain patients the respiratory depressant effect of opioids is compensated by the stimulating effect of pain on respiration, with the result that the risk of respiratory depression is low in these patients.

Whenever possible, analgesics for chronic pain should be given orally or in stable conditions transdermally and not injected. This provides the patient with the highest possible degree of independence and comfort, enhances quality of life and prevents side effects such as addiction and dependence. If oral or transdermal administration is not an option, opioids may alternatively be administered sublingually, by the oral transmucosal route, rectally, by feeding tube, or parenterally.

Short-acting analgesics are the treatment of choice for acute pain states requiring immediate treatment.

Table 12.27 - Treatment routes for administering opioids.

– Oral (tablets, capsules, sustained-release and non-sustained-release formulations)
– Intramuscular
– Intravenous
– Subcutaneous
– Sublingual
– Transmucosal
– Transdermal (patches)
– Epidural/intrathecal

Anorexia and cachexia

Anorexia, the loss of appetite or desire to eat, may occur early in the disease process or later, in cases where the cancer progresses. Anorexia and cachexia, a wasting condition in which the patient has weakness and a marked and progressive loss of body weight, fat, and muscle, frequently occur together. In patients with advanced cancer, cachexia is primarily due to alterations in protein, carbohydrate and lipid metabolism caused by inflammatory cytokines released by the tumour.

There is no satisfactory drug therapy for cachexia. Corticosteroids may reduce anorexia but have no effect on the metabolic abnormalities of cancer cachexia. Megestrol acetate may exert an anabolic effect and reduce or prevent weight loss.

Enteral and parenteral nutrition will not reverse or prevent cancer cachexia, but it may be appropriate for patients who are temporarily unable to eat for two weeks or more because of anticancer treatment (Muscarotili *et al.*, 2006). Dronabinol may be effective in maintaining weight for some patients.

The family needs to be dissuaded from trying to force the patient to eat, as this will only cause physical distress and guilt.

Complementary and alternative therapies

Complementary and alternative medecine (CAM) use by lung cancer patients, especially women, is increasing. CAM use is greatest for difficult breathing and pain and perhaps prayer is the most commonly used CAM for all symptoms (Wells *et al.*, 2007). There is some support for the use of several modalities as potential complements to conventional cancer care, particularly for the quality of life issues associated with lung cancer symptoms (table 6.24).

For example, there is much support for the use of hypnosis in managing pain associated with medical procedures and some support for its use in managing chronic cancer pain. There is less evidence to support the use of modalities such as acupuncture, meditation and massage for management of chronic pain. However, there is some compelling data to support the use of acupuncture for nausea and vomiting associated with cancer treatments, and there are some data suggesting that qigong, neuro-emotional techniques, meditation techniques, and massage can decrease pain levels and improve the sense of well- being.

So far no scientific study has proven any tumour-inhibiting effects of mistletoe preparations. The assertion that the patient's quality of life can be improved through its use is very difficult to confirm. Yet these mistletoe preparations are not only used by those practicing alternative and nature-oriented forms of medicine, but also by some oncologists. The reason for this is less the belief in its effectiveness, but rather the possibility of being able to offer the patient a further therapy option. Experience has shown not only that "faith can move mountains", but that it can also improve the quality of life. One should not shatter these patients' faith in a particular therapy form with evidence-based arguments.

Quality assurance and rehabilitative measures

As with acute therapy, certain guidelines and quality assurance procedures should also apply to rehabilitation and palliation (Barat and Franchignoni, 2004). Unfortunately, there are only few guidelines on this subject in rehabilitation and palliation of lung cancer patients. There are guidelines for general pulmonary diseases (AACR, 2002) and guidelines for physiotherapy but none regarding rehabilitative needs of lung cancer patients and how to secure quality of the different rehabilitative and palliative measures.

To guarantee quality of rehabilitation and palliation you have to ensure quality of structures, quality of rehabilitative and palliative measures and to evaluate the outcome.

Quality of structural features

Therapies needed in rehabilitation and palliation should be provided by specialized rehabilitation services with a team of patient care specialists. Rehabilitation services include critical components of assessment, physical reconditioning, skill training, and psychosocial support. They may include vocational evaluation and counselling.

Special experience and a specialised infrastructure are essential for lung cancer rehabilitation services. They are overseen by a medical director to assure appropriate performance by the program staff and to assure proper service delivery. The team should be coordinated by a physician experienced in rehabilitation and palliation with demonstratable oncological and pulmonary knowledge. Physiotherapists play an important role in this team (fig. 1.4). The collaboration of psycho-oncologists is very useful. Social workers are essential because of the social aids that are often needed. Cooperation and the exchange of information with the previously and subsequently treating physicians are important.

A lung cancer rehabilitation service necessitates special rehabilitative equipment as well as qualified and experienced personnel. Due to the experience necessary, the rehabilitative institution should care for at least fifty lung cancer patients per year (Schmidt, 2001).

The physical area for pulmonary rehabilitation can vary greatly, depending upon program structure, patient population, needs, and resources. The site should provide an appropriate environment with adequate space, few interruptions or other distractions. There needs to be sufficient lighting, temperature control, and comfortable seating. It is essential to have adequate parking and handicap access.

Quality of medical and therapeutic processes

Verifiability of the quality of rehabilitation and palliative therapies must be guaranteed.

All members of the pulmonary rehabilitation team should participate in the patient's assessment. The initial evaluation should include the medical history, diagnostic tests, current symptoms and complaints, physical assessment, psychological, social and vocational needs, nutritional status, exercise tolerance, determination of educational needs, the patient's ability to carry out activities of daily living and the patient's interests and compliance.

The rehabilitation program must be tailored to meet the needs of the individual patient, addressing age-specific and cultural variables, and should contain patient-determined goals, as well as goals established by the individual team. Both patients and families participate in this training administered by health care professionals.

Outcome assessment and evaluation

The evaluation of rehabilitative measures in lung cancer patients is directed not at survival time, but rather at quality of life criteria. This includes subjective parameters such as improvement of pain, dyspnea, physical fitness, appetite, overcoming fears, etc. (table 12.28). In general these parameters are not found in **outcome assessment and evaluation** of primary therapy (response, remission and length of remission).

Outcome assessment in most clinical trials is affected by a purely medical understanding of the disease. This is reflected in the predominant use of pneumologic and oncologic symptoms as the content of outcome measures. The assessment of other health aspects like psychological symptoms, interpersonal or social consequences of the disease, seems to be similarly, if not more, important and should be considered in quality control of rehabilitation (table 12.28, 12.29).

Activities of daily life play an important role in rehabilitation. Widely used measures to assess activities of daily life are the functional independence measure or the Barthel Index (Mahoney and Barthel, 1965).

Rehabilitative care can be offered either on inpatient or outpatient basis. Carcinoma sufferers who have undergone surgery and chemotherapy are often weakened. For this reason, patients in Germany – as opposed to most other countries – are usually offered inpatient rehabilitation in specialised hospitals following primary therapy.

Table 12.28 - Parameters and examinations to be evaluated.

– Effect on quality of life
– Pulmonary function assessment, including arterial blood gas analysis
– Use of medical resources such as hospitalizations, urgent care/emergency room visits, or physician visits
– Exercise ability
– Dependence versus independence in activities of daily living
– Impairment in occupational performance
– Psychosocial problems, such as anxiety or depression
– Oxygen saturation at rest, with activity, and possibly during sleep
– Comorbidity
– Smoking history
– Motivation for rehabilitation, including commitment to spending the time necessary for active program participation
– Current medications
– Appropriate blood tests
– Electrocardiogram
– Chest radiograph
– Potential need of assistive devices, e.g., walker, wheel-chair
– Adherence to recommended treatment modalities
– Physician support available to patient
– Availability of transportation and patient/family desire to use what may be available

Table 12.29 - Possible therapeutic aims and their effectiveness parameters in the rehabilitation of lung cancer patients

Therapy goal	Parameter of effectiveness
Reduction of disorders resulting from surgery/ chemotherapy/radiation therapy	WHO-Toxicity scale, CTC-classification, CIRS-G, FACT-L, EORTC QLQ-C30 and LC13, LCSS, DDC, assessment of organ function CCM
Improvement of lung functional capacity, improvement of breathlessness	Spiro-ergometry, bedside spirometry, maximum inspiratory pressure (MIP), arterial blood gases, shuttle-walking-Test (SWT), visual analogue scales of shortness of breath. Questionnaires: EORTC QLQ-LC13
Pain relief	Pain diary, reduction of analgesic drugs, pain sensitivity scales. Questionnaires: Pain Disability Index (PDI), EORTC QLQ-C30, SE36, SDS, RSCL, LCSS, FACT-L
Relief of pneumonitis	Reduction of symptoms, measurement of CO_2-diffusion, heart rate
To quit smoking	CO-Test
Improvement of physical fitness	KPS, ECOG, ergometry, KPS, WHO- and EORTC-Performance-Status, exercise capacity (symptom-limited bicycle ergometry), muscle force (hand-held dynamometry), walking distances, shuttle walking test. Questionnaires: : ADL, IADL, (EORTC) QLQ-LC-13, LC-13, CCM, Fact-L, Fact-An, QLQ-C30, LCSS, Nottingham Health Profile, ESAS.
Family member counselling	Questionnaires
Information on illness, follow-up examinations, signs of recurrence, therapy in the case of of recurrence, behaviour-influencing illness	Questionnaires, tests
Reduction of anxiety, depression, fatigue	Rating scales. Questionnaires: POMS, STAI, BDI, BFI, BSI, HADS-D, GDS, Symptom Checklist-90, SDS, MFI
Coping with illness	Questionnaires: FKV, FKV-LIS, BEFO, TSK, FIBECK
Clarification and improvement of vocational fitness	Resumption of vocation, length of time of inability to work, FLI-C
Reduction of necessity of nursing care	Questionnaires: Barthel Index, FIM, reduction of level of nursing care, ADL, CIRS-G, IADL, FLI-C
Relief of symptoms	Questionnaire: POS

ADL = Activities of Daily Life; BFI = Brief Fatigue Inventory; CCM = Cancer Care Monitor; CIRS-G = Cumulative Illness Rating Scale Geriatric; DDC = Daily Diary Card; EORTC-QLQ = European Organization for Research and Treatment of Cancer Quality of Life Questionnaire; ECOG = European Cooperative Oncology Group-Scale; ESAS = Edmonton Assessment Scale; Fact-G = Functional Assessment of Cancer Therapy (General); Fact-L = Functional Assessment of Cancer Therapy (Lung); Fact-An = Functional Assessment of Cancer Therapy (Anaemia); FIBECK = Freiburg Inventory on Coping with Chronic Illness; FIM = Functional Independence Measure; FLI-C = Functional Living Index-Cancer; GDS = Geriatric Depression Scale; HADS-D = Hospital Anxiety and Depression Scale; IADL = Instrumental Activity Daily Living; KPS = Karnofsky Performance Scale; MFI = Multidimensional Fatigue Inventory; LCSS = Lung Cancer Symptom Scale; PDI = Pain Disability Index; POMS = Profile of Mood Status; POS = Palliative Care Outcome Scale; RSCL = Rotterdam-Symptom Checklist; SDS = Symptom Distress Scale; STAI = Spiegelberger Trait Anxiety Inventory

Measurements of quality of life

Studies of quality of life in lung cancer patients have been performed mainly in therapeutic trials in order to assess the disease and treatment of specific symptoms. The studies mainly used performance status as a proxy regarding quality of life, even though there is only a weak association between the performance status such as the Karnofsky Performance Scale and the quality of life as measured by the EORTC QLQ-C30 (Montazeri *et al.*, 1998). Palliation of symptoms, psychosocial interventions, and understanding patient's feelings and concerns all contribute to improve quality of life in lung cancer patients.

The most widely used tools to measure quality of life include the European Organization for Research and Treatment of Cancer Quality of Life the quality questionnaire (EORTC QLQ-C30), (Aaronson *et al.*, 1993) and the Amrican equivalent, the functional assessment of cancer therapy (FACT) questionnaire (Bonomi *et al.*, 1999). These tools are self-reporting questionnaires designed for the patients.

Basically, improvement in quality of life is attained when there is less nursing care ("rehabilitation to combat the need of care"), when the patient can be vocationally reintegrated ("rehabilitation to combat early retirement"), when he/she feels secure ("rehabilitation to combat resignation and depression") and when the patient's physical handicaps and functional limitations are at a minimum ("rehabilitation to combat disability").

Bibliography

- AARC Clinical Practice Guideline (2002) Pulmonary rehabilitation. Respir Care 47(5): 617-25
- Abid SH, Malhotra V, Perry MC (2001) Radiation-induced and chemotherapy-induced pulmonary injury. Curr Opin Oncol 13: 242-8
- Abrahm J (2004) Assessment and treatment of patients with malignant spinal cord compression. J Support Oncol 2: 377-401
- Algar FJ, Alvarcz A, alvatierra A *et al.* (2002) Predicting pulmonary complications after pneumonectomy for lung cancer. Eur J Cardiothorac Surg 2003; 23: 201-8
- Ampil F, Caldito G (2006) Radiotherapy for palliation of lung cancer in patients with compromised hearts. J Pall Med 9, 2: 241-2
- Akira M, Ishikawa H, Yamamoto S (2002) Drug-induced Pneumonitis: Thin-Section CT Findings in 60 Patients Radiology 224: 852-60
- Arbeiter K, Prakash U, Tazelaar H *et al.* (1999) Radiation-Induced Pneumonitis in the "Non-Irradiated" Lung. Mayo Clin Proc. 74: 27-36
- Aspinal F, Hughes R, Higginson I *et al.* (2002) A user's guide to the palliative care outcome scale. Palliative care & policy publications. Kings College, London
- Barat M, Franchignoni F (2004) Assessment in physical medicine and rehabilitation. Maugeri Foundation Books, PI-ME Press Pavia
- Bausewein C, Fegg M, Radbruch L *et al.* (2005) Validation and clinical application of the German version of the palliative care outcome. J Pain Symptom Manage 30: 51-62
- Bergman B, Aaronson N *et al.* (1994) The EORTC QLQ-LC13: a modular supplement to the EORTC Core Quality of Life Questionnaire for use in lung cancer clinical trials. Eur J Cancer 30A, 635-42

- Bruera E, Ripamonti C (1998) Dyspnea in Patients with Advanced Cancer in Supportive Oncology. Berger A, Portenoy R, Weissman D, ed, Lippincott-Raven, 295-308
- Bundesarbeitsgemeinschaft für Rehabilitation (2003) Rahmenempfehlungen zur ambulanten onkologischen Rehabilitation. Bundesarbeitsgemeinschaft für Rehabilitation Frankfurt
- Bunn PA, Lilenbaum R (2003) Chemotherapy for elderly patients with advanced non-small-cell lung cancer. J Natl Cancer Inst, 5, 95: 341-3
- Cella D, Bonomi A et al. (1995) Reliability and validity of the functional assessment of cancer therapy-lung (Fact-L) quality of life instrument. Lung Cancer 12, 3: 199-220
- Cella D (1997) The functional assessment of cancer therapy anaemia (FACT-An) scale: A new tool for the assessment of outcomes in cancer anemia and fatigue. Semin Hematol 34 (suppl 2): 13-9
- Celli BR (2004) Chronic respiratory failure after lung resection: the role of pulmonary rehabilitation. Thorac Surg Clin 14, 3: 417-28
- Chanan A, Srinivasan S, Czuczman M (2004) Prevention and management of cardiotoxicity from antineoplastic therapy. J Support Oncol 2: 251-66
- Colchen A, Gonin F, Bonnette P (2004) The place of interventional endoscopy in the treatment of lung cancer. Rev Pneumol Clin 60, 3: 48-50
- Covey,A (2005) Management of malignant pleural effusions and ascites. J Support Oncol 3:169-76
- Delbrück H, Schmid L, Bartsch H et al. (2000) Zur Ergebnisqualität in der onkologischen Rehabilitation. Rehabilitation 39: 359-62
- De Gregorio Ariza MA, Gamboa P, Gimeno M et al. (2003) Percutaneous treatment of superior vena cava syndrome using metallic stents. Eur Radiol 8: 252-63
- Deschamps, Bernard A, Nichols C et al. (2001) Empyema and brochopleural fistula after pneumonectomy: Factors affecting incidence. Ann. Thorac Surg 72: 243-8
- Donner CF (2006) Vocational rehabilitation and pulmonary programs. In: Gobelet C, Franchignoni F (Edit) Vocational rehabilitation Springer Paris 185-194
- Dorman U, Weis J, Bartsch HH (2006) Qualitätssicherung in der onkologischen Rehabilitation. Der Onkologe, Heidelberg (in Press)
- Dubey S, Brown R, Esmond S et al. (2005) Patient preferences in choosing chemotherapy regiments for advanced non-small cell lung cancer. J Support Oncol 3: 149-54
- Dubois A, Schlaich M et al. (1999) Evaluation of neurotoxicity induced by paclitaxel second-line chemotherapy. Support Care cancer 7: 354
- Dunton JC (2002) Management of treatment-related toxicity in advanced ovarian cancer. Oncologist 7: 11-9
- Earle C, Tsai JS, Gelber RD (2001) Effectiveness of chemotherapy for advanced lung cancer in the elderly. J Clin Oncol 19, 4: 1064-70
- Edel H, Knauth K (1999) Grundzüge der Atemtherapie Urban & Fischer, München
- ESMO (2001) Minimum clinical recommendations for diagnosis, treatment and follow-up of small-cell cancer. Ann Oncol 12: 1051
- ESMO (2001) Minimum clinical recommendations for diagnosis, treatment and follow-up of non small cell cancer. Ann Oncol 12: 1049
- Estfan B, LeGrand S (2004) Management of cough in advanced cancer. J Support Oncol 2: 523-7
- Freitag L (2004) Interventional endoscopic treatment. Lung Cancer 45,2: 235-8

- Fromme E, Eilers KM, Mori M *et al.* (2004) How accurate is clinician reporting of chemotherapy adverse effects? J Clin Oncol 22, 17: 3485-90
- Fryback D, Craig BM (2004) Measuring economic outcomes of cancer. J Natl Cancer Inst Monographs 33: 134-41
- Gridelli C, Perrone F, Nelli F *et al.* (2001) Quality of life in lung cancer patients. Annals of oncology 12, 3: 21
- Harada H, Okada M, Sakamoto T *et al.* (2005) Functional advantage after radical segmentectomy versus lobectomy for lung cancer. Ann Thorac Surg 80, 6: 2041-5
- Hill K, Amir Z *et al.* (2003) Do newly diagnosed lung cancer patients feel their concerns are being met? Eur J Cancer Care 12, 1: 35-45
- Hollen P, Grall R *et al.* (1993) Quality of life assessment in individuals with lung cancer: Testing the Lung Cancer symptom Scale (LCSS). Eur J Cancer 29A, 1: 551-8
- Hopwood P, Stephens RJ (2000) Depression in patients with lung cancer: Prevalence and risk factors derived from quality of life data. J clin Oncol 18, 4: 893-903
- Huisman C, Smit EF, Giaccone G *et al.* (2000) Second--line chemotherapy in relapsing or refractory non-small cell lung cancer: A review. J Clin Oncol 18: 3722-30
- Kelly K, Bunn J (1998) Is it time to reevaluate our approach to the treatment of brain metastases in patients with non-small-cell lung cancer? Lung cancer 20: 85-91
- Korfee S, Gauler T, Hepp R *et al.* (2004) New targeted treatments in lung cancer – overview of clinical trials. Lung Cancer 45, 2: 199-208
- Licker M, Spiliopoulos A, Frey J *et al.* (2005) Risk factors for early mortality and major complications following pneumonectomy for non small cell carcinoma of the lung. Chest 121: 1890-7
- Limper AH (2004) Chemotherapy-induced lung disease. Clin Chest Med 25: 53-64
- Maguire P, Pitceathly C (2002) Key communication skills and how to aquire them. BMJ 325: 697-700
- Maini C, Sciutu R, Romano L, Bergomi S (2003) Radionuclide therapy with bone seeking radionuclides in palliation of painful metastases. J Exp Clin Cancer Res 22, 4: 71-4
- Mamon H, Wen PY, Loeffler JS (1999) Allergic skin reactions to anticonvulsant medications in patients receiving cranial radiation. Epilepsia 40 (3): 341-4
- Mancuso A, Migliorino M, de Santis S *et al.* (2006) Correlation between anemia and functional/cognitive capacity in elderly lung cancer patients treated with chemotherapy. Annals of oncoloy 17: 146-150
- Miller AB *et al.* (2004) Fruits and vegetables and lung cancer: Findings from the European Prospective Investigation into Cancer and Nutrition. Int J Cancer 108: 269-76
- Montazeri A, Gillis CR, McEwen J (1998) Quality of life in patients with lung cancer. Chest 113: 467-81
- Muscarotili M, Bossola M, Aversa Z *et al.* (2006) Prevention and treatment of cancer cachexia: New insights into an old problem. Eurp J Cancer 42: 31-41
- Mutee F, Jatoi A (2006) Megestrol aceatate for the palliation of anorexia in advanced, incurable patients. Clin Nutr 6
- Neuberger JS, Field RW (2003) Occupation and lung cancer in non smokers. Rev Environ Health 18, 4: 251--67
- Paice J (2003) Mechanisms and management of neuropathic pain in cancer. J support Oncol 1, 2: 107-14

– Pawel J, Schiller JH, Shepherd FA *et al.* (1999) Topotecan versus Cyclophosphamide, Doxorubicin, and Vincristine for the Treatment of Recurrent Small Cell Lung Cancer. J Clin Oncol 17, 2: 658

– Pezner RD, Bertrand M, Cecchi G *et al.* (1984) Steroid-withdrawal radiation pneumonitis in cancer patients. Chest 85: 816-7

– Ramsey SD, Howlader N, Etzioni RD *et al.* (2004) Chemotherapy use, outcomes, and costs for older persons with advanced non-small lung cancer. J Clin Oncol 22 (24): 4971-8

– Rizzo JD, Lichtin A *et al.* (2002) Use of epoetin in patients with cancer: Evidence-based clinical practice guidelines of the American society of clinical oncology and the American society of haematology. J Clin Oncol 20: 4083-4107

– Robnett T, Machtay M, Vines EF *et al.* (2000) Factors predicting severe radiation pneumonitis in patients receiving definitive chemoradiation for lung cancer. Int J Radiat Oncol Bio Phys 1, 48, 1: 89-94

– Ron IG, Stav O, Vishne T *et al.* (2004) The correlation between palliation of bone pain by intravenous strontium 89 and external beam radiation to linked field in patients with osteoblastic bone metastases. Am J Clin Oncol 27 (5): 5004

– Rosen LS, Gordon D, Tchekmedyian NS *et al.* (2004) Long-term efficacy and safety of zoledronic acid in the treatment of skeletal metastases in patients with non-small-cell lung cancer and other solid tumours. Cancer 100, 12: 2613-21

– Schofield P, Ball D, Smith JG *et al.* (2004) Optimism and survival in lung carcinoma patients. Cancer 100, 6: 1276-82

– Seegenschmidt M (1998) Nebenwirkungen in der Onkologie. Springer, Berlin, Heidelberg, New York, Tokyo

– Seute T, Leffers P, ten Velde GP *et al.* (2004) Neurologic disorders in 432 consecutive patients with small-cell lung carcinoma. Cancer 100: 801-6

– Shepherd F, Pereira J, Ciuleanu T *et al.* (2005) Erlotinib in previously treated Non-small-cell lung cancer. N Engl J Med 353: 123-32

– Sleijfer S (2001) Bleomycin-induced pneumonitis. Chest 120, 2: 617-24

– Spruit MA, Janssen PP, Willemsen SC *et al.* (2006) Exercise capacity before and after an 8-week multidisciplinary inpatient rehabilitation program in lung cancer patients. Lung Cancer (Mar)

– Stanley H, Kelley K (2004) CNS home visits following diagnosis of lung cancer. Cancer Nursing Practice 3, 2: 33-9

– Stinnett H, S, Williams C, Johnson D (2007) Role of chemotherapy for palliation in the lung cancer patient. J Support Oncol 5, 1: 19-24

– Sugimura, Yang H (2006) Long-term Survivorship in Lung Cancer*Chest. 129: 1088-97

– Tamburini M. (2001) Health related quality of life measures in cancer. Ann Oncol 12 (suppl 3): 7

– Thomas J, von Gunten C (2003) Management of dyspnea. J Support Oncol 1: 23-32

– Von Pawel J, Gatzemeier U, Pujol JL *et al.* (2001) Comparator of oral versus intravenous Topotecan in patients with chemosensitive small-cell lung cancer. J Clin Oncol 19: 1743-9

– Wells M, Sarna L, Cooley M *et al.* (2007) Use of complementary and alternative medicine therapies to control symptoms in women living with lung cancer. Cancer Nurs 30, 1: 45-55

– Zatloukal P, Petrzelka L *et al.* (2004) Concurrent versus sequential chemo radiotherapy with cisplatin and vinorelbine in locally advanced non-small-cell lung cancer: A randomized study. Lung cancer 46, 1: 87-98

Rehabilitation and palliation of patients with prostatic cancer

Aims of rehabilitation and palliation: Definition as distinct from curative tumour follow-up care

The chief aim of all medical, potentially **curative follow-up care** measures (recurrence prophylaxis, early detection and therapy of disease recurrence) is to lengthen survival time (fig. 1.3). The cancer disease thus represents the focus of curative follow-up care.

Rehabilitative and palliative measures, on the other hand, are not carried out in order to influence the disease, but rather to reduce the severity of the disabilities due to the tumor and implemented therapies. A significant improvement in the quality of life is the goal and the aim of all therapeutic procedures. All measures are necessary in order to alleviate the negative effects of the cancer disease and therapy, not only physically, but also psychologically, socially and vocationally (fig. 1.2). It is not so much the survival time as the quality during the time remaining and the activities of daily living which are to be positively influenced.

The nature and extent of the therapeutic measures necessary in rehabilitation (tables 3.1, 3.2) are determined primarily by the severity of the impairments. This is very different in comparison with curative follow-up care which considers, for the most part, the extent and the prognosis of the malignancy.

In theory, the aims of curative follow-up care can be differentiated simply and clearly from those of rehabilitation and palliation. In practice, however, there is much overlapping. This involves in particular tumour recurrence therapy and palliative measures. Potentially curative recurrence therapy does not only serve to prolong survival time, but also to alleviate symptoms.

Since it is well-known that complete elimination of a recurrence can not be attained by means of routine diagnostics, even if it has been detected at an asymptomatic stage, the value of routine follow-up diagnostics must be questioned. The value of prophylactic forms of therapy (adjuvant hormone-, chemo- and radiation therapy) is controversial, and therapy of disease recurrence brings marginal gains in survival time, if any at all. As long as the potentially curative measures (recurrence prophylaxis, early detection and therapy of recurrence) have failed to show a significant survival benefit, rehabilitative and palliative measures in the follow-up care of patients with carcinoma of the prostate gland will continue to be a main focus.

Rehabilitative measures in follow-up care

Rehabilitative measures can be considered for patients undergoing potentially curative as well as palliative treatment. There may be different problems and different rehabilitation measures according to the extent of the disease, according to the prior therapy, the comorbidity and the motivation of the patient as well. Comorbidity which is quite frequent in old men must also be treated during rehabilitation.

A certain minimum amount of information about the patient's disease status is required (table 13.1) before initiating and administering rehabilitative and palliative forms of therapy. Without this information, valuable time is wasted, thus threatening the success of rehabilitation. A rehabilitative assessment has to be conducted, including rehabilitation planning and documentation of the goals to be achieved (Barat and Franchignoni, 2004).

Table 13.1 - Minimum amount of information prior to rehabilitation in prostatic cancer patients.

– Extent of tumour (TNM) including grading of the tumour?
– Curative or palliative approach? R0, R1 or R2 resection of the tumour?
– Curative or palliative radiotherapy?
– Has prior hormone therapy and/or chemotherapy and/or radiotherapy taken place? (If yes, which drugs have been used, what dosages were prescribed and what were the results?)
– Has prior radiotherapy taken place? (External or internal? What dose and what were the results?)
– Curative or palliative approaches of prior surgery (i.e., radical prostatectomy, resection of the prostate gland)?
– Psychosocial information (for example, family structure, statements given pertaining to degree of patient information, problems with coping or compliance, support given by family members, social and occupational problems, etc.)?

Rehabilitation measures to reduce physical problems ("rehabilitation to combat invalidity")

The most frequently used treatments for prostatic cancer are surgery (e.g., radical retropubic prostatectomy, radical perineal prostatectomy), radiation therapy (e.g., brachytherapy, external beam radiation therapy, 3-dimensional conformal radiation therapy, intensity-modulated radiation therapy), cryoablative therapy and hormone/chemotherapies. Each of them may lead to physical impairments demanding rehabilitative interventions (Yablon, 2004).

The spectrum of possible physical impairments and deficiencies is large (table 13.2). Physical impairments are often present against a background of comorbidities and polypharmacy in older patients.

Table 13.2 - Therapy induced physical impairments and deficiencies in prostatic cancer patients demanding rehabilitative intervention.

– Urinary incontinence
– Urethral strictures
– Lymphedema
– Lymphocele
– Erectile dysfunctions
– Hormonal problems
– Complaints after orchiectomy
– Unwanted side effects of radiotherapy and/or chemotherapy
– Nutritional problems

Urinary incontinence and recommendations of treatment

Urinary incontinence has a significant negative impact on quality of life. The fear of urine leaking, having the scent of urine or to use diapers is humiliating for many men. There is a great risk of social withdrawal which is often mistaken for major depression. This situation, if disregarded, can lead to significant anxiety and depression, which may then need to be treated by anxiolytics or antidepressants.

Stress incontinence is more common after surgery, while irritative symptoms during urination and urge incontinence occurs more often after radiotherapy. In most patients, urine incontinence after surgery is caused by a sphincter defect, detrusor-hyperactivity and/or a mixed incontinence.

Urodynamics can help to evaluate the function of the bladder and the sphincter muscle to determine the exact cause of the postprostatectomy incontinence. Normally, as the bladder fills, there is very little change in bladder pressure and the sphincter remains closed. When incontinence occurs following prostatectomy, this normal balance of bladder and sphincter function is disturbed.

Up to half of all men develop urinary incontinence after radical prostatectomy for weeks to a few months. The symptoms range from the need to wear urinary incontinence pads, occasional dribbling to complete inability to store or control urinary leakage, independent of physical activity (total incontinence) (table 13.5).

Some experience no leakage and a small percentage will have continued long-term or permanent leaking. Studies show that one year after prostatectomy between 15% and 50% of men still report urinary problems. There is a 10% risk of stress incontinence lasting up to three years following surgery. Some of them experience long- term incontinence (Potasky *et al.*, 2000).

Patients who can stop the flow of the urine have a good prognosis (tables 13.3, 13.4) (Mc. Glynn *et al.*, 2004).

Table 13.3 - Increased risk for development of urinary incontinence following radical prostatectomy.

- Prior transurethral resection of the prostate
- Preoperative micturition disorders
- Extensive tumour
- Malignant invasion of external sphincter
- Prostatectomy after prior radiotherapy
- Presence of prostatic adenome and prior incontinence problems
- Advanced age
- Combination of radiotherapy and surgery

Table 13.4 - Favourable prognostic factors for reduction of continence recovery time.

- No incontinence at rest
- Capacity to stop urine flow
- Occasional dribbling

Table 13.5 - Graduation of severity in urine incontinence.

- Grade I: Involuntary dribbling when coughing or lifting up goods
- Grade II: Incontinence when walking, moving, standing up
- Grade III: Complete inability to store or control urinary leakage; total incontinence at rest

Conservative management is the primary rehabilitative measure and consists mainly of lifestyle adjustments including reduction in caffeine consumption, physical exercise, cessation of smoking, and bladder retraining. Urinary incontinence can be alleviated with symptomatic treatments (e.g., catheters, pads, clamps, drip collectors, condom catheter devices) and/or causal treatments (e.g., pelvic floor muscle training, biofeedback assisted pelvic floor exercises, electrical stimulation using a rectal electrode, transcutaneous electrical nerve stimulation, or a combination of these methods). Anticholinergic medications, serotonin and norepinephrine reuptake inhibitors (duloxetin) may help. Effective surgical therapies are the endo-urethral injection of bulking agents, the placement of a male sling or an artificial urinary sphincter (table 13.6).

Table 13.6 - Possible measures to regain urinary control after prostatectomy; treatments for urinary incontinence.

- Catheters
- Absorption products (pads or underwear)
- Conservative management (pelvic floor muscle training, biofeedback, electrical stimulation using a rectal electrode, transcutaneous electrical nerve stimulation, or a combination of methods)
- Compression devices
- Medications
- Artificial sphincters
- Collagen injections to narrow the urethra

Indwelling urethral catheters (**Foley catheters**) should be used only for a short period (usually overnight) to ensure that there will be no problems. **Condom catheters** are only for short-term use, because long-term use increases the risk of urinary tract infections, damage to the penis from friction with the condom, and urethral blockage. They are attached to the outside drains leaking urine into a bag that is worn under the man's clothing. They must be changed at least every other day, to protect the skin of the penis and prevent urinary tract infections. **Suprapubic catheters** are more comfortable, less prone to infection and most likely will not fall out or leak. They need to be changed just like an indwelling catheter at least every four weeks. A suprapubic catheter is preferable to an indwelling catheter in persons who require chronic bladder drainage.

A wide variety of **pads** are available for managing the leakage of urine associated with urinary incontinence. To control leakage, men can wear an absorbent pad inside the underwear or a disposable undergarment. There are pads available for all degrees of severity. Possible complications are: Irritations, allergic reactions, eczema and infections. They are not indicated in severe forms of incontinence. Men with urinary incontinence are often at risk for skin rashes and breakdown. Good skin care and preventing skin breakdown is very important.

Several types of **incontinence clamps** are available but many problems such as skin breakdown, swelling, strictures (scarring) can occur inside of the urethra if they are left in place too long. The Cunningham Clamp is the one most often used. Clamps must be taken off at least every one to two hours to urinate. Otherwise the bladder becomes full and can cause severe infections. They can cause problems such as prolonged compression of the penis that can lead to urethral stricture, decreased blood flow to the penis causing necrosis of the penis, or skin breakdown.

Men who have problems with constant leakage of small amounts of urine may find that a **drip collector** is sufficient. A drip collector is a small pocket of absorbent padding with a waterproof back side. The drip collector is worn over the penis and is held in place by close fitting underwear.

Men can also use a **condom catheter device**. This product is placed over the penis similar to a condom. It has a tube on the end and connects with a collection bag tied to the leg. This device can handle small or large volumes of urine with little odor, minimal skin irritation, and easy use. Apart from the risk of infections and allergic reactions, the disadvantage is that the devices will prevent muscle control development necessary to regain continence. Men with a small penis often do have to wear these condoms.

Pelvic floor rehabilitation

The treatment of stress incontinence has a high success rate using measures such as pelvic floor exercises which significantly reduce continence recovery time (van Kampen et al., 2000; Filocamo et al., 2005). Success can be evaluated by the use of pads daily (Mathewson-Chapman, 1997; van Kampen et al., 2000).

Training the pelvic floor musculature can be done by active or by passive strengthening. Active rehabilitation of the pelvic floor includes pelvic floor exercises (Kegal exercises). These exercises work by strengthening the muscles that control urination. Individuals are instructed to do the pelvic muscle exercises three times daily and, optimally, to perform the exercises in three positions – lying, sitting and standing. Results may not occur until after six-eight weeks of exercise, and optimal results usually take longer. Pelvic floor exercises should not be practised by men with a catheter in place.

Passive strengthening of the pelvic floor includes pelvic floor stimulation (PFS) by electrical stimulation of pelvic floor muscles using either a probe wired to a device for controlling the electrical stimulation, or, more recently, extracorporeal pulsed magnetic innervation. It is thought that pelvic floor stimulation of the pudendal nerve will improve urethral closure by activating the pelvic floor musculature. In addition, PFS is thought to improve partially denervated urethral and pelvic floor musculature by enhancing the process of reinnervation.

Biofeedback is a training program that can be used to reinforce the proper performance of pelvic floor muscle training. Biofeedback uses measuring devices to help the patient become aware of his body's functioning. By using electronic devices or diaries to track when urethral muscles contract, the patient can gain control over these muscles. Biofeedback can be used with pelvic muscle exercises and electrical stimulation to relieve stress and urge incontinence.

Serotonin and norepinephrine reuptake inhibitors (duloxetin) can be taken in conjunction with a regime of pelvic floor exercises. Duloxetin works by increasing the strength of the sphincter in the urethra. The most common side – effect is nausea but this usually wears off within a month.

There is a variety of medications that may be used to treat urinary incontinence. Decongestants may tighten up the muscles of the urethra and are used for stress incontinence. Anticholinergic drugs, which block messages to the bladder nerves and prevent bladder spasms, are sometimes recommended for urge incontinence.

To note is that some drugs can cause or contribute to urinary incontinence (table 13.7).

In the case of a long-lasting and therapy-resistant incontinence, an urge incontinence, a chronic infection and a damage to the sphincter should be ruled out as causes.

Neither drugs nor conservative treatments are indicated in total incontinence. Two surgical procedures may be used. One is the insertion of an artificial urinary sphincter and the other treatment consists of peri-urethral collagen injections.

In the case of small defects, a **collagen injection** may be sufficient. Many men consider the use of trans-urethral collagen injections as a more appealing alternative than placement of an artificial sphincter or a sling, as it is a simple, low-risk, non-surgical procedure. Series of collagen injections may be given to narrow the bladder neck and reduce leakage in case of incomplete closing of the urinary sphincter. Peri-urethral collagen injections have a reported success rate of approximately 40% in cases of severe stress incontinence and persistent leakage.

Implantation of an **artificial sphincter** (Amarenco and Chantraine 2006) has been successful in relieving incontinence in up to 90% of men. It is a treatment method that is generally reserved for patients whose other treatment options have failed.

An artificial sphincter has an inflatable cuff that fits around the urethra close to the point where it joins the bladder. A balloon regulates the pressure of the cuff, and a bulb controls inflation and deflation of the cuff. The balloon is surgically placed within the pelvic area, and the control bulb is placed in the scrotum. The cuff is inflated to keep urine from leaking. When urination is desired, the cuff is deflated, allowing urine to drain out. Since complications may occur, this is a treatment method that is generally reserved for people for whom all other treatment options have failed (Smith *et al.*, 2002). Patients should be informed that complications (e.g., revision because of mechanical malfunction, erosions, infections, casting off) necessitating device revision and/or explantation may appear later.

In well-selected candidates, the **male sling** is an effective treatment (Haab *et al.*, 1997). The bulbo-urethral sling procedure has emerged as a less invasive and less costly option for men with severe postprostatectomy incontinence. Functional or structural damage to the urethra that can occur during surgery renders the urethra vulnerable to abdominal pressures, which the sling, composed of either synthetic materials or human fascia or dermis, seeks to combat by compressing and elevating the urethra.

Table 13.7 - Drugs that can cause or contribute to urinary incontinence.

Drug class	Mechanism of incontinence
Drugs causing overflow incontinence	
Anticholinergics	
Antidepressants	Decreased bladder contractions with retention
Antipsychotics	Decreased bladder contractions with retention
Sedative-hypnotics	Decreased bladder contractions with retention
Antihistamines	Decreased bladder contractions with retention
Nervous system depressants	
Narcotics	Decreased bladder contractions with retention
Alcohol	Decreased bladder contractions with retention
Calcium channel blockers	Decreased bladder contractions with retention
Alpha-adrenergic agonists	Sphincter contraction with outflow obstruction
Beta-adrenergic blockers	Sphincter contraction with outflow obstruction
Drugs causing stress incontinence	
Alpha-adrenergic antagonists	Sphincter relaxation with urinary leakage
Drugs causing urge incontinence	
Diuretics	Contractions stimulated by high urine flow
Caffeine	Diuretic effect
Sedative-hypnotics	Depressed central inhibition of micturition
Alcohol	Diuretic effect and depressed central inhibition

Urethral strictures and recommendations of treatment

Up to 4% of patients being treated by surgery and/or by external radiotherapy experience urethral stricture. Urethral stricture is the most common late complication of trans-urethral prostatectomy and cryotherapy. A stricture of the urethra caused by scar tissue can block the flow of urine and result in overflow incontinence.

The decreased urinary stream can be confirmed by uroflowmetry and postvoid residual urine by ultrasonography. Subsequently, retrograde urethrography can be performed to confirm anastomotic stricture in patients with a weak urinary stream.

Strictures can be treated by incising the scar tissue surgically or by dilating (stretching) the urethra. It can be done on an outpatient basic

To note is that blocking of the urine flow can be due to tumour growth as well.

Lymphedema and recommendations of treatment

After a radical prostatectomy or pelvic radiation, there is an increased risk for developing lymphedema resulting from surgical incisions, removal of lymph nodes and the radiation scarring. Additionally, advancing prostate cancer can block or reduce lymphatic or venous outflow from the lower extremities and pelvis leading to lower extremity edema.

A swollen leg can be a challenge to move. It is possible for the swollen tissues to press on nerves causing pain. Genital edema can limit mobility and make use of the penis for urination difficult.

Early diagnosis (table 13.8) and manual lymphdrainage is required in order to prevent progression of lymphedema. If left untreated, changes in tissues in the affected parts of the body take place which makes treatments more difficult.

Table 13.8 - Early symptoms and warning signs of lymphedema.

- Feeling of tightness in the skin
- Feeling of tightness around the leg
- Achy feeling in a leg
- A tight sensation foot
- Noticeable swelling in thighs, legs or feet when physical effort is exerted
- Decreased flexibility
- Legs of the trousers feel tight
- Sudden increase in weight, not associated with overeating
- Pitting is positive (occurs when a finger pressed against the skin indents and holds the indentation)
- Paresthesia in the upper leg

The usual treatment is to initiate "complex decongestive therapy" (**manual lymphdrainage**) plus **bandaging** plus education plus fitting of special garments. Lymphdrainage must be repeated at regular intervals. Meanwhile bandaging and compressing stockings are indicated in severe edema.

Manual lymphdrainage should not be used over areas of active or potential cancer (however, in the case of palliative care and generalized metastasis lymphdrainage may be allowed). It is contraindicated in the presence of active infection or deep vein thrombosis in the limb. It is contraindicated during radiotherapy (however, lymphdrainage is possible during chemotherapy). Lymphedema may be exacerbated in saunas, steam baths or hot tubs, in hot climates or travel.

Diuretics may help in the short term as they remove excess fluid from the body via urination. They do not remove the excess protein deposits found in lymphedema and there is evidence that long-term use can be harmful by leading to connective tissue fibrosis.

Having a **compression sock** on only the lower leg is a bad idea. A whole leg swelling needs a full leg length compression stocking with sufficient compressive strength to hold the swelling down over the whole leg with the highest compression in the calf/ankle area and a less amount for the thigh. This aids fluid flow out of the leg.

Skin care is important. Scratches, sunburn, punctures or other injuries should be avoided. A skin moisturizer should be applied to prevent dryness and prevent the skin from cracking.

In the case of advancing cancer disease, chemotherapy and/or radiation therapy may help by shrinking the tumours in the lymph system (nodes). Lymphdrainage is contraindicated in patients with edema caused by tumour blockage. This could possibly induce distant metastases. However, in the case of palliative care and generalized metastasis lymphdrainage may be allowed.

Lymphocele and recommendations of treatment

Lymphoceles are relatively common in patients after pelvic lymph node dissection (Pepper *et al.*, 2004).

Ultrasonography and occasionally CT are used to diagnose lymphoceles. Cytological and biochemical analysis of the aspirate can be used to aid in their diagnosis (Yablon 2004).

Symptomatic lymphoceles may become quite debilitating and may necessitate surgical or less invasive intervention. They can block the lymph flow causing distention, pain, infection, or compression of adjacent structures.

Treatment options depend on factors such as size, infection risk, loculation and the recurrence of the collection. Most lymphoceles are small and asymptomatic. They do not require treatment and eventually resolve spontaneously.

Therapeutic objectives in symptomatic lymphoceles are to remove the fluid collection and to prevent its reaccumulation as a result of persistent leakage of lymph from the transected lymphatic channels (Caliendo *et al.*, 2001). They can be treated by single or recurrent percutaneous aspiration of lymphatic fluid, percutaneous drainage, sclerotherapy or open surgical methods.

Sclerotherapy adds a substantial advantage to drainage alone by enhancing the inflammatory reaction to achieve adhesion and fibrosis. Numerous therapeutics have been implemented in sclerotherapy, e.g., tetracycline, doxycyclin, bleomycin, ethanol.

Low dose percutaneous radiotherapy (up to 10 to 12Gy) is effective in healing lymphatic fistulas and lymphoceles without complications.

Problems of sexual intercourse and sexual counselling

Sexual counselling is important. Disorders of sexual experience and behaviour often occur. They usually lead to a considerable loss of quality of life for the patients and their partners.

In many cases the development of severe neurotic behaviour disorders can be avoided with prompt and adequate counselling (Dahn *et al*, 2004). Experience has shown that only a small number of those affected raise the subject of sexuality themselves. The vast majority wait to be asked by the doctor or nurse (Black, 2004).

Erectile dysfunction is just one of the common sexual problems men experience after prostate cancer treatment; sexual rehabilitation needs to focus also on decreased sexual desire, difficulty reaching orgasm, pain with ejaculation, and dismay at reduced penile size.

The effect of **surgery** on the ability to achieve an erection is related to a man's age and whether nerve-sparing surgery was performed (table 13.9). Erectile dysfunction is less frequent after radiotherapy and more often after surgery, in particular after radical prostatectomy. Up to 80% of men experience erection problems after radical prostatectomy. The nerves that control a man's ability to have an erection lie next to the prostate gland. They often are damaged or removed during surgery. Erectile dysfunction can begin immediately following the removal of the entire prostate and surrounding tissues. If the nerve-sparing technique is used, recovery from erectile dysfunction may occur within the first year following the procedure. Recovery of erectile function after a non-nerve-sparing technique is unlikely but is possible.

Table 13.9 - Bad risk factors for reduction of erectile dysfunction after radical prostatectomy.

- No nerve-sparing prostatectomy
- Extensive tumour
- Erection problems before surgery
- Advanced age
- Coexistant medical conditions (i.e., diabetes mellitus)
- Hypertension
- Coronary heart disease
- Arteriosclerosis

After surgery, men experience dry orgasms in which there is no ejaculation. The **vas deferens**, the tube which transports sperm from the testicles, has been shut off. This lack of fluid emission has no connection to and does not interfere with a man's ability to feel sexual desire and arousal, or achieve orgasm.

The onset of erectile dysfuction following **radiation therapy** is gradual and usually begins about six months following treatment. The main cause of erectile dysfunction following radiation is damage to the blood vessels supplying the nerves responsible for erections. External beam radiation therapy appears to cause more problems with potency than brachytherapy.

Table 13.10 - Treatment options for erectile dysfunction.

- Pelvic floor exercises
- Oral agents: PDE5 inhibitors like sildenafil (Viagra®), tadalafil (Cialis®) or vardenafil (Levitra®) and yohimbine
- Vacuum erection devices
- Vasoactive agents (self-injection, intra-urethral therapy)
- Surgical interventions (penile prosthesis)
- Dildos

When **hormone therapy** is used, erectile dysfuction may occur approximately two-four weeks following the initiation of the therapy and is usually accompanied by a decreased desire for sex. Some men can still achieve erection after orchiectomy, but there is almost always a decline in sexual drive

To note is that many **medical therapies** (e.g., antidepressants, medicaments against hypertension, etc.) induce erectile dysfunction.

Nerve-sparing surgery

The easiest way to prevent erectile dysfunction is to avoid damage to the nerves when doing radical prostatectomy. As long as some nerves are present the chances for spontaneous improvement are quite good (Walsh, 2000; Schover, 2005). The benefits of nerve-sparing surgery may be limited by fibrosis after surgery or by concomitant injury to the vascular bed of the penis.

Vacuum devices

Vacuum devices work best in men who are able to achieve partial erections on their own. They are easy to use at home, require no other procedure, and typically improve erections regardless of the cause of impotence. Vacuum devices work by manually creating an erection. The penis is inserted into a plastic tube, which is pressed against the body to form a seal. A hand pump attached to the tube is used to create a vacuum that draws blood into the penis, causing the penis to become engorged. After one to three minutes in the vacuum, an adequate erection is created. The penis is removed from the tube and a soft rubber O-ring is placed around the base of the penis to trap blood and maintain the erection until removed. The ring can be left in place for twenty-five to thirty minutes. The band can be left on safely for up to thirty minutes to allow successful intercourse. The device works for almost everyone, regardless of nerve damage. It can be used as often as desired, as long as the ring is removed every thirty minutes. Treatment compliance with the vacuum devices is low, with up to 50% to 70% discontinuing treatment after one year (table 13.11).

Table 13.11 - Possible side effects of vacuum constriction or vacuum erection device.

– Men who are able to achieve but not maintain erections may use the ring only.

– An erection obtained by the vacuum constriction device is not the same as an erection achieved naturally. Since the penis is flaccid between the ring and the body, the erection may be somewhat floppy.

– The penis tends to be purplish in color and can be cold or numb. A black and blue mark or small area of bleeding may appear on the shaft of the penis. This is usually painless and will generally resolve in a few days.

– Some men experience a numbing feeling after placing the O-ring.

– Decrease in the force of the ejaculation. The constriction band traps the ejaculate or semen at the time of orgasm. This is not dangerous and usually does not cause pain. The semen will usually dribble out once the constriction band is removed. Generally, this does not interfere with the pleasure of a climax or orgasm.

– It may be harmful to men who use blood thinners or have blood clotting problems.

Vasoactive agents (self-injection, intra-urethral therapy)

Although more invasive, the use of vasoactive agents such as alprostadil (prostaglandin E1 [PGE1]) is another effective secondary therapy. Prostaglandin (alprostadil, Caverject®, Edex®) and phentolamine (Regitine®) cause vascular dilation and a relaxation of smooth muscle. Self-injection involves using a short needle to inject medication through the side of the penis directly into the corpus cavernosum, which produces an erection that lasts from thirty minutes to several hours.

These drugs have been shown to produce erections in 80% of men who inject them. Some men claim that they produce erections that feel natural and improve sex. The injections are relatively painless and create an erection that begins about five to fifteen minutes after the injection. It is recommended that self-injection be performed no more than once every four to seven days.

Prostaglandin can be given either by injection or as a urethral suppository containing prostaglandin. Injections should be limited to once or twice a week to minimize risks of scars or penile damage.

When given as a suppository, the medicine is placed into the opening at the tip of the penis. When injected, a needle and syringe is used to inject the medicine in the penis. Prostaglandin delivered via a suppository is not as effective as when it is delivered by penile injection; it produces an erection in approximately 30-40% of men with erectile dysfunction.

Table 13.12 - Possible side effects associated with injection of prostaglandin.

– Bleeding at the site of injection.
– Infection at the site of injection.
– Pain at the site of injection (common).
– Painful erection.
– Bruising or clotted blood in the area of the injection. (usually caused by an incorrect injection).
– Dizziness, heart palpitations, and flushing.
– Repeated injection may cause scarring of erectile tissue, which can further impair erection.
– There is a small risk for priapism.

PDE5 inhibitors

Many men are quite resistant to penile injections with vasodilating agents, vacutainers, penile suppositories or penile implants. They are more willing to try medications such as sildenafil (Viagra®), tadalafil (Cialis®) or vardenafil (Levitra®). Patients respond well to PDE5 inhibitors if the nerve bundles on both sides of the prostate have been spared. However, they are not effective when one or both nerve bundles have been damaged (Montorsi, 2005).

They all work by increasing the flow of blood into the penis so that, when a man is sexually stimulated, he can get an erection. There are subtle differences in how long the drug works and how quickly it works. Levitra® works a little longer than Viagra®. They both take effect in about thirty minutes. With Levitra®, the effects last for about fice hours. With Viagra®, the effects last approximately four hours. Cialis® works a bit faster (within about fifteen minutes), and the effects last much longer (up to thirty-six hours in some cases).

Table 13.13 - Possible side effects of PDE5 inhibitors.

– Headache
– Upset stomach
– Flushing
– Nasal congestion
– Changes in vision
– Back pain

Yohimbine improves erections for a small percentage of men. It stimulates the parasympathetic nervous system, which is linked to erection, and may increase libido. It is necessary to take the medication for six to eight weeks before determining whether it will work or not.

Yohimbine has a stimulatory effect and side effects include elevated heart rate and blood pressure, mild dizziness, nervousness, and irritability. Yohimbine's effects have not been studied thoroughly, but some studies suggest that 10% to 20% of men respond to treatment with the drug.

Surgical interventions (penile prostheses)

When the above-mentioned strategies do not achieve the desired result, surgical options should be considered in motivated patients. Penile prostheses provide the most reliable and predictable way to achieve erectile function, but they are typically not considered unless natural erections have not been achieved with other treatment approaches at two years following surgery.

About 85% of men report satisfaction with this approach. With the advent of more modern devices and when the surgery is performed in high-volume centres, the potential for infection or urethral disruption has diminished considerably.

In cases when the neurovascular bundles cannot be spared during radical prostatectomy, a technique called sural nerve grafting, or nerve interposition grafting, has shown some promise in helping men to regain erectile function that would be otherwise permanently lost. The technique involves grafting the sural nerve (harvested through the ankle) between the remaining portions of the excised neurovascular bundles; in theory, the presence of the sural nerves would stimulate regeneration of the neurovascular bundles.

Penile implants are either malleable or inflatable. The simplest type of prosthesis consists of a pair of malleable rods surgically implanted within the erection chambers of the penis. With this type of implant the penis is always semi rigid and merely needs to be lifted into the erect position to initiate sex. Today, many men choose a hydraulic, inflatable prosthesis, which allows a man to have an erection whenever he chooses and is much easier to conceal.

Satisfaction rates with the prosthesis are very high, and typically 80-90% of men are satisfied with the results and say they would choose the surgery again. Surgery carries the risk of complications including bleeding, scarring, or problems with anesthesia (table 13.14).

Table 13.14 - Complications associated with penile implants.

- Uncontrolled bleeding after the surgery possibly leading to re-operation
- Infection
- Scar tissue formation
- Erosion (tissue around the implant may break down)
- Mechanical failure

Dildos

Dildos are a simple and inexpensive strategy for dealing with impotence; in certain circumstances they can work better than more established medical treatment. Use of a dildo potentially removes the fear of erectile failure, allows for increased stimulation of the glans, facilitates full-body contact between partners, and offers potential satisfaction to one's partner (Gray, 2004).

Hormonal problems and recommendations of treatment

Table 13.15 - Complaints and complications of androgen deprivation therapy in men with Prostate Cancer.

- Hot flashes
- Intense perspiration
- Insomnia
- Reduction of physical fitness
- Irritability
- Loss of libido
- Fatigue
- Troubles of dark-adaptation
- Osteoporosis with increased risk of bone fracture

Years ago, first-line treatment of extensive prostatic cancer consisted of **high dose estrogens**. Tumour response hereafter was sometimes dramatic but cardiovascular morbidity was high. Complications such as blood clots, lethal cardiovascular failures were not rare. Because of these side effects, estrogens have been largely replaced by LHRH analogs and anti-androgens.

Side effects of **antiandrogens** in patients who already have been treated by orchiectomy or with LHRH agonists are usually not serious. Diarrhea is the major side effect; nausea, liver problems, and tiredness can also occur. The major difference from LHRH agonists is that anti-androgens have fewer sexual side effects. Libido and potency can be maintained on these drugs if they are used alone. Liver function tests have to be performed regularly. Sometimes there is a deterioration of diabetes. Although not dangerous, many patients are disturbed by the green-yellow discoloration of the urine after ingestion of flutamide.

LHRH-analoga are considered to have only minor side effects. Possible side effects of LHRH analoga (e.g., hot flashes, loss of bone density, and others) are similar to those of orchiectomy. They are largely due to low testosterone levels. Loss of testicular function may contribute to osteoporosis by decreasing hormone levels with subsequent bone weakness and/or fractures. This problem necessitates the use of calcium, vitamin D, and possibly bisphosphonate therapy.

Osteoporosis and recommendations for prevention

Osteoporotic bone loss and associated fractures can occur in patients on androgen deprivation therapy. Benign skeletal complications (osteopenia and fractures) occur at significantly increased rates among patients with prostate carcinoma. The incidence increases with longer durations of therapy (Kruspski *et al.*, 2004; Shahininan *et al.*, 2005). The risk for osteoporosis may be higher with orchiectomy than with hormonal drugs (Shahininan *et al.*, 2005).

In postmenopausal women, the risk for osteoporosis and associated fractures is traditionally expressed by T-score, representing the number of standard deviations (SD) by which the patient's BMD is below that of the mean for healthy young white adult women. A T-score superior to -1 is normal, a T-score of -1 to -2.5 indicates osteopenia, and a T-score superior to -2.5 indicates osteoporosis. Although using these reference measurements in men with prostate cancer may be questionable, it has been estimated that each SD decrease in BMD confers an increase in fracture risk of over 2.5%. The necessity for a clear identification of patients at risk for osteoporosis and patients with a low BMD is a pressing problem.

Patients at risk for bone loss should have an assessment of their bone mineral density so that prevention or therapeutic interventions are instituted at an early enough stage to prevent fractures.

Physical activity, less alcohol and a diet rich in vitamin D and calcium should be recommended to prevent osteoporosis.

Bisphosphonates may play a role in preventing osteopenia and, potentially, bone metastases among men with prostate carcinoma. However, whether or not prophylactic prescription of bisphosphonates is reasonable is being discussed controversially. The use of bisphosphonates seems to be associated with the risk of osteonecrosis of the jaw. Previous dental procedures may be a precipitating factor for the development of such problems (Bamias *et al.*, 2005).

Oncologists should consider referring all patients already receiving bisphosphonates to a dentist or oral and maxillofacial surgeon for an examination and a surveillance schedule. The dental team should carefully evaluate the oral cavity for exposed bone in the areas most commonly affected, such as the posterior lingual area of the mandible, and for radiographic evidence of osteolysis, osteosclerosis, widened periodontal membrane spaces, and furcation involvements.

Hot flashes and recommendations of treatment

Hot flashes, similar to symptoms that women have during menopause, are caused by many of the hormonal therapies and after orchiectomy. Symptoms include diaphoresis and feelings of intense heat and chills. At times, hormonal therapy must be stopped because of the drenching sweats and discomfort caused by hot flashes, especially when sleep is disturbed. This has led to a strategy of intermittent hormonal use to decrease the side effect burden.

Conservative treatment consists of physical therapies. Kneipp showers have a stabilizing effect on the circulation and immune system. They help to relax the muscles and the autonomic nervous system. Sage extracts and tea may reduce the frequency and intensity of perspiration.

Cyproteronacetat (50mg/d) or low doses of gestagens (2 x 5mg/d), low doses of clonidin (0,1mg/d) or low doses of estrogens (e.g., estrogen patches 0,05-1mg, twice a week) may redress grievances. Antidepressants, particularly selective serotonin reuptake inhibitors such as sertraline, venlafaxin (e.g., paroxetine 10mg/d) and gabapentine 900mg/d may reduce the frequency and intensity of hot flashes (Barton and Loprinzi, 2004).

Gynecomastia and recommendations for prevention and treatment

Breast tenderness with growth of breast tissue is a troublesome complication after orchiectomy and some hormone therapy. Gynecomastia is not only a cosmetic problem. Although gynecomastia is not directly harmful, the enlargement of the breast and the associated pain and tenderness may cause psychological and social problems, often severe enough to lead to the discontinuation of the therapy.

There are several treatments available to alleviate or prevent the development of gynecomastia, including medical treatment with anti-estrogens and aromatase inhibitors.

The development of breast pain and gynecomastia may be prevented by prophylactic irradiation of the breast. Radiotherapy may provide effective relief from the breast pain associated with gynecomastia.

An alternative option is surgery, which has proved to be effective. The three most frequently used procedures are mastectomy with excision of the gland, liposuction, and a hybrid therapy with a combination of the two techniques. Surgical liposuction is effective in particular in the very early stages because the breast becomes irreversibly fibrous as the disease progresses (Precioso et al., 2004).

Complaints after orchiectomy and advice

Loss of libido and erectile dysfunction after surgical castration are irreversible in contrast to chemical/hormonal castration. Possible side effects of orchiectomy (table 13.16) are generally related to changing levels of hormones in the body. Even cognitive problems may occur.

Many men can still achieve erection after orchiectomy, but there is almost always a decline in sexual drive. Patients do not experience a reversal of sex characteristics: The voice does not change and body hair is not affected.

It is important for clinicians to anticipate the side effects and to initiate measures to prevent or minimize them in order to maintain quality of life in prostate cancer survivors (Chen *et al.*, 2004). Hot flashes may go away with time. Antidepressants may reduce the intensity of hot flashes. Substitution by testosterone is contraindicated.

Gabapentine (900mg/d) is a promising non-hormonal therapy for hot flashes. It was originally approved by the FDA to control epileptic seizures, but has since become more widely used to reduce pain. Gabapentine effectively reduces both the frequency and severity of hot flashes. Other non-hormonal treatments for hot flashes include such drugs as venlafaxine (e.g., paroxetine 10mg/d) and low dose of clonidine (0.1mg/d).

To prevent psychological problems arising from the cosmetic appearance patients should be offered a testicular prosthesis.

Physical activity, less alcohol and a diet rich in vitamin D and calcium should be recommended to prevent osteoporosis. Whether or not prophylactic prescription of bisphosphonates is reasonable is being investigated in several studies.

Table 13.16 - Possible side effects of orchiectomy.

– Reduced or absent libido and impotence
– Hot flashes
– Breast tenderness and growth of breast tissue
– Osteoporosis and increased risk of bone fractures
– Changes in body composition
– Anemia
– Decreased mental acuity
– Loss of muscle mass
– Weight gain
– Fatigue
– Decrease in HDL cholesterol
– Depression

Unwanted side effects of radiotherapy and recommendation of treatment

The adverse effects of **external beam radiotherapy** are grouped into three major categories: **sexual, bowel and urinary** (Pisansky, 2005). Adverse effects may be acute (occurring during or shortly after external beam RT) or may persist or appear several months after treatment is completed.

The incidence and severity of adverse effects is influenced by several factors, including coexistent medical conditions, treatment technique, dose conformity to the prostate, and the radiotherapy dose level and volume of the structure that is irradiated.

The likelihood of maintaining **erectile function** after radiotherapy ranges from 20% to 86%, depending on the definition of potency. It appears that the primary aetiology of radiotherapeutic-induced erectile dysfunction is from a disruption in the vascular system of the penile corporal structures. It does not appear that external beam radiotherapy diminishes erectile function in men who undergo nerve sparing prostatectomy.

Between 13-38% of patients record moderate or severe **bowel stress** (blood per rectum, flatulence, bowel cramps after conventional radiotherapy) and grade 3 or 4 urinary complications. Long-term follow-up of patients undergoing radical prostatectomy, brachytherapy, and external beam radiotherapy indicate that most of the symptoms gradually decline over the course of one-two years

Urge incontinence (overactive bladder) may occur as a result of prostate infection, such as **prostatitis**, or as a result of bladder lining irritation caused by radiation therapy. Moderate **proctopathy** or chronic **cystitis** may occur in up to one in six patients after postoperative external beam radiotherapy. Most cases are mild and improve spontaneously. Sucralfat suppositories may help in proctitis. There is no clear association between external beam radiotherapy and the development of bladder neck or urethral stricture.

Stress urinary incontinence, which is frequently seen following prostatectomy but rarely seen following radiotherapy, can improve over time but often does not resolve completely.

Potential adverse effects of brachytherapy are summarized in table 13.17. Urinary incontinence is present in 5-6% of patients but is much more common (13%) after trans-urethral resection of the prostate (TURP). Potency is maintained in 86-96% of patients for two-three years after implantation. Complications can manifest several years after completion of therapy. Peri-anal eczema can badly influence quality of life.

Table 13.17 - Potential adverse effects of brachytherapy in prostate cancer patients (Yi Su *et al.*, 2004).

Acute side effects
– Irritative urinary symptoms (grade 1-2): 40-50%
– Urinary retention: 1-14%
– Proctitis: 1-2%

Chronic side effects
– Urinary symptoms: 29% at 12 months and 14% at 24 months
– Incontinence: 5-6%
– Incontinence after TURP: 13%
– Hematuria: 1-2%
– Stricture: 1-2%
– Proctitits: 1-3%
– Impotence: 4-14%
– Peri-anal eczema: 2-5%

Nutritional problems and counselling

Cancer survivors often receive dietary advice from family, friends, and health care providers, as well as from the media, health food stores, and the nutritional supplement industry. Magazine articles, books, Internet, family, and friends present cancer survivors with a wide range of options and choices about what to eat and what types of supplements or herbal remedies might improve the outcome of standard cancer therapy. The value of this information is at best minimal.

For many of the most important nutrition questions faced by cancer survivors, the scientific evidence of recommendations for special diets comes only from *in vitro* and laboratory animal data or anecdotal reports from poorly designed clinical studies. Moreover, the findings from these studies are often contradictory. Very few controlled clinical trials have been done to test the impact of diet, nutritional supplements, or nutritional complementary methods on cancer outcomes among cancer survivors.

Special dietary recommendations are not necessary. Neither dietary modifications nor nutritional supplements such as vitamins, anti-oxidants, retinol, and garlic alter the disease course of patients with prostatic cancer.

On the other hand, "encouraging a healthy diet" is certainly important because many patients with prostatic cancer will live a long time and may die of other diseases related to nutrition (table 13.18). Older men with early-stage prostate cancer are actually at higher risk of death from heart disease than from prostate cancer, so it is especially wise for prostate cancer survivors to follow a heart-healthy diet that is low in saturated fat, high in fruits and vegetables, and accompanied by regular physical activity.

High-fat diets can increase testosterone levels, which may account for their apparent stimulatory effect on prostate cancer growth. Less red meat intake, particularly processed meat, and physical activity may have beneficial effects on the course of the disease, protect against diabetes and cardiovascular diseases (Stoeckli, 2004; Key *et al.*, 2004).

An unhealthy weight may not only influence the risk of progression; it is a bad risk factor for urine incontinence and for other impairments and diseases as well. Sometimes fat in the abdomen can put pressure on the bladder; losing weight may help improve bladder control.

Table 13.18 - Recommendations for a healthy diet for men with prostatic cancer.

– Food rich in omega-3 fatty acids
– To be physically active to help achieve and maintain healthy weight. Primarily a plant-based diet.
– Limit single sugars
– Adequate fluids
– Limit alcohol and caffeine intake (may help to control urine leakage)

Necessity of information and patient education (health training and discussion groups)

Many patients are concerned with being diagnosed with prostate cancer, with the treatment decisions, and most importantly, with the impact of prostate cancer and its treatment on their quality of life. Some of them have been called the "walking worried": Anxious about slow-rising PSA test results, the recurrence of cancer, and the need for knowledge and training regarding the disease.

One of the tasks in rehabilitation is to inform, to instruct and to train patients (table 2.12). Information promotes self-help. Self-help (empowerment) is an important goal of training. Explanation and information are important aids in helping to cope with the disease and overcome illness. This involves the patient's understanding of what is happening in his body and why a certain form of therapy has been suggested. The majority of patients do not wish to decide about tumour therapy themselves, but like to know the reasons for pursuing a certain treatment strategy. Wives have a wide range of information needs.

In the case of recurrence it is the aim of health training to inform the patient of the possibilities and limitations of standard medicine, to protect them from harmful alternative forms of therapy and to convey to them the significance of medical surveillance (table 13.19).

Table 13.19 - Subjects of education counselling programmes for patients with prostatic cancer.

– Information about the disease, the various possibilities of treatment, the prevention of recurrences, the various prognosis criteria
– Information about aftercare, content and timetable of follow-up examinations
– Information about symptoms of recurrences
– Information about therapies in the case of recurrences
– Information about alternative therapy forms and complementary therapies
– Measures to improve general physical and mental performance
– Significance of physical activity
– Information about pain and possible pain therapies
– Information about postorchiectomy complaints and possible therapies.
– Information about urinary incontinence and possible therapies; significance of pelvic floor muscle training, biofeedback, bladder diary, etc.
– Information about sexuality, erectile dysfunction, erectile aids
– Dietary recommendations
– Information about adverse effects of radio-, hormone-, chemotherapy; prevention and therapy of side effects
– Information about interpersonal and social consequences of the disease.
– Information about questions concerning medical care, nursing care, socio-legal issues, and practical issues
– Effects of cancer and cancer therapies on restrictions of working incapacity; measures for the protection and maintenance of workplaces; aids and measures for vocational reintegration; information about vocational consequences
– Recommendations how to cope with fears, depression and fatigue symptoms
– Recommendations how to deal with family members

Health education takes place in discussion groups in which psychologists, physicians and social workers all take turns moderating the groups. Education counselling programmes comprise general information on prostatic cancer, its causes, and different therapeutic approaches including alternatives and complementary treatment. Consequences of therapy on sexuality (Black, 2004), prevention of recurrent disease, aftercare, coping with anxiety, how to cope with pain and treatment of relapsing disease, will be discussed and information on entitlement to social care, legal aspects and career consequences will be given.

Besides questions relating to nutrition, urinary incontinence (Mathewson-Chapman, 1997) and other side effects of therapy and hormonal symptoms, social provisions and psychological strategies for relaxation and to combat fear are important topics.

It has been proven to be helpful for those patients who have undergone surgery recently to meet with others who have had the same cancer treatment several years earlier. The "more experienced" patients function as positive models encouraging the recently diagnosed patients.

Patients are more and more often finding information for themselves, using literature, Internet and other media. Further, explanatory information and, in particular, assistance in dealing with this information are necessary. This may be done in a one-to-one setting or in group discussions.

Interested patients and their families should be advised on Internet resources, which in the physician's opinion are informative, useful and provide well-founded information.

It is useful for patients and their family members also to have access to printed versions of the information which they have received in health education sessions. This printed material should of course never take the place of consultations with a physician, but it should rather provide the basis for productive discussions with the attending physician.

Rehabilitation measures to avoid psychological problems ("rehabilitation to combat resignation and depression")

See also the chapter: "Psychological support in cancer rehabilitation and palliation".

Depressions and distress

Causes of psychological problems can be very complex (table 13.20) (Norton *et al.*, 2004). Patients often have anxiety, depression, psychological distress, loss of control, and fear. Issues such as chronic fear of follow-up diagnostic tests, fear of progression or recurrence, fear of sexual dysfunction, of urinary incontinence, PSA hypervigilance, fatigue, pain, hot flashes, economic and social problems, the uncertain future and forced lifestyle changes lead to psychological distress. Hormonal changes cause vegetative disturbances with depressive cases, insomnia, distress and nervousness.

Table 13.20 - Frequent psychological problems to be considered in prostatic cancer patients.

– Depression
– Distress
– Anxiety
– PSA hypervigilance
– Fear of disease progression
– Partner problems
– Fatigue
– Passivity and lack of motivation

Assessment of these problems is not easy, particularly in distinguishing between physical and psychological aetiologies of distress.

Increased attention, conversations, "taps on the shoulder", and social activities on their own are often not sufficient to solve psychological problems. It may be necessary to involve a psycho-oncologist.

Psychological and psychiatric interventions provide avenues for decreased stress and improved quality of living. Supportive and cognitive-behavioural therapy can assist a man in coping with changes in life style.

Psychosocial support includes one-on-one psychological therapy sessions as well as topic-oriented group support, such as life goals, sexuality, relationships, helps to cope with illness and impairments (tables 2.3, 2.6). How to reduce fear (table 2.5) and depression are, how to cope with feelings of helplessness and hopelessness are other topics. It also includes the instruction of various relaxation techniques (such as autogenic training, progressive muscle relaxation, imaginative and hypnotherapeutic procedures), and art therapies (such as music therapy, art therapy, dance therapy) (table 2.4).

Helping patients to reorganize their schedule and set realistic goals may result in less distress. Apart from classic psychological therapies (autogenic training, progressive muscle relaxation, imagery, qigong, tai chi, yoga, behaviour therapies within the context of a one-on-one meeting or in a group discussion, etc.) a stay in a rehabilitation clinic may be indicated.

One of the pros for inpatient rehabilitation measures is the experience that rehabilitation is greatly helped by an appropriate environment, in which the patient's fears and anxieties may be relatively limited. Patients can share their experiences with one another in this environment and are given social care around the clock.

Psychostimulants are sometimes effective. It should be noted, however, that many medicaments (e.g., antidepressants, medicaments against hypertension, etc.) induce erectile dysfunction.

Anxiety and PSA hypervigilance

The PSA tumour marker that is used to follow treatment outcomes can be a significant source of anxiety. Many patients become hypervigilant about their PSA tests, equating any change in their PSA test with "being a dead man". This PSA anxiety can lead to panic symptoms and insomnia.

It may be relieved with instruction, support and anxiolytic medications, if needed (Roth *et al.*, 2003; Roth, 2006).Education about PSA levels as well as acknowledging some of the fears of what a rising PSA might mean, while recognizing how constant worry about the future negates the whole reason these men fear losing their lives, can help to reduce this worry.

Partner problems

Prostate cancer is often a "couple's disease". There are considerable inhibitions associated with the subject of sexuality and particularly with "sexual failure". Fears and feelings of guilt play a central part. These can be reduced in discussion.

Cancer can cause considerable distress for the healthy partners of cancer patients. Plans for a "peaceful retirement" are shattered, prospects for their life in old age must be reconsidered and redeveloped. The physical exertion involved in caring for the patient as well as the financial costs of old and new burdens pose substantial problems for the family. The transition in role allocation from "being provided for" to "being the provider" places high demands on the family's ability to adapt to the new situation.

Fatigue and lack of motivation

See also chapter: "Psychological support and self help groups in cancer rehabilitation and palliation".

Fatigue (extreme tiredness and exhaustion, lack of motivation) is a prominent complaint in patients with cancer and multifactorial in origin (2.8, 2.9, 2.10). In contrast to normal exhaustion, cancer-related fatigue does not improve with rest, adequate nutrition, and sleep (Watson, 2004). Somatic factors contributing to fatigue include anemia, hydronephrosis, weight loss, pain, medication, infections and dysbalance between endogenous cytokine levels and their natural antagonists. Frequently, hormonal changes cause fatigue.

Fatigue symptoms are particularly upsetting to men who have led active and independent lives. They usually result in increased dependence on family or friends, which are further reminders of the contrast with how patients lived before the cancer. Because of the possible overlap in symptoms between a fatigue syndrome and depression and anxiety syndromes, these entities must be identified as completely as possible and distinguished from each other, as they each require different treatment strategies.

The positive influence of erythropoietin on fatigue symptoms with low Hb level has been proved in a series of international studies. Hemoglobin levels of 12g/dL should be the aim. Thromboembolic complications after erythropoietin treatment may happen, when Hb levels are superior to 12g/dL. If no somatic cause can be found and treated, non-medication measures should be used first (e.g., physiotherapy, ergometric training, conversation therapy, behavioural therapy, diet, change of environment) (Watson, 2004).

If depression is present, activating antidepressants can be used. Sometimes, however, fatigue symptoms are linked to the antidepressant medications themselves. Some antidepressant drugs can affect sexual desire and function (tables 5.34, 5.35).

Physical exercise has benefits both physically and psychosocially in cancer patients over time (Watson, 2004; Windsor et al., 2004). Many studies indicate the positive effects of physical activity on fatigue syndrome. Bicycle ergometer training, walking, weight training, aerobic exercises, and athletic activity are shown to have not only a positive effect on physical fitness and psychological well-being, but also on fatigue symptoms (Oldevoll, 2004; Spruit et al., 2006). A gradual increase in the training intensity is recommended, starting with fifteen to thirty minutes three to five days a week. It is important to clarify to both the patient and to family that physical inactivity which may be intended as rest, will be more likely to promote symptoms of fatigue than to alleviate them (Watson, 2004).

Particularly in Germany group activities such as "sport after cancer" are supported by public health insurance. Apart from the positive effects on fatigue syndrome and general health these physical activities are expected to have positive repercussions on social integration.

Some patients experience a feeling of relief when informed about the somatic causes of fatigue syndrome. They are often distraught because they believe they are suffering from depression with mental causes. When it is explained to them that the symptoms can emerge in conjunction with, for example, chemo- or hormone therapy, they are very relieved and motivated to begin with physical training.

A balanced and vitamin-rich diet is important, since fatigue symptoms are occasionally caused by improper and unbalanced nourishment. Some centers successfully use megestrol acetate for the treatment of both emaciation and fatigue symptoms.

Sometimes fatigue symptoms are the consequence of hydronephrosis, urinary stasis and renal failure. In this case drainage of urine or elimination will improve fatigue symptoms.

Insomnia

Insomnia is a frequent problem associated with prostate cancer. Sleeplessness influences the level of pain sensitivity. It often occurs independently of anxiety and depression.

In prostatic cancer patients insomnia is often influenced by the presence of physical and psychological symptoms associated with side effects of hormonal therapies, including orchiectomy. PSA anxiety (PSA hypervigilance) can lead to panic symptoms and insomnia. Because hot flashes often occur during the night, their presence has been frequently associated with insomnia.

Rehabilitative measures to avoid social problems ("rehabilitation to combat the need of care")

See also chapter: "Social support in rehabilitation and palliation".

Securing adequate care at home

The planning of further **care** must be arranged with both the patient's and the family's consent. The patient and his family are confronted with a complexity of problems. One of the aims of rehabilitative measures is to strengthen the patient's own resources and to prevent the risk of the need of care, or at least reduce such a need.

If the patient is no longer able to care for himself, support must be organized. In patients with prostate cancer this situation arises particularly frequent. Early organisation of assistance and support is crucial in patients with poor prognosis and rapidly progressive disease. The planning of further care must be done with the patients' family. Patients themselves are often not aware of social deficits or do not declare them. Assistance such as "meals on wheels", household assistance, home nursing care, care assistance, and under certain circumstances nursing home or hospice care need to be arranged. Providing contact addresses (self-help groups, counselling centres, etc.) is helpful.

Rehabilitation hospitals

If home care cannot or cannot yet be guaranteed, the time spent in hospital can be followed up by a temporary stay in an institution for follow-up care. In Germany there are rehabilitation hospitals which are designed especially to meet the needs of patients with urologic cancers and in which plans are made for the patients' social assistance, in addition to medical and psychological guidance (AHB hospital). Adjuvant and additive cancer therapies, supportive therapies, psychological support, counselling of the patients and their families are some of the tasks of these AHB hospitals.

Experienced physicians, psychologists and representatives of self-help groups share their experiences, information and helpful advice in these AHB hospitals. Some of the *maisons de repos* in France, and the bridge clinics in Italy have similar functions.

A subsequent **stay in a rehabilitation hospital**, directly following the standard hospital stay, is recommended for all patients being prostatectomized in Germany. In Germany every cancer patient has a legal claim to a three-five week stay in such an institution. 20 to 30% of all German cancer patients who have had a radical prostatectomy prefer staying at such a rehabilitation hospital.

Self-help groups

Providing contact addresses of self-help groups is helpful.

In addition to psychological support, self-help groups often provide their members with specific knowledge about medications and resources as well as social laws. Self-help groups play an important role with regard to the aims of follow-up on the social level; their impact is often limited, however, by the complexity of problems patients are facing. A support group may help to cope with the practical and emotional aspects of the disease. Talking with other people with prostatic cancer may also help ease feelings of isolation.

The concept behind self-help groups is based on the idea that mutual experience and situations offer a person strength. The participants discover that they are not alone in their experiences and emotions, and that other patients experience the same things. These common experiences and feelings are intended to strengthen the patient's feeling of self-worth. Self-help groups for prostatic cancer patients and groups for patients with urine incontinence exist in most countries. The prostate cancer charity is the largest and most comprehensive of the charities in the UK working in the field of prostate cancer (www.prostate cancer.org.uk).

There are various motives for becoming and remaining member of a patient association. Motives for membership reflect both benefits for the individuals and the welfare of others. The idea "wanted to use the association's information and activities" is very common in members of a prostatic cancer association (Carlsson *et al.*, 2005).

Rehabilitative measures to reduce problems at work. ("rehabilitation to combat early retirement")

See also chapter: "Vocational integration in cancer rehabilitation".

Every cancer patient of working age must be advised on eventual effects of cancer and cancer therapies and restrictions of working capacity, workloads to be avoided and measures for the protection and maintenance of workplaces.

Restrictions of working capacity

Whether or not the patient is capable of working depends on tumour spread and on side effects of therapy. It also depends on severity of concurring diseases, whether additional therapies were undertaken and, last not least, subjective ability to work plays a role.

Restrictions refer especially to patients with extensive cancer and to those suffering from stress urinary incontinence after prostatectomy or urge incontinence after radiotherapy. They refer especially to jobs that are associated with physical strain. Blue collar work is no longer possible in the case of osseous metastases in contrast to white collar work.

Continuation of vocational activity is still possible in patients having tumour activity. Biochemical recurrences are not identical with incapacity for work. Many patients with tumour activity do not have any symptoms, any physical complaints and can accomplish all work.

Harmful occupational substances

They are no known links between harmful occupational substances and prostatic cancer.

Type of work to be avoided

For prostatic cancer patients who have been treated potentially curatively, there are professional limitations, which are mainly due to urine incontinence and hormonal changes.

Desks jobs are entirely feasible for patients with incontinence grade I. Today a wide variety of products are available to control leakage and smell of urine. Patients with incontinence grade III (total incontinence) are generally not fit for work. They should submit applications for work incapacity pension as soon as possible unless they get an artificial sphincter which controls leakage.

Many manual activities being associated with physical strain in particular with abdominal stress (including lifting, working above head height, jobs connected with severe vibrations and in which more than 5kg have to be frequently lifted), unfavourable working posture (e.g., squatting or lying), extreme climatic situations (e.g., working in the heat) are not possible in the case of stress urine incontinence grade II. In contrast, office work and non-physical activities are quite feasible.

Irregular working hours are not possible for patients with urge incontinence. Pollakisuria requires the opportunity to take individual breaks in the case of irregular evacuation without interfering with colleagues' work flow.

How to return to work

It can be expected that work can be fully resumed two-three months after radical prostatectomy unless there is adjuvant hormone- or radiotherapy and still problems with urine continence, lymphedema and other complications. In the USA men diagnosed with prostate cancer missed an average of 27 days (median days = 20) from work. The median days missed for men treated surgically without hormone or radiation therapy was 25. Men treated with hormone and/or radiation therapy or who were not treated missed fewer days from work relative to men undergoing surgery (Bradley *et al.*, 2006).

In many countries assistance is available for returning to work. Gradual resumption of work is particularly recommended. The particular advantage of this arrangement is the work load can be matched to the fitness level of the patient without financial disadvantages. Unfortunately this sensible vocational rehabilitation measure is possible only in a few countries and often only in large companies and the civil service.

Palliative measures

Many clinicians find it difficult to give patients negative information about their prognosis and many battle with their own emotions during these exchanges.

Despite the unfavourable prognosis in the case of tumour recurrence, there are more points in favour than against patient information. This does not mean however that the patient should be confronted with the full implications of the illness. Information without the simultaneous offering of prospects and assistance is never constructive. Many fears associated with the illness originate from the fact that the affected person does not know how the situation should be assessed or what he/she should expect. It is better in any case for the patient to be informed by the attending physician than by prayer healers, moneymakers, or by random information found on the internet. Even when prognosis is desperate, positive aspects have to be mentioned (e.g., references to progress in palliative therapy, better pain control, provision of constant medical/psychological service, better supportive care, etc.). In the discussion, the seriousness and also the extent of the findings should be communicated to the patient but a time scale regarding the prognosis should never be made, all the more because diseases can commonly follow an unpredictable course.

Answering the question: "How much therapy, and which one?" not only requires oncological expertise. Ethical competence and communication skills are just as important. Under no circumstances should therapeutical decisions be made exclusively depending on response in terms of likelihood of remission or reduction of PSA level; goals such as reduction of physical symptoms, emotional stabilisation, and maintenance of daily activities are pre-eminent.

Altered pharmacodynamics mainly in old or patients with over- or under weight, may influence therapeutic strategies; comorbidity, quality of life scores and toxicity have to be taken into account (Earle et al., 2001; Ershler, 2003). Treatment must be tailored to the individual patient.

Response rates, remission rates and survival time may be a quantifiable and reproducible criterion for demonstrating effectiveness of primary therapy, but it is only one of many evaluation criteria within the context of therapy in progressive prostatic cancer.

The evaluation of palliative measures in prostatic cancer patients is directed not at survival time, but rather at quality of life criteria. This involves primarily subjective parameters such as pain, mobility, overcoming fears, etc. (table 13.21) and not such parameters as are found in association with primary therapy (response, remission and length of remission).

Table 13.21 - Symptoms hinting towards possible tumour progression.

– Irregular bowel movement
– Hematuria
– Bone pain, "rheumatic pain"
– Sciatica-like complaints
– Bone fractures
– Pain in the lumbar spine/sacrum
– Urinary tract infections, back pain and other complaints associated with hydronephrosis
– Unilateral lymphedema
– Paresthesia

A rising PSA can cause significant anxiety not only for the patient but also for the physician (Roth, 2003) as there are few clearly defined therapeutic standards for the treatment of a rising PSA in the absence of any other objective measures of disease progression.

Because PSA changes can precede clinical disease progression by months or even years, the question of when and if to initiate therapy in patients with a rising PSA and no evidence of clinical disease can be challenging. PSA levels can fluctuate in response to a variety of factors unrelated to tumour growth. Furthermore elevated levels of PSA do not demand urgent therapeutic consequences. Salvage radiotherapy may delay disease progression in patients with a rising PSA following radical prostatectomy and "unfavourable" risk factors (PSA doubling time inferior to 6 months, Gleason 2-7, and positive surgical margins). Treatment is not necessary in patients with elevated level of PSA but without substantial tumour evidence.

Androgen deprivation therapy should be initiated first in patients with a rising PSA following radical prostatectomy despite salvage radiotherapy. Secondary hormonal manipulation in patients with a rising PSA despite androgen deprivation therapy can be effective.

Pros and cons of possible tumour therapies and possible alternatives must be discussed with the patient. Comorbidity and psychosocial factors should be included in the therapeutic considerations (Charlson et al., 1987).

Local and regional problems and palliative therapies

Clinical manifestations of prostate cancer result from the effects of recurrence of the tumour, local growth, spread to regional lymph nodes, and/or dissemination to distant metastatic sites. Although patients with advanced prostate cancer may be asymptomatic, in patients with local tumour growth into the urethra or bladder, bladder obstructive or irritative voiding symptoms may be present (table 13.21). Bone metastatic disease may present itself with symptoms of continual pain in the lower back, pelvis, or upper thighs, while disease that has spread to the ureters may present itself with symptoms of uremia. It is important to distinguish symptoms caused by the disease from those caused by benign conditions or by prior therapy. Bone pain associated with metastatic disease may be similar to pain present in arthritis or degenerative disease; in men who are initially diagnosed with advanced disease and who do not undergo local treatment, the symptoms of urinary obstruction caused by the spread of disease into the urethra can be similar to those seen with benign prostatic hyperplasia.

Metastases to the bones, pelvis, spine and ribs are especially common (85%). About 10% to 15% of patients are found to have soft tissue lesions. About 9% have lung metastases and 3% liver metastases.

Hydronephrosis

Hydronephrosis is a common complication to advanced prostatic carcinoma. The cause of the obstruction that has led to hydronephrosis may be intravesical or retrovesical. Ureter obstruction and hydronephrosis are usually due to tumour compression rather than infiltration. Long-standing hydronephrosis may be associated with obstructive nephropathy and renal failure. Urinary stasis may result in infection, renal scarring, calculus formation, and sepsis. Renovascular hypertension may result from renin secretion from the hydronephrotic kidney.

In general, any signs of infection within the obstructed system warrant urgent intervention because infection with hydronephrosis may progress rapidly to sepsis. Prompt drainage for hydronephrosis is indicated if renal function is compromised. In acute hydronephrosis, urine that has accumulated above the obstruction is drained as soon as possible, usually with a needle inserted through the skin into the kidney. The goals of this urgent drainage are to prevent loss of kidney function or prevent further loss if function is already impaired. The obstruction must also be relieved quickly. Complications of acute hydronephrosis, such as urinary tract infections and kidney failure, if present, are treated promptly.

Lower obstructive uropathy may require catheter drainage or urinary diversion. Indwelling pigtail ureteral catheters can be placed for acute or long-term drainage in selected patients. Stents can bypass an obstruction and dilate the ureter for subsequent endoscopic treatment. Surgery should be considered in a patient with pain and a positive diuretic renogram.

Advances in endoscopic and percutaneous instrumentation have limited the role of open or laparoscopic surgery for hydronephrosis. Urologists or interventional radiologists can place a percutaneous nephrostomy tube.

No therapy is necessary in an asymptomatic patient with a positive diuretic renogram but normal renal function or with a negative diuretic renogram. Urgent treatment of chronic unilateral hydronephrosis is usually not required (Zaak et al., 2003).

Chronic bilateral hydronephrosis is corrected by draining urine above the obstruction. For example, soft tubes (ureteral stents) may be inserted into the ureter to bypass an obstruction. Complications of ureteral stents can include movement of the tube, infection, irritation, and discomfort.

The cause of the obstruction that led to hydronephrosis is treated whenever possible. Treatment consists of eliminating of the obstruction by hormonal or chemotherapy, endoscopy or surgery. Diethylstilbestrol diphosphate is recommended in the treatment of soft tissue metastases. The tumour responses outweigh the side effects of the drug.

Be aware of the altered kinetics of some drugs in the case of impaired renal function. In particular the dose of opioids needs to be adjusted to the degree of renal function disorder in order to avoid tolerability problems. Buprenorphine, which is mainly excreted via the faeces, can be administered to patients with renal impairment up to renal failure without the need of dose adaption.

Osseous metastases

Up to 80% of patients with advanced prostate cancer develop bone metastases that account for a vast majority of disease-related mortality and is associated with significant morbidity. Metastases to the bones of the pelvis, spine and ribs are especially common.

Patients with lung cancer metastatic to bone have median survivals of less than six months; however, patients with prostate cancer can have prolonged survival with bone metastases. In patients who fail radical prostatectomy, the median time from PSA rise following local therapy with curative intent to the onset of bone metastases is approximately eight years, and the median survival following establishment of metastatic disease is five years (Ward et al., 2003).

It is important to distinguish symptoms caused by the disease from those caused by benign conditions or by prior therapy. Bone pain associated with metastatic disease may be similar to pain present in arthritis or degenerative disease; in men who are initially diagnosed with advanced disease and who do not undergo local treatment, the symptoms of urinary obstruction caused by the spread of disease into the urethra can be similar to those seen with benign prostatic hyperplasia.

Radionuclide (technetium-99m) bone scan is the standard test for diagnosis of bone metastases. Although a sensitive technique, false-positive bone scans are not unusual in areas of previous injury or arthritis, and an abnormal scan should be followed up by a plain X-ray film to document the presence of a benign condition. As it is true for CT scans, bone scans are of limited utility in the setting of early biochemical failure and are generally recommended only if the patient has bone pain symptoms, rapid rise in PSA (PSA velocity superior to 0.5ng/mL/month or PSA doubling time before 6 months), or a significantly elevated PSA value (superior to 10-20 ng/mL).

If X-ray shows a metastatic lesion in a long bone with cortical destruction, particularly the femur or humerus, pathologic fracture must be prevented if possible. Generally this will require local irradiation and **internal fixation**. If the patient has or develops a pathologic fracture, internal fixation followed by radiotherapy is a most effective approach, assuming the patient can undergo the operative procedure. If bone metastases are not complicated by pathologic fracture or do not involve the spinal cord or nerve roots, treatment is dictated by symptoms, by the risk of pathologic fracture, and by the potential for effective systemic therapy. Prostate cancer patients will achieve substantial palliation from hormonal manipulation.

In symptomatic bone metastases **percutaneous cement injection** and **thermal ablation** are alternative or additive treatment options to standard therapy. Thermal ablation could achieve spontaneous pain relief due to the destruction of sensitive nerves surrounding the tumour. Thermal ablation and percutaneous cement injection seem to be a reasonable combination as thermal ablation destroys sensitive nerve ends, whereas cement injection increases stability.

Prophylactic **orthopedic/surgical stabilization** is required if there is an increased risk of fracture. An increased risk of fracture of the long bones can be anticipated with 50% destruction of the cortex and a defect size superior to 2.5cm. There is a risk of vertebral fracture if there is destruction of the middle/central or anterior and posterior pillar of over 60% in the axial plane.

The use of local hemibody radiotherapy, which targets the lower half of the body with a single dose of radiation, has demonstrated significant improvements in pain scores and significant delays in the development of new sites of pain. However, the high rates of toxicity seen with these therapies resulting from the destruction of normal tissue make them a less than optimal strategy.

Bisphosphonates emerged in the 1990s as an effective strategy to target bone metastases secondary to prostate cancer. Clinical trial data with zoledronic acid, a potent third-generation bisphosphonate, demonstrated significant reductions in pain and time to first occurrence of any skeletal complication, and skeletal morbidity rate in patients with metastatic lesions. Parenteral administration of bisphosphonates is indicated in symptomatic and oral administration in asymptomatic bone metastases. They should be given in an asymptomatic stage because of reducing the risk of pathologic fractures, hypercalcaemia, immobilisation, spinal cord compression and last not least need of care.

Radio-isotopes such as strontium-89 and samarium-153 have been shown to decrease pain in patients with osteoblastic metastases resulting from prostate cancer.

Brain metastases, spinal cord compression syndrome and recommendations for treatment

Brain metastases from prostatic carcinoma are considered rare. Usually they are diagnosed at postmortem examination.

Neurosurgical resection and the ablation by gamma knife or total brain radiation can be considered in the case of **single brain metastasis**. The role of surgery in patients with **multiple brain metastases** is usually limited to resection of large lesions or symptomatic lesions or life-threatening lesions. In asymptomatic multiple brain metastases many authors start with whole brain radiation only in the case of symptomatic progression.

The main goal of radiation therapy is to improve neurological deficits caused by the tumour deposit. Symptoms such as headache, focal neurological dysfunction, cognitive dysfunction, and seizures will improve.

Symptomatic therapy includes the use of corticosteroids for the treatment of peritumoural edema, anticonvulsants for control of seizures, and anticoagulants for the management of venous thromboembolic disease. External beam radiotherapy and supportive therapies, such as corticosteroids, anticonvulsants, and anticoagulants are necessary for patients with symptomatic metastases.

Acute spinal cord compression syndrome requires prompt treatment within a few hours. Paralysis is inevitable unless radiotherapy is initiated within two or three days. Patients with corresponding symptoms (progressive back pain, spinal cord compression syndrome) should be promptly referred to a centre which can offer complete diagnostic tests and has the appropriate departments (neurosurgery, radio-oncology, orthopedics, and hematology). Meanwhile the patient should get corticosteroids.

Liver and lung metastases

Solitary liver and lung metastases are rare. Therefore, neither surgical removal of metastases nor isolated regional chemotherapy or embolisation can be expected to bring about any significant benefit in survival time.

In the case of multiple liver metastases hormonal therapy should be considered. Chemotherapy should be applied only if hormonal therapy is no more possible.

Systemic palliative therapies in advanced prostate cancer

Role of hormonal therapies

Hormonal therapy usually becomes ineffective within three to five years in men with widespread prostate cancer.

When hormonal therapy fails (hormone resistance), alternative hormone drugs or chemotherapy may be tried.

Most hormonal approaches have been based on blockade of adrenal androgens. Responses have been noted in as many as 20% of such patients but usually remissions last less than six months in duration and do not significantly alter survival. Flutamide may be used in patients who have failed monotherapy with surgical castration, or LHRH agonists. Hydrocortisone alone, given at replacement doses, can provide significant relief of pain to patients with metastatic disease. Ketoconazole alone or in combination with hydrocortisone can result in a response in up to 25% of all patients.

Role of chemotherapies

Cytotoxic chemotherapy has demonstrated activity and palliative benefit in patients with hormone-refractory prostate carcinoma (William, 2000; Gilligan et al., 2002). However, response rates of monotherapy are less than 20%. Polychemotherapies may have higher response rates but this is not identical with a prolongation of survival. Unfortunately, the grade 3 and 4 toxicities of polychemotherapy schedules are significantly greater demanding more supportive measures.

Chemotherapy should be applied only if hormonal therapy is no more possible and when symptoms have appeared. Chemotherapy is not indicated at an asymptomatic stage. Quality of life data should be considered when choosing and evaluating the chemotherapy regime. Prostate-specific antigen (PSA) response is not sufficient to evaluate the response of chemotherapy.

Promising results have been shown when bevacizumab is combined with docetaxel, estramustine, and prednisone, but the toxicity profile of this schedule is high. Increasing evidence is supporting the benefit of thalidomide in the management of metastatic prostate cancer. Its mechanism of action has yet to be defined, but it has been shown to have strong anti-angiogenic, immunomodulatory, and antitumour effects.

Thromboembolic occurrences tend to complicate the progressive disease frequently. Thrombophlebitis with fatal pulmonary embolism is a common problem. Low molecular weight heparin is suitable for therapeutic and prophylactic purposes. In the case of low grade D.I.C. mitoxantrone may be indicated.

Anemia and recommendations for treatment

Anemia has a negative impact on the majority of organs; in an elderly cancer population the consequences of anemia can be even more invalidating due to its contribution to the "fragility syndrome". Anemia is the reason for many objective and subjective functional declines of capacities.

Considerable improvement of physical condition and functional/cognitive capacities and quality of life can be achieved when the hemoglobin level is raised.

If anemia is tumour-growth-associated tumour therapy is indicated. Unfortunately hormone-, chemo- and radiotherapy are often no longer feasible. In this case blood transfusions or erythropoietin should be given.

The beneficial effects of erythropoietin on quality of life and functional cognitive capacities have been proven (Mancuso et al., 2006). The treatment should be started at Hb levels inferior to 9/dL and continued as long as Hb level remains below 12g/dL. When Hb level is superior to 12g/dL there is a greater risk for thrombo-embolism.

Erythropoietin is effective in cases of anemia due to bone marrow infiltration as well; however, in this case cytostatic or radiation therapies would generally be the preferred treatment.

Characteristics of pain therapy

See also chapter: "Pain management in cancer rehabilitation and palliation".

Pain can lead to depression, loss of appetite, irritability, anger, loss of sleep, withdrawal from social interaction, and inability to cope. All these symptoms lower the pain threshold and result in more severe pain and a higher analgesic requirement. If uncontrolled, pain can destroy relationships with loved ones and the will to live. Fortunately, pain can almost always be controlled.

The first step in reducing pain is to evaluate the cause and source of pain. It is important to differentiate malignant from non-malignant aetiology. It is important to evaluate how much of the patient's complaints are, in fact, fear of malignant pain (table 5.4).

Pharmaceutical therapy of bone pain includes **non-steroidal analgesics and opiates**. (fig. 5.5). Non-steroidal anti-inflammatory drugs are often more effective for bone pain than are opioids (table 5.18). However, in a long term they are associated with more side effects, and tolerance to these agents necessitates treatment with other modalities (table 5.32). Morphine preparations have fewer side effects in the long run (tables 5.37, 5.38, 5.39). In several studies it has been shown that the physical and mental fitness of patients with tumour-related pain tends to increase with opioids. Periphery-acting pain medications should be administered very early together with long-term morphine preparations.

A requirement for successful therapy with morphine preparations is using a controlled-release formula. Drugs should be administered "by the clock" and not as needed. Long-acting morphines should be preferred. The advantages of using transdermal application are fewer problems and potentially fewer side effects. Pain peaks can be covered with short-acting morphine preparations (e.g., Sevredol®, Temgesic sublingual® or Actiq®). The patches only have to be changed every 48 to 72 hours (table 5.23).

The analgesic effect of **sexual hormone therapy** depends mainly on the hormone sensitivity of the primary tumour and its metastases (table 5.14). Pain relief occurs just a few days after initiation of hormone therapy in subjects with these hormone sensitive cancers. Estrogens are very effective but take care of side effects. Recent studies in advanced prostate cancer have shown that the high risk of cardiovascular morbidity associated with oral estrogens may be avoided by parenteral estrogen administration (e.g., intramuscular polyestradiol phosphate and transdermal estradiol).

Corticoids are indicated in painful peritumoural edema but are effective for a limited period only.

Bisphosphonates are excellent painkillers in osteolytic metastases. The rationale for the use of bisphosphonates in metastastatic prostate cancer is not commonly obvious, given the predominantly osteoblastic nature of the metastatic process. Clinical experiences show however beneficial effects in osteoblastic metastases as well. Parenteral administration of bisphosphonates is indicated in symptomatic and oral administration in asymptomatic bone metastases. They should be given in an asymptomatic stage because of reducing the risk of pathologic fractures, the need of bone irradiation. hypercalcaemia, immobilisation, spinal cord compression and last not least need of care (Saad, 2004; Smith, 2003; Rosen et al., 2004).

Percutaneous (external) radiotherapy is effective in palliating pain from solitary bone metastases. Two different mechanisms apply (table 5.15). The first mechanism is that of reducing tumour volume (curative radiotherapy), involving elevated cumulative therapeutic doses and fractionation (e.g., 5 x 4Gy or 10 x 3Gy). The analgesic effect of fractionated radiotherapy correlates with cancer cell kill and occurs after several days or weeks of treatment.

The second mechanism is that of symptomatic radiotherapy, requiring lower doses and only one shot (e.g., 1 x 8Gy). Pain relief is rapid. The "only" effect is reduction of peritumoural inflammatory acidosis, i.e., reduction of tumour swelling but not of actual tumour size.

Both regimens are equivalent in terms of pain and narcotic relief at three months and are tolerated with few adverse effects (Hartsell et al., 2005).

Systemic **beta-emitting, bone-seeking radiopharmaceuticals** represent a good alternative or adjuvant to external beam radiotherapy for palliation of painful osteoblastic bone metastases. Documented response rates in prostatic cancer patients with painful bone metastases range from 40% to 95%. Pain relief starts within one-four weeks after the initiation of treatment, continues for up to eighteen months, and is associated with a reduction in analgesic use in many patients (Finlay et al., 2005; McEwan, 2000; Hamdy 2001).

The most frequently used radio-isotopes in pain management are P-32-labelled phosphate, strontium-89, samarium-153, rhenium-186 and rhenium-188. Radio-isotopes have mainly been used in patients with bone metastases from prostatic cancer because these metastases are in most cases osteoblastic (sclerotic). The majority of radiocompounds accumulate where new bone is formed. Pain patients with refractory bone metastases and a positive technetium 99m methylene diphosphonate bone scan are ideal candidates for treatment.

Toxicity is mostly hematological. Thrombocytopenia is significant and protracted. Any concomitant myelosuppressive chemotherapy should be carefully monitored. Thrombocytopenia is the main toxicity of relevance in limiting further chemotherapy.

Radionuclides should not be given to patients with suspected disseminated intravascular coagulation (McEwan, 2000).

Relative contraindications for treatment include osteolytic lesions, pending spinal cord compression or pathologic fracture, pre-existing severe myelosuppression, urinary incontinence, inability to follow radiation safety precautions, and severe renal insufficiency.

The effect of **chemotherapy** (e.g., mitoxantrone in combination with corticoids) on pain is surprising as chemotherapy has generally only limited effect on tumour growth in bone metastases due to prostate cancer. A possible explanation is this chemotherapy has an inhibitory activity on the inflammatory component of metastases (Nilsson *et al.*, 2005).

Some **antidepressants** can be used for their analgesic effect alone or in combination with other analgesics (mainly opioids). The doses used for pain management are considerably lower than those used for psychiatric treatment. In addition to their antidepressant and analgesic effect, some antidepressants (amitriptyline and doxepine, for instance) also have sedative effects and may be indicated for patients with sleep disorders. Some antidepressants are associated with weight gain (e.g., amitriptyline, doxepine, maprotiline, mirtazapine) while others are used for weight loss (e.g., sibutramine, fluoxetine) (tables 5.34, 5.35).

Anorexia and cachexia and recommendations for treatment

Anorexia and cachexia (wasting condition in which the patient has weakness and a marked and progressive loss of body weight, fat, and muscle) frequently occur together. In patients with advanced cancer, cachexia is primarily due to alterations in protein, carbohydrate and lipid metabolism caused by inflammatory cytokines released by the tumour.

There is no satisfactory drug therapy for cachexia. Corticosteroids and alcohol may reduce anorexia but have no effect on the metabolic abnormalities of cancer cachexia. Megestrol acetate may exert an anabolic effect and reduce or prevent weight loss (Mateen and Jatoi, 2006).

Enteral and parenteral nutrition will not reverse or prevent cancer cachexia, but it may be appropriate for patients who are temporarily unable to eat for two weeks or more because of anticancer treatment. Dronabinol may be effective in maintaining weight for some patients.

The family needs to be dissuaded from trying to force the patient to eat, as this will only cause physical distress and guilt.

Role of complementary and alternative therapies

Numerous therapy forms are offered by various industries to which are ascribed the qualities of improving unspecific immune functions and activating the body's own immune defenses against the tumour (**immunostimulants or immune modulators**). Examples of such substances are mistletoe extract, enzyme and thymus preparations, snake venom, oxygen multistep therapy, phototherapy, symbiosis control, microbiological therapy, vitamins, among many others. All these therapy options are based on widely speculative assumptions, do not appear very plausible from a theoretical standpoint and are not recognized by standard medicine. Their therapeutic effects on tumours are at best only minimal.

So far there has been no scientific study that might have proven the tumour-inhibiting effects of **mistletoe preparations**. The assertion that the patient's quality of life can be improved through its use is very difficult to confirm. Yet these mistletoe preparations are not only used by those practicing alternative and nature-oriented forms of medicine, but also by some oncologists. The reason for this is less the belief in its effectiveness, but rather the possibility of being able to offer the patient a further therapy option. Experience has shown not only that "faith can move mountains", but that it can also improve the quality of life. One should not shatter these patients' faith in a particular therapy form with evidence-based arguments.

Pain is a major problem for many prostatic cancer patients. There is much support for the use of hypnosis in managing pain associated with medical procedures and some support for its use in managing chronic cancer pain. There is less evidence to support the use of modalities such as acupuncture, meditation and massage for management of chronic pain. However, there is some compelling data to support the use of acupuncture for nausea and vomiting associated with cancer treatments, and there are some data suggesting that qigong, neuro-emotional techniques, meditation techniques, and massage can decrease pain levels and improve the sense of well-being.

PC-SPES is a patented mixture of eight herbs. It was sold as a dietary supplement to support and promote healthy prostate function. Evidence from clinical trials has shown that PC-SPES lowers PSA and testosterone levels in humans, but it is not known whether these results were caused by contaminants, the herbs in PC-SPES, or their combination.

Ensuring the quality of rehabilitation and palliative measures

To guarantee quality of rehabilitation and palliation you have to ensure quality of structures, quality of rehabilitative and palliative measures and to evaluate outcome.

As with acute therapy, guidelines and quality assurance procedures should also apply to follow-up care, including rehabilitation and palliation of patients with prostatic cancer. The progress and results of rehabilitation and palliation must be recorded and evaluated (Barat and Franchignoni, 2004). Unfortunately there are only few guidelines on this subject.

There are guidelines for general urologic diseases (AACR 2002), guidelines for treatment of prostatic cancer, but no guidelines about what to do in the event of rehabilitative needs and how to secure quality of the different rehabilitative and palliative measures.

Quality of structural features

Therapies needed in rehabilitation and palliation should be provided by specialised rehabilitation services with a team of patient care specialists.

Urologic rehabilitation services include critical components of assessment, physical reconditioning, skills training, and psychological support. Special experience and a specialised infrastructure are essential. Appropriate performance by the program staff and proper service delivery has to be assured. The team should be coordinated by a physician experienced in rehabilitation and palliation with demonstrable oncological knowledge. Incontinence nurses and physiotherapists play an important role in this rehabilitation team. The collaboration of psycho-oncologists is very useful. Social workers are essential because of the social aids that are often needed. Cooperation and the exchange of information with the previously and subsequently treating physicians are important.

To rehabilitate prostatic cancer patients demands many experiences. Due to the experience necessary, the rehabilitative institution should care for at least fifty prostatic cancer patients per year. This is not necessary for the palliative institution caring prostatic cancer patients. The site should provide an appropriate environment with adequate space, few interruptions or other distractions (Schmidt, 2001).

Quality of medical and therapeutic processes

Verifiability of the quality of rehabilitation and palliative therapies must be guaranteed.

All members of the rehabilitation team should participate in the patient's assessment. The initial evaluation should include the medical history, diagnostic tests, current symptoms and complaints, physical assessment, psychological, social, or vocational needs, nutritional status, exercise tolerance, determination of educational needs, the patient's ability to carry out activities of daily living and his interests and compliance.

The rehabilitation program must be tailored to meet the needs of the individual patient, addressing age-specific and cultural variables, and should contain patient-determined goals, as well as goals established by the individual team discipline. Both patients and families participate in this training administered by health care professionals.

Outcome assessment and evaluation

The evaluation of rehabilitative measures in prostatic cancer patients is directed not at survival time, but rather at quality of life criteria. This involves primarily subjective parameters such as improvement of urine incontinence, pain, mobility, overcoming fears, etc. and not such parameters as are found in association with primary therapy (response, remission and length of remission).

Outcome assessment in most clinical trials is affected by a purely medical understanding of the disease. This is reflected in the predominant use of urologic and oncologic symptoms as the content of outcome measures. The assessment of other health aspects like psychological symptoms, interpersonal or social consequences of the disease, seems to be similarly, if not more, important and should be considered. Some of therapy goals and evaluation criteria are listed in table 13.22. Patient satisfaction – as measured by the patient him-/herself – can be evaluated most readily by questionnaires.

Different outcome scales in palliative care of cancer patients have been developed (Aspinal *et al.*, 2002; Bausewein *et al.*, 2005). The scales cover physical and psychological symptoms, spiritual considerations, practical concerns, emotional concerns of the patient and family, and psychosocial needs of the patient and family. The Palliative Care Outcome Scale (POS) is a multidimensional instrument covering these physical, psychosocial, spiritual, organizational, and practical concerns.

Measurements of quality of life

Quality of life in prostatic cancer patients has been performed mainly in therapeutic trials in order to assess disease- and treatment-specific symptoms. Performance status as a proxy of quality of life has mainly been used although there is only a weak association between the performance status such as the Karnofsky performance scale (table 3.4) and quality of life as measured by the EOTC QL PR25 (Montazeri *et al.*, 1998). Palliation of symptoms, psychosocial interventions, and understanding patient's feelings and concerns all contribute to improve quality of life in prostatic cancer patients.

Basically, improvement in quality of life is attained when there is less nursing care ("rehabilitation to combat the need of care"), when the patient can be vocationally reintegrated ("rehabilitation to combat early retirement"), when he/she feels secure ("rehabilitation to combat resignation and depression") and when the patient's physical handicaps and functional limitations are at a minimum ("rehabilitation to combat disability").

Table 13.22 - Possible therapeutic aims and their parameters for effectiveness in the rehabilitation of pancreatic cancer patients.

Therapy goal	Parameter of effectiveness
Urine continence recovery	Urinstatus, ultrasound measurements of residual urine, number of pads, urometry, Biofeedback, Uroflowmetrie, length of micturation intervals, bladder diary. Questionnaires: QLQ-PR25
Reduction of complaints resulting from hormonotherapy	Reduction of symptoms (e.g., hot flashes, insomnia, sexual satisfaction, osteodensitometry etc.), y
Pain relief	Pain diary, reduction of analgesic drugs, pain sensitivity scales, questionnaires: PDI, EORTC QLQ-C30, SE36, SDS, RSCL
Reduction of lymphedema, lymphocele	Volume measurements, reduction of symptoms, abdominal ultrasound
Sexual helps	Questionnaires: QLQ-PR25, IIEF, diary
Improvement of physical condition	Ergometry, Karnofsky-Index, WHO- und EORTC-Performance-Status, walking distance, Harvard-step-test, vigorimeter, muscle force (hand held dynamometry), exercise capacity (symptom limited bicycle ergometry). Questionnaires: (EORTC) LC-13, FACT G, Fact P, EORTC-QLQ-C30, Nottingham Health Profile
Reduction of disorders resulting from surgery/chemotherapy/radiotherapy	WHO-toxicity scale, CTC-Classification, assessment of organ function, vibration test
Information on illness, follow-up care, signs of recurrence, therapies in the case of recurrence, behaviour-influencing illness etc.	Questionnaires, tests
Reduction of anxiety, depression, fatigue	Rating scales. Questionnaires: STAI, POMS, BDI, BSI, HADS-D, PAF, MFI,MAX-PC
Coping with cancer disease	Questionnaires: FKV, BEFO, TSK, Fibeck
Clarification and improvement of vocational fitness	Resumption of work, length of time of inability to work
Reduction of necessity of nursing care	Reduction of level of care, Barthel Index, FIM, ADL
Relief of physical and psychological symptoms	Questionnaire: POS

Abbreviations of questionnaires

ADL = Activities of Daily Life; BDI = Beck-Depressionsinventar; DDC = Daily Diary Card; EORTC-QLQ = European Organization for Research and Treatment of Cancer Quality of Life Questionnaire; ECOG = European Cooperative Oncology Group-Scale; Fact G = Functional Assessment of Cancer Therapy (General); Fact-An = Functional Assessment of Cancer Therapy (Anemia); Fact F = Functional Assessment of Cancer Therapy (Fatigue); FACT-Ct = Functional Assessment of Anorexia and Cachexia; Fact P = Functional Assessment of Cancer Therapy (Prostate); FIBECK = Freiburg Inventory on Coping with Chronic Illness; FIM = Functional Independence Measure; FLI-C = Functional Living Index-Cancer; IIEF = International Index of Erectile Function; HADS-D = Hospital Anxiety and Depression Scale; KPS = Karnofsky Performance Scale; MAX-PC = Memorial Anxiety Scale for Prostate Cancer; MFI = Multidimensional Fatigue Inventory; PDI = Pain Disability Index; POMS = Profile of Mood Status; POS = Palliative Care Outcome Scale; RSCL = Rotterdam Symptom Checklist; SF-36 = SF-36 Health Survey; SIP = Sickness Impact profile; SIRO = Stress Index Radio Oncology; STAI = Spiegelberger Trait Anxiety Inventory

Bibliographie

- Amarenco G, Chantraine A (edit) (2006) Les fonctions sphinctériennes. Springer Paris
- Aspinal F, Hughes R, Higginson I *et al.* (2002) A user's guide to the palliative care outcome scale. Palliative care & policy publications. Kings College, London
- Barat M, Franchignoni F (2004) Assessment in physical medicine and rehabilitation. Maugeri Foundation Books, PI-ME Press Pavia
- Bartsch HH, Delbrück H, Kruck P *et al.* (2000) Zur Prozessqualität in der onkologischen Rehabilitation. Rehabilitation 39; 355-8
- Bamias A, Kastritis E, Bamias C (2005) Osteonecrosis of the jaw in cancer after treatment with bisphophonates: Incidence and risk factors J Clin Oncol 23, 34: 8580-7
- Barton D, Loprinzi CL (2004) Making sense of the evidence regarding nonhormonal treatments for hot flashes. Clin J Oncol Nurs 8, 1: 39-42
- Bausewein C, Fegg M, Radbruch L *et al.* (2005) Validation and clinical application of the German version of the palliative care outcome. J Pain Symptom Manage 30: 51-62
- Bradley C, Oberst K, Schenk M (2006) Absenteeism from work: The experience of employed breast and prostate cancer patients in the months following diagnosis. Psycho-oncology 15, 8: 739-47
- Bundesarbeitsgemeinschaft für Rehabilitation (BAR) (2004) Rahmenempfehlungen zur ambulanten onkologischen Rehabilitation. Schriftenreihe der Bundesarbeitsgemeinschaft für Rehabilitation, Frankfurt
- Caliendo MD, Lee E, Queiroz R *et al.* (2001) Sclerotherapy with Use of Doxycycline after Percutaneous Drainage of Postoperative Lymphoceles. Journal of Vascular and Interventional Radiology 12: 73-7
- Carlsson C, Baigi A, Killander D *et al.* (2005) Motives for becoming and remaining member of patient associations. Support Care Cancer 20
- Charlson M, Pompei P, Ales K *et al.* (1987) A new method for classifying prognostic comorbity in longitudinal studies. J Chronic Dis, 40: 373-83
- Chen A, Petrylak D (2004) Complications of Androgen Deprivation Therapy in Men with Prostate Cancer. Current Oncology Reports 2004, 6: 209-15
- Dahn JR, Penedo FJ, Gonzalez JS *et al.* (2004) Sexual functioning and quality of life after prostate cancer treatment: Considering sexual desire. Urology 63, 2: 273-7
- Delbrück H, Schmid L, Bartsch H *et al.* (2000) Zur Ergebnisqualität in der onkologischen Rehabilitation. Rehabilitation 39: 359-62
- Ershler N (2003) Cancer: A disease of the elderly. J support Oncol 1, 2: 5-10
- Esper P, Redman BG (1999) Supportive care, pain management and quality of life in advanced prostate cancer. Urol Clin North Am 26: 375
- Finlay IG, Mason M, Shelley M (2005) Radioisotopes for the palliation of metastatic bone cancer: A systematic review. Lancet Oncol 6, 6: 392-400
- Gilligan T, Kantoff P (2002) Chemotherapy for prostate cancer. Urology 60 (suppl. 3A): 94-100
- Gray RE, Klotz LH (2004) Restoring sexual function in prostate cancer patients: An innovative approach. Can J Urol 11, 3: 2285-9
- Gontero P, Fontana F, Bagnasacco A *et al.* (2003) Is there an optimal time for intracavernous prostaglandin E1 rehabilitation following nonnerve sparing radical prostatectomy? Results from a hemodynamic prospective study. J Urology 169: 2166-9

- Haab,F, Trockman B, Zimmern P *et al.* (1997) Quality of life and continence assessment of the artificial urinary sphincter in men with minimum 3,5 years of follow-up. J Urology 158: 435-9
- Hamdy NA, Papapoulos SE (2001) The palliative management of skeletal metastases in prostate cancer: Use of bone-seeking radionuclides and bisphosphonates
- Hartsell WF, Scott CB, Brunner DW *et al.* (2005) Randomized trial of short-versus long-course radiotherapy for palliation of painful bone metastases. J Natl Cancer Inst 97, 11: 798-804
- Key TJ *et al.* (2004) Fruits and vegetables and prostate cancer: No association among 1104 cases in a prospective study of 130,544 men in the European Prospective Investigation into Cancer and Nutrition (EPIC). Int J Cancer 109: 119-124
- Krupski T, Smith MR, Lee WC *et al.* (2004) Natural history of bone complications in men with prostate carcinoma initiating androgen deprivation therapy. Cancer 101, 3: 541-9
- Lawton CA, Won M, Pilepich M *et al.* (1991) Long-term treatment sequelae following external beam irradiation for adenocarcinoma of the prostate: Analysis of RTOG studies 7506 and 7706. Int J Radiat Oncol Biol Phys 21: 935-9
- Lilleby W, Fossa SD, Waehre HR *et al.* (1999) Long-term morbidity and quality of life in patients with localized prostate cancer undergoing definitive radiotherapy or radical prostatectomy. Int J Radiat Oncol Biol Phys 1, 43, 4: 735-43
- Mason T (2005) Information needs of wives of men following prostatectomy. Oncol Nurs Forum 10, 32, 3: 557-63
- Mathewson-Chapman M (1997) Pelvic muscle exercise/biofeedback for urinary incontinence after prostatectomy: An education program. J Cancer Educ 12,4: 218-23
- McEwan AJ (2000) Use of radionuclides for the palliation of bone metastases. Semin Radiat Oncol 10, 2: 103-14
- McGlynn B, Al-Saffar N, Begg H *et al.* (2004) Management of urinary incontinence following radical prostatectomy. Urol Nurse 24, 6: 475-82
- Montorsi F, Salonia A, Briganti A *et al.* (2005) Vardenifil for the treatment of erectile dysfunction: A critical review of the literature based on a personal clinical experience. Eur Urol 47, 5 : 612-21
- Nishimura K, Yamaguchi Y, Yamanaka M *et al.* (2005) Climacteric-Like Disorders in Prostate Cancer Patients Treated with LHRH Agonists. Arch of Andrology 51,1: 41-8
- Nilsson S, Strang P, Ginman C *et al.* (2005) Palliation of bone pain in prostate cancer using chemotherapy and strontium-89. A randomized phase II study. J Pain Symptom Manage 29, 4: 352-7
- Pepper R, Pati J, Kaisary A (2004) The incidence and treatment of lymphoceles after radical retropubic prostatectomy: BJU International 95: 772-5
- Pisansky T (2005) External Beam Radiotherapy as Curative Treatment of Prostate Cancer. Mayo Clin Proc 80: 883-98
- Pomfret I, Haslam J (2002) To exercise or not to exercise? Journal of Community Nursing 16: 08
- Potosky AL, Legler J, Albertsen PC *et al.* (2000) Health outcomes after prostatectomy or radiotherapy for prostate cancer: Results from the prostate cancer outcomes study. J Natl Cancer Inst 92: 1582-92

- Potosky AL, Davis WW, Hoffman RM *et al.* (2004) Five-year outcomes after prostatectomy or radiotherapy for prostate cancer: The Prostate Cancer Outcomes Study. J Natl Cancer Inst 96: 1358-67
- Prezioso D, Piccirillo G, Galasso R *et al.* Gynecomastia due to hormonte therapy for advanced prostate cancer. Tumouri 90, 4: 410-5
- Riechers FA (2004) Including partners into the diagnosis of prostate cancer: a review of the literature to provide a model of care. Urol Nurse 24, 1: 22-9
- Roth AJ, Rosenfeld B, Kornblith AB *et al.* (2003) The memorial anxiety scale for prostate cancer: Validation of a new scale to measure anxiety in men with prostate cancer. Cancer 97, 11: 2910-8
- Roth A (2005) Improving Quality of Life: Psychiatric Aspects of Treating Prostate Cancer. Psychiatric Times Vol. XXII: 5
- Saad F, Gleason DM *et al.* (2004) Long term efficacy of zoledronic acid for the prevention of skeletal complications in patients with metastatic hormone-refractory prostate cancer. J Natl Inst 96: 879-82
- Schmid L, Delbrück H, Bartsch H *et al.* (2000) Zur Strukturqualität in der onkologischen Rehabilitation. Rehabilitation, 39: 350-4
- Schover LR (2005) Sexuality and fertility after cancer. Hematology 1: 523
- Shahininan *et al.* (2005) N Engl J Med 352: 154-64
- Smith JJ, Barrett D (2002) Implantation of the artificial genito-urinary sphincter. In PC Walsh *et al.*, eds., Campbell's Urology, 8th ed., 2: 1187-94. Philadelphia: WB.Saunders.
- Smith M *et al.* (2003) Randomised controlled trial of zolendronic acid to prevent boneloss in men receiving androgen deprivation therapy for non metastatic prostate cancer. The Journal of Urology, 169: 2008-12
- Stoeckli R, Keller U (2004) Nutritional fat and the risk of type 2 diabetes and cancer. Physiol Behav 83, 4: 611-5
- Tanvetyanon T (2005) Long-term efficacy of zoledronic acid fort he prevention of skeletal complications in patients with metastatic hormone-refractory prostate cancer. J Natl Cancer Inst 5, 97, 1: 70-1
- Yablon CM, Banner MP, Ramchandani P *et al.* (2004) Complications of prostate cancer treatment : Spectrum of imaging findings. Radiographics 24, suppl. 1: 181-94
- Yi Su, Davis B, Herman M *et al.* (2004) Prostate brachytherapy seed localization by analysis of multiple projections: Identifying and addressing the seed overlap problem. Medical Physics 31, 5: 1277-87
- Van Kampen M, de Weerdt W, van Poppel H *et al.* (2000) Effect of pelvic-floor reeducation on duration and degree of incontinence after radical prostatectomy: A randomized controlled trial. Lancet 355: 98-102
- Watson T, Mock V (2004) Exercise as an intervention for cancer- related fatigue. Phys Ther 84: 736-43
- Walsh PC, Marschke P, Ricker D *et al.* (2000) Patient-reported urinary continence and sexual function after anatomic radical prostatectomy. Urology 55(1): 58-61
- Ward JF, Blute ML, Slezak J *et al.* (2003) The long-term clinical impact of biochemical recurrence of prostate cancer 5 or more years after radical prostatectomy. J Urol 170: 1872-6
- William K (2000) Chemotherapy for patients with advanced prostate carcinoma. A new option for therapy. Cancer 88: 3015-21

- Windsor PM, Nicol KF, Potter J (2004) A randomized, controlled trial of aerobic exercise for treatment-related fatigue in men receiving radical external beam radiotherapy for localized prostate carcinoma Cancer, 101, 3: 550-7
- Zaak D, Hungerhuber E, Müller-Lisse U *et al.* (2003) Urological emergencies. Urologe (A) 42: 849-63
- Zeegers MP, Friesema IH, Goldbohm RA *et al.* (2004) A prospective study of occupation and prostate cancer risk. J Occup Environ Med 46, 3: 271-9

Palliation of cancer patients in terminal care

Terminal care refers to the care of the dying patient in the last hours or days of life. Principles of care in terminal care are symptom control, avoidance of unnecessary interventions, a regular control of drugs and symptoms, continuity of regular communication, and support of relatives and carers. Clinical issues that commonly arise in the last hours of living include the management of feeding and hydration, changes in consciousness, delirium, pain, breathlessness, and secretions. All drugs necessary for symptom control must continuously be given in the terminal phase.

Table 14.1 - Frequent symptoms in the advanced stage of cancer that require palliative intervention (meta-analysis of 10 studies, based on Zech, Grond *et al.* 1994).

– Pain (70%)
– Dry mouth (68%)
– Anorexia (61%)
– Weakness (47%)
– Constipation (45%)
– Difficulty breathing (42%)
– Nausea, vomiting (36%)
– Insomnia (34%)
– Sweating (25%)
– Problems swallowing (23%)
– Urinary symptoms (21%)
– Neuropsychiatric symptoms: disorders of consciousness, cramps, dizziness, restlessness (20%)
– Skin problems: itching, allergic reactions, infections, decubitus ulcers (16%)
– Dyspepsia (11%)
– Diarrhea (70%)

Management principles are the same at home or in a healthcare institution (table 1.15). However, death in an institution requires accommodations to assure privacy, cultural observances, and communication that may not be customary

Clinical competence, willingness to educate, and calm and empathic reassurance are critical to help patients and families in the last hours of living.

Particularities in pharmaceutical medication

As patients approach death, the need for each medication has to be reassessed. The number of drugs that the patient is taking should be minimized.

The oral route is generally preferred when patients are capable of and enteral absorption is not problematic. In the palliative care setting, alternative routes of administration must be available for patients who can no longer swallow or when other dynamics preclude the oral route. Enteral feeding tubes can be used to access the gut when patients can no longer swallow. The rectum can be used to deliver medication, although fecal contents, mucosal dryness, thrombocytopenia, or painful lesions may preclude the use of these routes.

Only those medications should be continued which are needed to manage symptoms such as pain, breathlessness, excess secretions, and terminal delirium and to reduce the risk of seizures. Choose the least invasive route of administration: The buccal mucosa or oral routes first, the subcutaneous or intravenous routes only if necessary, and the intramuscular route almost never. Rectal administration can also be considered, especially if the oral route is not possible (Twycross, 1998; MacDonald, 1998; Storey, 1998).

In the terminal stage **tricyclic antidepressants** are of little use. Side effects, e.g., sedation and xerostomia, may predominate.

Benzodiazepine therapy should be administered cautiously in patients with delirium due to the possibility of paradoxical agitation that can aggravate the patient's pre-existing distress. Alternatively, sedated patients who have been taking benzodiazipines for months or years and who then stop swallowing should have their dose continued, sublingually or rectally, to prevent agitation from benzodiazepine withdrawal (Levy and Cohen, 2005). Benzodiazepines may paradoxically excite some patients (Feldmann, 1986). These patients require neuroleptic medications to control their delirium. Haloperidol 0.5-2.0mg intravenously, subcutaneously, or rectally every hour (titrated to effect, then nightly to every six hours to maintain) may be effective. Chlorpromazine 10-25mg orally, rectally, or intramuscularly nightly to every six hours and titrated to effect intravenously or rectally is a more sedating alternative.

Knowledge of **opioid** pharmacology becomes critical during the last hours of life. The liver conjugates codeine, morphine, oxycodone, and hydromorphone into glucuronides. Some of their metabolites remain active as analgesics until they are renally cleared, particularly morphine. As dying patients experience diminished hepatic function and renal perfusion, and usually become oliguric or anuric, routine dosing or continuous infusions of morphine may lead to increased serum concentrations of active metabolites, toxicity, and an increased risk of terminal delirium. The dose of opioids needs to be adjusted to the degree of renal function. To minimize this risk, discontinue routine dosing or continuous infusions of morphine when urine output and renal clearance stop. Titrate morphine breakthrough (rescue) doses to manage expressions suggestive of continuous pain. Consider the use of alternative opioids with inactive metabolites such as fentanyl or hydromorphone

Pain

While many people fear that pain will suddenly increase as the patient dies, there is no evidence to suggest that this occurs. Pain is seldom a problem as death approaches. Do not confuse pain with the restlessness, agitation, moaning, and groaning that accompany terminal delirium. If the diagnosis is unclear, a trial of a higher dose of opioid may be necessary to judge whether pain is driving the observed behaviours.

For morphine, commercially prepared suppositories, compounded suppositories, or microenemas can be used to deliver the drug directly to the rectum or stoma.

Parenteral administration in palliative care is usually limited to subcutaneous and intravenous delivery because repeated intramuscular opioid delivery is excessively noxious. The intravenous route provides rapid drug delivery but requires vascular access, which may not be easily obtained or maintained in a home or long-term care setting. In the absence of intravenous access, it must be remembered that subcutaneous boluses, although effective, have a slower onset and lower peak effect when compared with intravenous boluses. Subcutaneous infusions as much as 10mL/hour are usually absorbed, although most patients tolerate 2-3mL/hour with least difficulty.

Intraspinal routes, including epidural or intrathecal delivery, may allow administration of drugs, such as opioids, local anesthetics, and/or a-adrenergic agonists. However, the equipment used to deliver these medications is complex, requiring specialized knowledge for healthcare professionals and potentially greater caregiver burden. Risk of infection and other complications along with upfront and maintenance costs are significant concerns when contemplating high-technology procedures. Selection should be based on greater than six months life expectancy for implanted programmable pumps, and adequate organizational infrastructure to manage these devices should be in place.

Despite the importance of pain management at the end of life, there are often substantial roadblocks to overcome in getting patients the treatment that they need. Professional healthcare workers may have unsubstantiated but strong beliefs about analgesic use, especially opioid use, that lead to underprescribing. Several surveys show that physicians, nurses, and pharmacists express concerns about addiction, tolerance, and side effects of morphine and related compounds. These fears are pervasive among patients and family members as well. Studies have suggested that these fears lead to undermedication and increased pain intensity. Concerns about being a "good" patient or belief in the inevitability of cancer pain lead patients to hesitate in reporting pain. In these studies, less educated and older patients were most likely to express these beliefs.

Food intake

It is very common that the person is too weak to swallow. Once the patient is unable to swallow, cease oral intake. Warn families and professional caregivers of the risk of aspiration. Most dying patients lose their appetite. Unfortunately, families and professional caregivers may interpret cessation of eating as "starving to death". Yet, studies demonstrate that parenteral or enteral feeding of patients near death neither improves symptom control nor lengthens life (Bruera, 1998). Anorexia may be helpful as the resulting kctosis can lead to a sense of well-being and diminish discomfort.

Clinicians should help families understand that loss of appetite is normal at this stage. Remind them that the patient is not hungry, that food either is not appealing or may be nauseating, that the patient would likely eat if he or she could, that the patient's body is unable to absorb and use nutrients, and that clenching of teeth may be the only way for the patient to express his/her desire not to eat.

Whatever the degree of acceptance of these facts, it is important for professionals to help families and caregivers realize that food pushed upon the unwilling patient may cause problems such as aspiration and increased tension.

Fluid intake

It is particularly important in the last days and hours of life to decide in the best interest of the patient, especially when the termination of or non-use of life prolonging measures are considered (Twycross, 1998; MacDonald, 1998; Storey, 1998).

Most dying patients stop drinking (Billings, 1985). Most experts feel that dehydration in the last hours of living does not cause distress and may stimulate endorphin release that promotes the patient's sense of well-being. Low blood pressure or weak pulse is part of the dying process and not an indication of dehydration. Patients who are not able to be upright do not get light-headed or dizzy. Patients with peripheral edema or ascites have excess body water and salt and are not dehydrated.

Provision of parenteral fluids is still controversially discussed when the patient is incapable of drinking or can drink only little. Parenteral fluids, given either intravenously or subcutaneously using hypodermoclysis, are sometimes considered, particularly when the goal is to reverse delirium. However, intravenous lines can be cumbersome and difficult to maintain. Changing the site of the angiocatheter can be painful, particularly when the patient is cachectic or has no discernible veins. Excess parenteral fluids can lead to fluid overload with consequent peripheral or pulmonary edema, worsened breathlessness, cough, and orotracheobronchial secretions, particularly if there is significant hypoalbuminemia.

To maintain patient comfort and minimize the sense of thirst, even in the face of dehydration, maintain moisture on mucosal membrane surfaces with meticulous oral, nasal, and conjunctival hygiene (Lethen, 1993). Treat oral candidiasis with topical nystatin or systemic fluconazole if the patient is able to swallow. Coat the lips and anterior nasal mucosa hourly with a thin layer of petroleum jelly to reduce evaporation.

Urine output falls as perfusion of the kidneys diminishes. Oliguria or anuria is normal.

Cardiac dysfunction and renal failure

As cardiac output and intravascular volume decrease at the end of life, there will be evidence of diminished peripheral blood perfusion. Tachycardia, hypotension, peripheral cooling, peripheral and central cyanosis are normal. Venous blood may pool along dependent skin surfaces.

Parenteral fluids will not reverse this circulatory shut down.

Terminal restlessness

Terminal restlessness is an agitated delirium that occurs in some patients during the last few days of life. Clinical features are agitation, restlessness, impaired conscious state, muscle twitching, multifocal myoclonus, seizures, and distressed vocalizing. After having excluded restlessness due to dyspnea, brain metastasis, dehydration, anxiety, fear, unrelieved pain, urinary retention, faecal impaction, drug, alcohol or nicotine withdrawal, benzodiazepines should be given. For benzodiazepine failure haloperidol 5mg s.c., followed by 20-30mg/24h or levomepromazine 12.5-50mg s.c. every 4-8h can be given. Be aware that restlessness can be the result of medications, e. g. opioids, steroids, etc.

When moaning, groaning, and grimacing accompany the agitation and restlessness, these symptoms are frequently misinterpreted as physical pain. However, it is a myth that uncontrollable pain suddenly develops during the last hours of life when it has not previously been a problem. While a trial of opioids may be beneficial in the unconscious patient who is difficult to assess, clinicians must remember that opioids may accumulate and add to delirium when renal clearance is poor (Zaw Tun, 1992). If the trial of increased opioids does not relieve the agitation or makes the delirium worse by increasing agitation or precipitating myoclonic jerks or seizures (rare), then pursue alternative therapies directed at suppressing the symptoms associated with delirium.

Dyspnea

The etiology of dyspnea is often multifactorial as anxiety is almost always associated (table 12.25). The condition can result from impairment of one or more body systems. In addition to pharmacologic interventions and oxygen, there are a number of non pharmacologic strategies that can be beneficial in the management of dyspnea (Thomas et al., 2003). General measures – reassurance and explanation, upright positioning, good ventilation, chest physio and relaxation exercises – may be beneficial. Dyspnea occurs in many patients with terminal cancer and is perceived as one of the most devastating symptoms by the patient and the family (Dudgeon et al., 1999). Families and professional caregivers frequently find changes in breathing patterns to be one of the most distressing signs of impending death. Many fear that the comatose patient will experience a sense of suffocation. Knowledge that the unresponsive patient may not be experiencing breathlessness or "suffocating" and may not benefit from oxygen (which may actually prolong the dying process) can be very comforting.

Low doses of opioids or benzodiazepines are appropriate to manage any perception of breathlessness.

Controlled single-dose trials have suggested that opioids are effective in chronic obstructive lung disease. However, opioids are poorly tolerated in these patients during repeated administration, mostly because of sedation and nausea. These side effects usually disappear with the development of tolerance and are rarely a cause for discontinuing treatment among approximately 80% of terminal patients who receive opioids for pain.

While it is true that patients are more likely to receive higher doses of both opioids and sedatives as they get closer to death, there is no evidence that initiation of treatment or increases in dose of opioids or sedatives is associated with precipitation of death. In fact, the evidence suggests the opposite.

Terminal respiratory congestion (death rattle)

In the terminal phase rattling or gurgling sounds while breathing is frequent. It may be caused by secretion in the lower pharynx and trachea during inspiration and expiration in unconscious terminal patients. It has to be differentiated from congestive heart failure, air flow obstruction, and pneumonia.

Anticholinergic drugs can suppress the production of secretions and alleviate death rattle. Scopolamine (0.2-0.4mg subcutaneously every 4 hours) or glycopyrrolate (0.2 mg subcutaneously every 4-6 hours) will effectively reduce the production of saliva and other secretions. Bronchodilators may be indicated if there is a reversible element to the bronchial obstruction.

Therapy of death rattle is often more for the comfort of the relatives and other patients, as most of the patients are no longer aware of their surroundings. Relatives should be reassured that the noisy breathing is not causing any added suffering for the patient. If the patient is able to swallow, ice chips may help. In addition, a cool mist humidifier may help make the patient's breathing more comfortable.

Loss of sphincter control

Fatigue and loss of sphincter control in the last hours of life may lead to incontinence of urine and/or stool. Both can be very distressing to patients and family members, particularly if they are not warned that these problems may arise. If they occur, attention needs to be paid to cleaning and skin care. A urinary catheter may minimize the need for frequent changing and cleaning, prevent skin breakdown, and reduce the demand on caregivers. However, it is not always necessary if urine flow is minimal and can be managed with absorbent pads or surfaces. If diarrhea is considerable and continous, a rectal tube may be similarly effective.

Sedation

A variety of drugs can be used for sedation, many of which are used in lowered doses or administered during the various phases of palliative care. A typical drug is midazolam, a short acting benzodiazepine. Opioids such as morphine are not used as tolerance to sedation develops rapidly (unlike pain relief to which tolerance does not occur), and the doses of opioids needed for sedation can cause increased agitation (unlike the doses needed for pain relief). However, if a patient was already on an opioid for pain relief, this is continued subcutaneously at the same dose as before.

Extraordinary sedation with continuous infusions of midazolam, thiopental, and propofol can relieve refractory symptoms in most patients in their final days of life.

Psychiatric symptoms

Psychiatric symptoms include depression, anxiety and delirium. Neurological symptoms include symptoms affecting the central and peripheral nervous system. They can be caused by the actual tumour, by the treatment or by complex disturbances.

Confusion, disorientation and/or hallucinations tend to occur most commonly during the terminal phase (Ljubisavljevic, 2003). Neuroleptics are suitable for symptomatic therapy and in delirium syndrome (e.g., haloperidol); benzodiazepines are suitable in extreme anxiety as well as in agitation and in restlessness (e.g., lorazepam, midazolam).

A variety of drugs can be used for sedation, many of which are used in lowered doses or administered during the various phases of palliative care. Routine sedation is achieved by increasing the doses of opioids, benzodiazepines and neuroleptics. Extraordinary sedation with continuous infusions of midazolam, thiopental, and propofol can relieve refractory symptoms in most patients in their final days of life.

Benzodiazepines are used widely to treat terminal delirium. They are anxiolytics, amnestics, skeletal muscle relaxants, and antiepileptics. Common starting doses are: Lorazepam 1-2mg as an elixir, or a tablet predissolved in 0.5-1.0mL of water and administered against the buccal mucosa every hour as needed will settle most patients with 2-10mg/24 hours. It can then be given in divided doses, every 3-4 hours, to keep the patient settled. For a few extremely agitated patients, high doses of lorazepam, 20-50+mg/24 hours, may be required.

Benzodiazepines may paradoxically excite some patients. These patients require neuroleptic medications to control their delirium. Haloperidol 0.5-2.0mg intravenously, subcutaneously, or rectally every hour (titrated to effect, then nightly to every 6 hours to maintain) may be effective. Chlorpromazine 10-25mg orally, rectally, or intramuscularly nightly to every 6 hours and titrated to effect intravenously or rectally is a more sedating alternative.

Barbiturates have been suggested as alternatives. Seizures may be managed with high doses of benzodiazepines. Other antiepileptics such as intravenous phenytoin, subcutaneous fosphenytoin, or phenobarbital 60-120mg rectally, intravenously, or intramuscularly every 10-20 minutes as needed may become necessary until control is established. Alternatively, carbamazepine 200mg rectally 3-4 times per day can be used.

Pastoral care

Spiritual and psychological issues are confronted by cancer patients and their families, staff members, and the community at large; therefore, effective pastoral care is an integral part of relating to such issues.

Table 14.2 - The role and necessary competences of pastoral care in rehabilitational oncology.

– Pastoral care is supervised by a qualified professional chaplain with appropriate education (college and accredited theological school) and clinical training (units of clinical pastoral education are preferred).
– Spiritual needs may be identified and referred to a professional chaplain by all members of the oncology team.
– Spiritual assessment by a professional chaplain is incorporated into basic patient assessment.
– A clearly defined and functional referral system is established and maintained.
– Pastoral care involves sacramental, liturgical, and counselling services in keeping with the beliefs of patients and their families.
– Spiritual guidance in decisio-making related to patient care and biomedical ethics is available to patients and their families as well as caregivers.
– Ongoing multidisciplinary staff education and support is provided.
– Pastoral care recognizes diversities of faith, culture, and race. Pastoral care staff communicates with and supports clergy in the community.
– Pastoral care is available to staff members through individual counselling and group sessions.

Bibliography

– Bausewein C, Fegg M, Radbruch L et al. (2005) Validation and clinical application of the German version of the palliative care outcome. J Pain Symptom Manage 30: 51-62
– Billings JA (1985) Comfort measures for the terminally ill: Is dehydration painful? J Am Geriatr Soc 33: 808-10
– Bruera E, Fainsinger RL (1998) Clinical management of cachexia and anorexia. In: Doyle D, Hanks GWC, MacDonald N, eds. Oxford Textbook of Palliative Medicine. 2nd ed. Oxford, England: Oxford University Press; 548
– Dudgeon D, Lertzmann M (1999) Dyspnea in the advanced cancer patient. J Pain Symptom Manage. 18, 5: 313-5
– Feldman MD (1986) Paradoxical effects of benzodiazepines. NC Med J 47: 311-2

Mise en page : Graficoul'Eure (27)

Achevé d'imprimer sur les presses de l'Imprimerie BARNÉOUD
B.P. 44 - 53960 BONCHAMP-LÈS-LAVAL
Dépôt légal : octobre 2007 - N° d'imprimeur : 704072
Imprimé en France

– Lethen W (1993) Mouth and skin problems In: Saunders C, Sykes N. The Management of Terminal Malignant Disease, 3rd ed. Boston: Edward Arnold, 139-42
– Levy MH, Cohen SD (2005) Sedation for the relief of refractory symptoms in the imminently dying: A fine intentional line. Semin Oncol 32: 237-46
– Ljubisavljevic V, Kelly B (2003) Risk factors for development of delirium among oncology patients. Gen Hosp Psychiatry 25: 345-52
– Storey P (1998) Symptom control in dying. In: Berger A, Portenoy RK, Weissman D, eds. Principles and Practice of Supportive Oncology Updates. Philadelphia, Pa: Lippincott-Raven Publishers, 741-8
– Thomas J, von Gunten C (2003) Management of dyspnea. J Support Oncol. 1: 23-32
– Twycross R, Lichter I (1998) The terminal phase. In: Doyle D, Hanks GWC, MacDonald N, eds. Oxford Textbook of Palliative Medicine. 2nd ed. Oxford, England: Oxford University Press, 985-6
– Zaw-Tun N, Bruera E (1992) Active metabolites of morphine. J Palliat Care 8: 48-50